Bariatric and Metabolic Surgery

Guest Editor

SHANU N. KOTHARI, MD, FACS

SURGICAL CLINICS OF NORTH AMERICA

www.surgical.theclinics.com

Consulting Editor
RONALD F. MARTIN, MD

December 2011 • Volume 91 • Number 6

SAUNDERS an imprint of ELSEVIER, Inc.

W.B. SAUNDERS COMPANY

A Division of Elsevier Inc.

1600 John F. Kennedy Blvd., Suite 1800, Philadelphia, PA 19103-2899

http://www.surgical.theclinics.com

SURGICAL CLINICS OF NORTH AMERICA Volume 91, Number 6
December 2011 ISSN 0039-6109, ISBN-13: 978-1-4557-1044-7

Editor: John Vassallo, j.vassallo@elsevier.com

Developmental Editor: Donald Mumford

Surgical Clinics of North America (ISSN 0039–6109) is published bimonthly by Elsevier Inc., 360 Park Avenue South, New York, NY 10010-1710. Months of publication are February, April, June, August, October, and December. Business and Editorial Offices: 1600 John F. Kennedy Blvd., Suite 1800, Philadelphia, PA 19103-2899. Periodicals postage paid at New York, NY and additional mailing offices. Subscription prices are $311.00 per year for US individuals, $532.00 per year for US institutions, $152.00 per year for US students and residents, $381.00 per year for Canadian individuals, $661.00 per year for Canadian institutions, $429.00 for international individuals, $661.00 per year for international institutions and $210.00 per year for Canadian and foreign students/residents. To receive student/resident rate, orders must be accompanied by name of affiliated institution, date of term, and the *signature* of program/residency coordinator on institution letterhead. Orders will be billed at individual rate until proof of status is received. Foreign air speed delivery is included in all *Clinics* subscription prices. All prices are subject to change without notice. POSTMASTER: Send address changes to *Surgical Clinics*, Elsevier Health Sciences Division, Subscription Customer Service, 3251 Riverport Lane, Maryland Heights, MO 63043. **Customer Service (orders, claims, online, change of address): Telephone: 1-800-654-2452 (U.S. and Canada); 314-447-8871 (outside U.S. and Canada). Fax: 314-447-8029. E-mail: journalscustomerservice-usa@elsevier.com (for print support); journalsonline support-usa@elsevier.com (for online support).**

Reprints. For copies of 100 or more, of articles in this publication, please contact the Commercial Reprints Department, Elsevier Inc., 360 Park Avenue South, New York, New York 10010-1710. Tel. (212) 633-3812, Fax: (212) 462-1935, e-mail: reprints@elsevier.com.

The Surgical Clinics of North America is also published in Spanish by McGraw-Hill Interamericana Editores S.A., P.O. Box 5-237 06500 Mexico D.F. Mexico; and in Portuguese by Interlivros Edicoes Ltda., Rua Comandante Coelho 1085, CEP 21250, Rio de Janeiro, Brazil; and in Greek by Paschalidis Medical Publications, Athens Greece.

The Surgical Clinics of North America is covered in *MEDLINE/PubMed (Index Medicus)*, *EMBASE/Excerpta Medica*, *Current Contents/Clinical Medicine*, *Current Contents/Life Sciences*, *Science Citation Index*, and *ISI/BIOMED*.

Printed and bound by CPI Group (UK) Ltd, Croydon, CR0 4YY

Transferred to Digital Print 2011

Contributors

CONSULTING EDITOR

RONALD F. MARTIN, MD
Staff Surgeon, Department of Surgery, Marshfield Clinic, Marshfield, Wisconsin; Clinical Associate Professor, University of Wisconsin School of Medicine and Public Health, Madison, Wisconsin; Colonel, Medical Corps, United States Army Reserve

GUEST EDITOR

SHANU N. KOTHARI, MD, FACS
Department of General and Vascular Surgery, Gundersen Lutheran Health System, La Crosse, Wisconsin

AUTHORS

AYMAN B. AL HARAKEH, MD
Department of General and Vascular Surgery, Gundersen Lutheran Health System, La Crosse, Wisconsin

MOHAMED R. ALI, MD
Associate Professor of Surgery, Chief of Bariatric Surgery, Director of Minimally Invasive and Robotic Surgery, University of California Davis Medical Center, Sacramento, California

MATTHEW T. BAKER, MD, FACS
Department of Surgery, Gundersen Lutheran Health System, La Crosse, Wisconsin

ALEC C. BEEKLEY, MD, FACS
Department of Surgery, Thomas Jefferson University, Philadelphia, Pennsylvania

STACY A. BRETHAUER, MD
Assistant Professor of Surgery, Cleveland Clinic Lerner College of Medicine; Staff Surgeon, Bariatric and Metabolic Institute, Cleveland Clinic, Cleveland, Ohio

KRISTOFFEL R. DUMON, MD, FACS
Assistant Professor, Department of Surgery, Perelman School of Medicine, University of Pennsylvania, Philadelphia, Pennsylvania

ADOLFO Z. FERNANDEZ Jr, MD, FACS
Associate Professor of Surgery, Department of General Surgery, Wake Forest University School of Medicine, Winston-Salem, North Carolina

JORGE ZELADA GETTY, MD
Fellow in Minimally Invasive and Bariatric Surgery, University of California Davis Medical Center, Sacramento, California

ISAM N. HAMDALLAH, MD
Fellow in Minimally Invasive and Bariatric Surgery, University of California Davis Medical Center, Sacramento, California

ANNA R. IBELE, MD
Fellow, Minimally Invasive and Bariatric Surgery, Department of Surgery, Indiana University School of Medicine, Indianapolis, Indiana; Fellow, Division of Pediatric Surgery, Department of Surgery, University of Louisville, Louisville, Kentucky

DANNY O. JACOBS, MD, MPH
David C. Sabiston, Jr. Professor of Surgery, Chair, Department of Surgery, Duke University Medical Center, Duke University School of Medicine, Durham, North Carolina

ASHUTOSH KAUL, MD, MS, FACS, FRCS(Edin), FASMBS
Director of Minimally Invasive and Robotic Surgery, Department of Surgery, Westchester Medical Center; Associate Professor of Surgery, New York Medical College, Valhalla, New York

TODD ANDREW KELLOGG, MD
Assistant Professor of Surgery, Division of Bariatric and Gastrointestinal Surgery, University of Minnesota, Minneapolis, Minnesota

VISHAL KOTHARI, MD
Assistant Professor of Surgery, University of Nebraska Medical Center, Omaha, Nebraska

SEAN M. LEE, MD
General Surgery Chief Resident, Department of Surgery, Duke University Medical Center, Durham, North Carolina

SAMER G. MATTAR, MD, FACS
Director, Indiana University Health Bariatrics and Weight Loss; Associate Professor of Surgery, Indiana University School of Medicine, Indianapolis, Indiana

CORRIGAN L. MCBRIDE, MD, FACS, FASMBS
Associate Professor of Surgery, Director of UNMC Bariatric Surgery, University of Nebraska Medical Center, Omaha, Nebraska

RACHEL L. MCKENNEY, MD
Internal Medicine Resident, Department of Internal Medicine, Gundersen Lutheran Medical Foundation, La Crosse, Wisconsin

KENRIC M. MURAYAMA, MD, FACS
Professor, Department of Surgery, Perelman School of Medicine, Penn Presbyterian Medical Center, University of Pennsylvania, Philadelphia, Pennsylvania

CHAN W. PARK, MD
Duke Endosurgery, Department of Surgery, Duke University Medical Center, Duke University, Durham, North Carolina

MYRON S. POWELL, MD
Minimally Invasive and Bariatric Surgery Fellow, Department of General Surgery, Wake Forest University School of Medicine, Winston-Salem, North Carolina

AURORA D. PRYOR, MD, FACS
Professor of Surgery and Director, Bariatric and Metabolic Weight Loss Center, Division of General Surgery, Department of Surgery, Stony Brook University Medical Center, Stony Brook, New York

NATHAN G. RICHARDS, MD
Department of Surgery, Thomas Jefferson University, Philadelphia, Pennsylvania

PAUL A. SEVERSON, MD, FACS
Co-Director, Minnesota Institute for Minimally Invasive Surgery; Co-Director, MIMIS Weight Loss Center, Crosby, Minnesota

HAZEM SHAMSEDDEEN, MD
Fellow in Minimally Invasive and Bariatric Surgery, University of California Davis Medical Center, Sacramento, California

JYOTI SHARMA, MD, MPH
Department of Surgery, Westchester Medical Center, Valhalla, New York

DANIEL K. SHORT, MD, PhD, FACP, FACE
Department of Endocrinology, Gundersen Lutheran Health System, La Crosse, Wisconsin

JAY MICHAEL SNOW, MD
MIS/Bariatric/Flexible Endoscopy Fellow, Minnesota Institute for Minimally Invasive Surgery, MIMIS Weight Loss Center, Crosby, Minnesota

RANJAN SUDAN, MD
Associate Professor of Surgery and Psychiatry, Vice Chair for Surgical Education, Department of Surgery, Duke University Medical Center, Durham, North Carolina

DAVID S. TICHANSKY, MD, FACS
Department of Surgery, Thomas Jefferson University, Philadelphia, Pennsylvania

ALFONSO TORQUATI, MD, MSCI
Duke Endosurgery, Department of Surgery, Duke University Medical Center, Duke University, Durham, North Carolina

Contents

Obesity plays a major role in the development of type 2 diabetes mellitus, and it has long been accepted that weight loss plays a significant role in diabetes therapy. This weight loss has traditionally been accomplished through lifestyle changes including diet and exercise. What has only more recently gained acceptance is that bariatric surgery may have a role to play in diabetes therapy as well. This article discusses the pathophysiology of type 2 diabetes mellitus and obesity and provides a basic understanding of these diseases, which forms the basis for understanding the importance of weight loss in their treatment.

The clinical outcomes achieved by bariatric surgery have been impressive. However, the physiologic mechanisms and complex metabolic effects of bariatric surgery are only now beginning to be understood. Ongoing research has contributed a large amount of data and shed new light on the science behind obesity and its treatment, and this article reviews the current understanding of metabolic and bariatric surgery physiology.

Obesity has become a major public health concern in the United States and the rest of the world. This disease carries significant health risks that encompass several organ systems. Type 2 diabetes mellitus is a major comorbidity of obesity that predisposes patients to significant end-organ damage. The prevalence of obesity and diabetes is increasing worldwide, and the economic impact of these diseases currently assumes a significant portion of health care expenditure. These factors mandate implementation of therapeutic medical and surgical strategies that target prevention and treatment of obesity and its related medical conditions.

The obesity epidemic has far-reaching implications for the economic and health care future in the United States. Treatments that show reduction in health care costs over time should be approved and made available to as many patients as possible. It is our opinion that bariatric surgery meets this criterion. However, bariatric surgery cannot provide the impact necessary for reduction in health care and economic costs on a national scale. The obesity epidemic must be addressed by policy efforts at the local, state, and national levels. As experts on obesity, bariatric surgeons must be prepared to guide and inform these efforts.

The search for the ideal weight loss operation began more than 50 years ago. Surgical pioneers developed innovative procedures that initially created malabsorption, then restricted volume intake, and eventually combined both techniques. Variations, alterations, and modifications of these original procedures, combined with intense efforts to follow and document outcomes, have led to the evolution of modern bariatric surgery. More recent research has focused on the hormonal and metabolic effects of these procedures. These discoveries at the cellular level will help develop possible mechanisms of weight loss and comorbidity reduction beyond the traditional explanation of reduced food consumption and malabsorption.

Over the past 20 years bariatric surgery proved to be a valid treatment for reduction and elimination of obesity-related diseases and long-term sustainable weight loss. Minimally invasive or laparoscopic techniques such as laparoscopic Roux-en-Y (LRNY) have replaced open procedures. Many factors play important roles in the small intricacies and variations of the procedure, chief of which is the creation and size of the gastrojejunostomy. Regardless of the variations in technique, the LRNY remains the gold standard for the surgical treatment of clinically severe or morbid obesity, with relatively low morbidity and mortality.

Despite the well-documented safety of laparoscopic RYGB, several short-term and long-term complications, with varying degrees of morbidity and mortality risk, are known to occur. Bariatric surgeons, all too familiar with these complications, should be knowledgeable in risk-reduction strategies to minimize the incidence of complication occurrence and recurrence. Bariatric and nonbariatric surgeons who evaluate and treat abdominal pain should be familiar with these complications to facilitate early recognition and intervention, thereby minimizing the associated morbidity and mortality.

This article reviews the use of laparoscopic adjustable gastric banding in the United States today. It comments on the history of the procedure as well as technical aspects of the operation. Short-term and long-term outcomes of the procedure are examined, and the advantages and disadvantages of this procedure in comparison with the laparoscopic gastric bypass are discussed.

Jay Michael Snow and Paul A. Severson

Adjustable gastric banding (AGB) has become increasingly used by bariatric surgeons and their patients as the surgical weight loss procedure of choice. The popularity of this procedure is in large part a result of the remarkable safety profile and low initial complication rate. Complications of AGB were initially believed to be minor and infrequent, but longer-term studies have increasingly described complications that lead to revisional surgery. In addition, a larger fraction of patients fail to lose weight than with other surgical weight loss procedures, frequently necessitating conversion to these other options.

Stacy A. Brethauer

Sleeve gastrectomy (SG) was originally performed as the restrictive component of the duodenal switch procedure. This partial vertical gastrectomy served to reduce gastric capacity and initiate short-term weight loss while the malabsorptive component of the operation (biliopancreatic diversion) provided the long-term weight loss. Some patients, however, could not undergo the intestinal bypass, and early investigations found that substantial weight loss occurred with the SG alone. The sleeve then developed into a risk management strategy for very large or high-risk patients who would not tolerate a longer or higher-risk procedure.

Ranjan Sudan and Danny O. Jacobs

The biliopancreatic diversion with a duodenal switch (BPD-DS) is a less commonly performed but very effective bariatric procedure that has been in existence for more than 20 years. It is particularly effective for the resolution of diabetes and is associated with the highest weight loss among other bariatric operations. Typically, the BPD-DS is not associated with postgastrectomy symptoms, such as dumping and marginal ulceration. Because of its complexity, it has usually been performed by laparotomy in the past; but, more recently, minimally invasive techniques are being used with acceptable risk.

Ashutosh Kaul and Jyoti Sharma

Published data show that bariatric surgery not only leads to significant and sustained weight loss but also resolves or improves multiple comorbidities associated with morbid obesity. Evidence suggests that the earlier the intervention the better the resolution of comorbidities. Patients with metabolic syndrome and comorbidities associated with morbid obesity should be promptly referred for consideration for bariatric surgery earlier in the disease process.

THE CLINICS ARE NOW AVAILABLE ONLINE!

Access your subscription at:
www.theclinics.com

Foreword
Bariatric and Metabolic Surgery

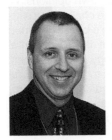

Ronald F. Martin, MD
Consulting Editor

The greater danger for most of us lies not in setting our aim too high and falling short; but in setting our aim too low, and achieving our mark.
—*Michelangelo*

It would seem to me that many of the major problems we face at all levels of society essentially involve a disagreement of how to distribute something; perhaps money, perhaps power (usually related to money), perhaps food, perhaps some natural resource such as petrochemicals or rare earth metals, or maybe even education. It doesn't really matter where you go, people seem to disagree, often fiercely and fundamentally, about who deserves what and who should pay for it or provide it. One can see it in our local communities, or watch it on television, or go to some remote village in Iraq or valley in Afghanistan or impoverished city in the Horn of Africa. It's all the same— people arguing and jockeying for position of control over something that is limited in availability, or at least perceived to be limited or valuable.

Then we have obesity. Actually, we have an epidemic of obesity. We have an epidemic of a disease of excess that is subsequently causing a shortage of resources—ironic, really. The contributors to this issue very nicely review the basis of this problem as well as some of its societal implications and provide a sound foundation for our current solutions such as they are. I commend any surgeon to read these reviews carefully as this is material that any surgeon, in particular any general surgeon, needs to be facile with whether she or he performs these operations or doesn't.

From a surgical standpoint, bariatric surgery is a bit of an intellectual enigma. We take perfectly working anatomy and physiology and we derange it to a point where we hope it solves the problem of calorie intake and absorption excess. All the while hoping that the problem we create, while solving the problem we encountered,

Surg Clin N Am 91 (2011) xiii–xv
doi:10.1016/j.suc.2011.09.002
0039-6109/11/$ – see front matter © 2011 Elsevier Inc. All rights reserved.

won't overshoot the target and cause starvation or create some new problem as a result of altered anatomy, like, for example, lose endoscopic access to the foregut for future concerns.

As a person responsible for training other surgeons, bariatric surgery presents me with other dilemmas as well. No matter how much of it one does, it doesn't help one become that much better at dealing with most other surgical problems. I can feel the backlash as I type this from some people but I'll let them write their own opinions. I'll grant you that one can develop better laparoscopic skills under some challenging situations and that is a plus. Also, one can see what happens when one's best performed technical efforts go awry—also a good learning experience. But the incremental benefit for diagnosing problems and understanding pathophysiology becomes fairly minimal after managing a few patients such as these. Largely due to the successful development of these procedures and the ample supplies of candidates for them, we have created an almost assembly-line approach to bariatric operations. And while that is necessary and good for the bariatric patient, it isn't necessarily all that useful for surgical education.

I hate to turn the conversation back to money but it is pretty near impossible not to do so. We physicians are an adaptable and creative bunch. If the people who pay us say they will reduce the unit reimbursement for something, then we crank up the utilization rates to make up for it. Then we have the "Well, if you think I am expensive, try the alternative argument." And it's a good argument; take, for example, renal transplant versus continued dialysis—good argument, financially. In particular regard to obesity surgery, some say these operations cost too much and some say it is cheap compared to treating diabetes and hypertension and obstructive sleep apnea and replacing joints. And both sides are right. The fact remains that we will much more likely pay for solutions to the problem of obesity than the prevention.

At this moment the big economic question facing us is, are we coming out of a recession or going into a double-dip recession? Some might even argue that there is an actual depression but I'll leave that to the economists to argue. No matter how you classify it, money is tight and getting tighter for the foreseeable future. Many clamor that health care costs have to be cut. Well they do, but doing it now would be really pretty counterproductive. Health care is one of the few "nongovernment" sectors of the economy that didn't tank. A ten percent reduction in health care spending all of a sudden would create an almost two percent reduction in gross domestic product: that would put huge brakes on any recovery or initiate a depression and it would further worsen the unemployment situation as most health care jobs in the United States are not readily outsourced and would mostly solely affect American workers. So while health care costs need to come back on line with reality as a percent of our total spending, especially value for costs, today just isn't the right time for that to happen. The passion to cut health care costs makes for good politics until you actually have to tell someone what goes away.

Obesity as a disease gives us a real chance to look in the mirror and see who we are (please forgive the metaphor). It shows us how our view of this disease is markedly altered by the prism through which we look. And it tells us how we respond to incentives—both as physicians and as patients. If you make your living as a bariatric surgeon, the obesity epidemic is the job security dreamscape. If you make your living as a grocer or a restaurateur, same deal. If you are a government planner, an insurance executive, health care administrator, or a physician who plans on practicing medicine in a capitated world—it is a real nightmare scenario; a disease that increases consumption on both sides of the scales, takes a long time to grow, and doesn't kill people quickly.

If ever there were a problem that we should look at from a pan-societal viewpoint, obesity is it: from childhood education, to food distribution, to early screening and management, to research and development into satiety and metabolism, to policy on funding and reimbursing for prevention and for treatment, and even for civil engineering and design to make our communities more conducive to human propulsion and less dependent on motorized propulsion.

As I said, it is hard to reconcile, at least for me, that in a world suffering from so much need that one of our biggest challenges is a disease of excess. My personal intellectual challenges aside, the case remains that it is true. As for us surgeons, we must once again do what we must to understand the disease and understand the role it plays and that we play in society. We must also do what we can to put ourselves out of business as much as possible with regard to obesity as we have with trauma and other diseases—realizing that we are at no risk for becoming completely unemployed as a result of our efforts to reduce the public's need for us. I suggest that we aim for a higher goal than just becoming proficient at the technical aspects of managing obesity. We need to lead the way out of this problem altogether.

The best tool to be an effective part of the solution to any problem is always a good knowledge of the fundamentals. Dr Kothari and his colleagues have provided us with an excellent review in this issue of the *Surgical Clinics of North America*. Once informed, we can all decide how to proceed with that information. As always, your readership of this series is valued and appreciated.

Ronald F. Martin, MD
Department of Surgery
Marshfield Clinic
1000 North Oak Avenue
Marshfield, WI 54449, USA

E-mail address:
martin.ronald@marshfieldclinic.org

Preface

Bariatric and Metabolic Surgery

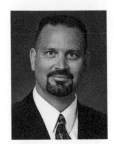

Shanu N. Kothari, MD
Guest Editor

Since the last publication of the *Surgical Clinics of North America* dedicated to Bariatric Surgery in 2005, several milestones have taken place:

- Laparoscopic bariatric procedures are now performed more frequently than their open counterparts.
- There have been significant advances in the understanding of the metabolic and hormonal mechanisms influenced by bariatric surgical procedures. Consequently, in 2007 the American Society for Bariatric Surgery became the American Society for Metabolic and Bariatric Surgery in recognition of the metabolic impact that bariatric surgical procedures have on conditions such as diabetes.
- The American Diabetes Association and International Diabetes Federation have recognized bariatric surgery as a treatment option for diabetes in the severely obese patient.

This issue of the *Surgical Clinics of North America* has 16 articles that encompass a variety of topics pertinent to both dedicated bariatric surgeons as well as general surgeons with an interest in the field.

I appreciate the opportunity to serve as the guest editor of this issue given to me by Dr Ron Martin. I also greatly appreciate the contributions of each of the authors and I hope that the reader finds their contributions to be as educational as I have.

Shanu N. Kothari, MD
Department of General and Vascular Surgery
Gundersen Lutheran Health System
1900 South Avenue
La Crosse, WI 54601, USA

E-mail address:
snkothar@gundluth.org

Surg Clin N Am 91 (2011) xvii
doi:10.1016/j.suc.2011.09.001
surgical.theclinics.com
0039-6109/11/$ – see front matter © 2011 Elsevier Inc. All rights reserved.

Tipping the Balance: the Pathophysiology of Obesity and Type 2 Diabetes Mellitus

Rachel L. McKenney, MD[a],*, Daniel K. Short, MD, PhD[b]

KEYWORDS

• Diabetes • Obesity • Pathophysiology • Lipocentric

Obesity is a disease of epidemic proportion in the United States. In 2007 and 2008, obesity affected 33.8% of the US population, and the combined prevalence of overweight and obesity (body mass index [BMI; calculated as weight in kilograms divided by height in meters squared] ≥ 25 kg/m^2) was 68%. Thus, this country has come to the point to which being of normal weight is no longer normal.[1] The cost of treating obesity was estimated to be $78.5 billion in the United States in 1998.[2] Obesity-related conditions such as type 2 diabetes mellitus have similarly skyrocketed in prevalence, with type 2 diabetes alone affecting 8.3% of the US population, at an estimated annual cost of $174 billion in health care expenditures.[3] Complications of type 2 diabetes mellitus include diabetic retinopathy, which is the leading cause of adult-onset blindness in the United States; diabetic nephropathy, which leads to chronic kidney disease and is the leading cause of kidney failure; diabetic peripheral neuropathy, which is the leading cause of nontraumatic lower limb amputations; as well as coronary artery disease and peripheral vascular disease, which are major sources of morbidity and mortality.[4] At any given age, a person with diabetes has a risk of dying that is twice that of age-matched peers without diabetes. In the United States, diabetes is the seventh leading cause of death.[3]

Obesity plays a major role in the development of type 2 diabetes, and it has long been accepted that weight loss plays a significant role in diabetes therapy. This weight loss has traditionally been accomplished through lifestyle changes including diet and exercise. It has only more recently gained acceptance that bariatric surgery may have a role to play in diabetes therapy as well.[5] This article discusses the pathophysiology

The authors have nothing to disclose.
a Department of Internal Medicine, Gundersen Lutheran Medical Foundation, 1836 South Avenue, La Crosse, WI 54601, USA
b Department of Endocrinology, Gundersen Lutheran Health System, 1836 South Avenue, La Crosse, WI 54601, USA
* Corresponding author.
E-mail address: RLMckenn@gundluth.org

of type 2 diabetes mellitus and obesity and provides a basic understanding of these diseases, which forms the basis for understanding the importance of weight loss in their treatment.

TYPE 2 DIABETES MELLITUS

Type 2 diabetes mellitus is caused by a combination of insulin resistance in peripheral tissues and a loss of beta cell function in the pancreas.[3] Insulin resistance occurs when the body cannot respond appropriately to normal or even high circulating levels of insulin and is usually related to underlying obesity. This condition then leads to hyperglycemia due to relative insulin deficiency. There is also a progressive loss of beta cell function over time, which contributes to the progression of the disease by decreasing the amount of insulin available in the circulation. Therefore, treatment usually includes insulin sensitizers such as metformin and thiazolidinediones, as well as medications such as sulfonylureas and insulin injections that increase the available amount of insulin.[6]

Diabetes develops due to a complex combination of environmental and genetic factors that together lead to the development of the disease. For example, for insulin secretion to occur, glucose must first be transported into the beta cell. The glucose transporter (GLUT) type 2 is central to this process.[2] In mouse models when this transporter has a genetic defect, glucose intolerance occurs. The same intolerance occurs when mice lacking the defect are fed a high-fat diet.[4] This suggests that not only genetic factors but also environmental influences can lead to disorders of glucose metabolism. In humans, obesity and the aging process predispose to the development of hyperglycemia in those who have an appropriate genetic background, and the genetics of type 2 diabetes is poorly understood. However, genes affecting the development of type 2 diabetes mellitus have only recently been identified.[7] The hyperglycemia associated with type 2 diabetes is frequently well tolerated for years until the relative insulin deficiency has become severe enough that symptoms of hyperglycemia develop. Thus, many patients are undiagnosed until they begin to experience the complications of the disease. It has been estimated that in 2010 there were approximately 7 million undiagnosed cases of diabetes.[1]

Of the 2 types of diabetes, type 2 has a much stronger genetic component than type 1.[3] Observational studies have repeatedly demonstrated the role genetics plays in the development of type 2 diabetes mellitus. It is known that more than one-third of patients with type 2 diabetes have at least 1 parent with diabetes,[8] and having a first-degree relative with type 2 diabetes increases the risk of developing the disease 10-fold. In twin studies, almost 90% of those with a monozygotic twin with type 2 diabetes mellitus will eventually develop the disease.[9] Several defects in single genes have been identified; however, several cases of type 2 diabetes mellitus are thought to be caused by polygenic defects.[10] The single gene defects tend to affect beta cell function and therefore the release of insulin. Examples include defects of glucokinase and hepatocyte nuclear factor 1α, which cause maturity-onset diabetes of youth 2 and maturity-onset diabetes of youth 3, respectively. Defects can also occur in genes that are involved in the regulation of insulin action on target cells, such as the insulin receptor, peroxisome proliferator-activated receptor γ, and adiponectin.[11] There have been several other genetic loci that have been recently identified that may shed further light on the process by which diabetes develops. Defects in the fat mass and obesity gene, FTO, have been shown to cause an increase in BMI, which then increases the risk of developing diabetes.[11] Another recently identified gene is HMGA1, which is an important regulator of insulin receptor gene expression. Defects in this gene have been associated with the development of insulin resistance and type 2 diabetes mellitus.[12,13] However, for most patients with diabetes, it is thought that the disease is polygenic in origin. There are currently at least 11 separate genetic regions that have been confirmed to be linked to an increased likelihood of developing type 2 diabetes mellitus.[7] These genes are involved in insulin secretion, beta cell function, beta cell development, and beta cell survival. One such gene is TCF7L2, which encodes for a transcription factor. Defects in this gene increase the risk for developing type 2 diabetes mellitus by 45%[14] and seem to decrease the beta cell response to glucose administration.[15]

Obesity has been shown to be an independent risk factor for the development of type 2 diabetes mellitus. The exact mechanism by which obesity causes insulin resistance is unknown. One theory is that high plasma concentrations of free fatty acids seen in obesity help to drive insulin resistance. High levels of free fatty acids are known to inhibit the secretion of insulin and decrease insulin-mediated glucose uptake in peripheral tissues.[16,17] Another explanation could involve adiponectin. Adiponectin is a cytokine that is released by adipose tissue that decreases insulin resistance.[18] Adiponectin levels are decreased in obesity, and this may lead to an increase in insulin resistance.[19,20] Other substances produced by adipocytes that may be related to the development of insulin resistance in obesity include tumor necrosis factor α (TNF-α), plasminogen activator inhibitor 1, retinol-binding protein 4, and resistin.[21–24] The increased amount of free fatty acids seen in obesity increases TNF-α expression, which may lead to an increase in insulin resistance.[25,26] In addition to its association with increased risk for cardiovascular disease, plasminogen activator inhibitor has been found in several studies to independently predict the development of type 2 diabetes mellitus.[22] Resistin is secreted by adipocytes and decreases insulin-mediated glucose uptake by adipocytes.[21]

OBESITY

One of the most important risk factors for the development of type 2 diabetes mellitus is obesity. Obesity is defined as a BMI of greater than 30 kg/m^2 and represents a degree of fat accumulation that is likely to affect health.[2] In general, weight tends to peak in the sixth to seventh decade of life and then tends to decrease after that. The World Health Organization indicated that in 2008 there were 1.5 billion adults aged at least 20 years who were overweight, and, of these, 200 million men and 300 million women were obese.[27] At present, it is estimated that at least 25% of children in the United States are either overweight or obese.[2] However, in industrialized societies, overweight and obesity are becoming more prevalent, particularly in children. This is especially true in urbanized cultures in which physical activity has diminished and high-fat, calorie-dense, convenience foods have become more common and accessible. It is projected that by 2015 this number will almost double.[3]

There are several factors that can lead to the development of obesity. These factors include genetics, insufficient exercise (sedentary lifestyle), and excess calorie consumption. Some medications such as steroids and antipsychotic drugs are also known to have significant weight gain as a common side effect. Psychosocial factors can also contribute to the development of obesity. Ultimately, these factors combine to form an imbalance between caloric intake and energy expenditure.

Metabolic syndrome (also called syndrome X) consists of a combination of abdominal obesity, hyperglycemia, abnormal serum lipid levels, and hypertension. It is thought that this syndrome is related to insulin resistance, a certain degree of which may be mediated by elevated levels of circulating fatty acids.[28] Like both obesity and diabetes, metabolic syndrome is associated with increased cardiovascular risk. Some of this risk may arise through the mechanism of a prothrombotic and proinflammatory state, as evidenced by elevated levels of C-reactive protein and interleukin 6.[29] Questions remain as to whether metabolic syndrome yields greater risk than the sum of its individual components, but it remains a useful marker for patients who are at an increased cardiovascular risk.[30]

Weight gain and adiposity are determined by the balance between energy expenditure and caloric intake. Caloric intake is determined by both the amount of food ingested and the nutritional composition of the food.[3] More than 30% of the calories in the diet of Western societies are from fat. Fat is more calorie dense than carbohydrates or protein. Fat also has less of an impact on satiety than carbohydrates or protein.[4]

Food intake is largely controlled by appetite, which is regulated through the hypothalamus in a complex manner through multiple different mechanisms. One hormone is leptin, which is produced in adipose tissue and is a potent appetite suppressant.[31] Glucagonlike peptide 1 is an incretin hormone that is produced in the gut. It has been shown to inhibit food intake when administered subcutaneously.[32] There are also several other hormones produced in the gut that seem to have a suppressive effect on hunger and induce satiety. These hormones include cholecystokinin, enterostatin, polypeptide Y 3–36, α melanocyte-stimulating hormone, corticotropin-releasing hormone, TNF-α, and obestatin.[2]

In addition to appetite suppressants, there are several hormones that are strong stimulants of hunger. Ghrelin is produced by the gut and seems to have 2 main effects: stimulating growth hormone secretion and increasing food intake.[33] When a person anticipates ingestion of food, serum concentrations of ghrelin increase. Conversely, after a meal has been consumed, ghrelin secretion is suppressed.[34] After diet-induced and exercise-induced weight loss, ghrelin levels increase. This increase stimulates appetite, thus potentially complicating efforts at dieting.[35] A decrease in serum ghrelin concentration was demonstrated after gastric bypass in one study and has been proposed as one mechanism by which bariatric surgery may induce weight loss and correct hyperglycemia[36]; however, similar decreases have not been seen in all studies.[37] Other appetite stimulators include neuropeptide Y, dynorphin, melanin-concentrating hormone, norepinephrine, growth hormone–releasing hormone, orexin-A, and orexin-B.[38,39]

There are several different areas in the brain that are important in appetite modulation, which respond to these signalizing molecules. These areas include the arcuate nucleus, where leptin acts; the nucleus of the tractus solitarius, where vagal signals are received; the paraventricular nucleus; and the lateral and ventromedial cites of the hypothalamus, as well as areas of the amygdala.[40] The sympathetic nervous system also has a role in modulating energy intake. Glucocorticoids stimulate food intake, whereas activation of the peripheral sympathetic nervous system decreases food intake via β_3-adrenergic receptors.[41–43]

Exercise and other caloric expenditures counterbalance the effects of food intake. Total energy expenditure (TEE) consists of both resting energy expenditure (REE) and calories burned through exercise. REE is the amount of energy needed by the body throughout the day to carry out basic chemical reactions and physiologic functions when the body is at rest. REE makes up 70% of TEE. The REE increases as fat mass increases; thus there is no evidence that people who are obese have a lower REE or basal metabolic rates.[2] Thermic response to food makes up another 15% to 20% of TEE. Physical activity constitutes only 10% to 15% of TEE,[44] which is the only readily modifiable component of the TEE.

Obesity has a strong familial component, as demonstrated by multiple twin studies. Identical twins have been found to be more alike in body weight than fraternal twins,[11] and the fat distribution of children who are adopted seems to follow that of their biological parents rather than their adoptive parents.[45] Some specific factors influencing the development of obesity also seem to have a hereditary basis. These factors include metabolic rate, spontaneous physical activity, and thermic response to food, of which all affect the TEE.[46] Obesity is also associated with several genetic disorders. The most commonly known disorders are Prader-Willi syndrome and Bardet-Biedl syndrome, but there are at least 22 other known disorders.[47]

One known genetic defect that causes obesity involves leptin, a hormone that is well known to be involved in the control of appetite. Mice that are deficient in leptin because of a defect in the leptin protein or in its receptor demonstrate infertility, hyperinsulinemia, hyperphagia, and insulin resistance.[48,49] It has been shown that giving leptin to these mice can reverse the features caused by the deficiency. Leptin deficiency also has been found in humans, having initially been discovered in 2 consanguineous families.[50] When these patients received leptin replacement, dramatic weight loss was noted, in addition to a decrease in food intake.[51] Although this discovery was very promising, several patients who are obese do not have a defect in the leptin gene. In fact, most patients with obesity have been found to have elevated levels of serum leptin.[52] Thus, the role of leptin in obesity therapy is unclear, although metreleptin is currently being developed as a possible weight loss agent.[53]

There are several other genes that have been implicated in the development of obesity. One such example is the TUB gene, which results in retinitis as well as hypothalamic damage, which in turn results in overstimulation of appetite.[54] Other genes implicated in the development of obesity code for enzymes such as prohormone convertase 1 that are involved in processing prohormones into mature hormones.[55] Loss of the α melanocyte-stimulating factor, which is a satiety factor, can also lead to severe obesity, as can the loss of its receptor (the melanocortin 4 receptor).[7] These genetic defects are of particular interest; however, more research needs to be accomplished before they will have therapeutic applications.

Genetic factors and deficiencies are only part of the explanation for why patients develop obesity and type 2 diabetes mellitus.[56] Environmental and behavioral influences also contribute significantly to the development of these conditions. The 2 main factors that cause weight gain include excessive caloric intake and low physical activity. Either of these conditions creates an imbalance of energy use, favoring energy accumulation and thus weight gain. Both conditions are favored by industrialized societies such as the United States. Excessive caloric intake is perpetuated by easy access to inexpensive convenience foods that are high in fat content.[11] In addition, advances in transportation as well as a decrease in employment requiring manual labor have both led to a dramatic decrease in the overall level of physical activity of the population as a whole. Behavioral factors also influence the development of obesity. For instance, there have been studies performed, specifically in the Framingham cohort, which have shown that obesity has a strong social component.[57] It is thought that people who are surrounded by obese individuals are influenced by the behaviors of those individuals. This influence in turn can lead to increased caloric intake and lower physical activity levels in close social contacts. In addition, it is thought that the intrauterine environment may play an important role in metabolic programming. For example, rodent studies have shown that gestational diabetes can lead to a syndrome of insulin excess. Likewise, in similar studies, insulin deficiency can develop after a period of undernutrition.[58] This finding suggests that the environment early in life may influence appetite patterns, physical activity, and even food preferences late in life.[11]

TYING IT TOGETHER

The development of diabetes and obesity is closely interrelated. Obesity predisposes the development of type 2 diabetes mellitus, whereas some of the genetic defects that have been discovered to be involved with type 2 diabetes mellitus are also involved in the development of obesity. Environmental influences and certain lifestyle choices can also simultaneously contribute to one or both of these disease states. The traditional idea that type 2 diabetes mellitus is solely a matter of hyperglycemia, insulin resistance, and relative insulin deficiency may now be overly simplistic. Treating diabetes with antihyperglycemic agents is not the only way to approach this disease, nor does it get to the root of the problem of the disorder. There is an alternative model that suggests that type 2 diabetes is caused more by abnormal lipid metabolism rather than abnormal glucose metabolism.

The lipocentric view of diabetes postulates that type 2 diabetes mellitus is caused by the ectopic deposition of excessive fatty acids.[5] This deposition then leads to insulin resistance, beta cell loss, and hyperglycemia.[59] The basic chain of events that is postulated by the lipocentric model begins with excess caloric intake, which then leads to hyperinsulinemia. This condition then causes increased expression of a lipogenic transcription factor, SREBP-1c, which causes increased lipogenesis. Increased lipogenesis leads to an increase in adipose tissue.[5] In addition to adipose tissue, excess fatty acids are also deposited in other tissues such as muscle and liver. There is evidence that excess fatty acids inhibit insulin-mediated glucose uptake into muscle cells by interfering with the translocation of the GLUT-4 to the plasma membrane.[60] In the liver, fatty acids inhibit suppression of insulin-mediated glycogenolysis and gluconeogenesis.[61] There is also evidence that these ectopic lipids can be deposited into the beta cells of the pancreas, leading to beta cell dysfunction and hyperglycemia.[62] This model predicts that hyperglycemia should be corrected by a reversal of lipid overload, through weight loss.

Regardless of which mechanism is more important, lipocentric or glucocentric, excess caloric intake is important in the development of type 2 diabetes mellitus. However, the lipocentric model places excess caloric intake as the root cause of hyperglycemia and type 2 diabetes mellitus and stresses the central importance of reducing caloric intake in those individuals who already have or are at risk for developing diabetes. The goal of reducing caloric intake is both to prevent further lipid overload as well as to yield a modest weight loss, thereby reducing the burden of adiposity and insulin resistance. Although lifestyle changes are widely recognized as being important in type 2 diabetes, the lipocentric view gives special emphasis to weight reduction in preference to traditional therapies such as oral hypoglycemic agents and insulin. This model also leads one to question the wisdom of using large amounts of insulin as the primary therapy for type 2 diabetes mellitus. One of the unfortunate side effects of insulin therapy is weight gain. The question is whether it is wise to continue treating these obese patients with a medication that could be potentially perpetuating the problem as the sole form of treatment. There are recent data showing that aggressive lowering of blood glucose level with hypoglycemic agents may actually be dangerous. A recent publication of results from the ACCORD (Action to Control Cardiovascular Risk in Diabetes) trial demonstrated that targeting hemoglobin A1C levels of less than 6% actually increased the 5-year mortality, specifically in high-risk patients with type 2 diabetes mellitus.[63] The lipocentric hypothesis could be used to argue that those patients might be better served with aggressive weight loss management, possibly including bariatric surgery. If the deposition of lipids is indeed one of the main mechanisms for development of diabetes, then the reversal of lipid deposition should be the primary goal of therapy. In that case, the main mode of treatment should be to focus on weight reduction, not just treating hyperglycemia. Weight reduction is not an easy task. Our society favors the consumption of fast food because of both economic reasons as well as the time constraints that come from living in a modern society. Physical activity has decreased with the increase in service versus labor jobs and with the advent of more sedentary leisure activities, such as television, computers, and video games. This trend is likely not going to change in the near future. For this reason, patients with obesity are turning to options such as weight-reduction surgery as a more definitive therapy.

A study published recently by Dixon and colleagues[64] demonstrated that patients undergoing bariatric surgery were more likely to obtain remission of diabetes mellitus than those treated with lifestyle modifications alone. Around 73% of patients who underwent weight reduction surgery had remission of diabetes as compared with only 13% in the group that received only conventional therapy. There have been various other studies demonstrating similar findings. These data are exciting because they seem to suggest that dramatic weight loss can not only improve control of diabetes but also reverse the disease. This finding supports the lipocentric view of lipid overload being the causative factor by which hyperglycemia and insulin resistance develop. These data do not mean that we should not use insulin or other antihyperglycemic agents to treat the hyperglycemia in diabetes but only suggest that there is another tool that can be used in addition to pharmacologic agents with their attendant side effects and lifestyle modifications, which oftentimes are ineffective due to poor patient compliance. If bariatric surgery succeeds as a primary form of diabetes therapy, then early recognition of patients who demonstrate clinical features of metabolic syndrome will be more important than ever. In these patients, if weight loss cannot be achieved by conventional methods, then weight reduction surgery may be the most beneficial form of therapy because the long-term effects of lipid overload can hopefully be prevented.

SUMMARY

Obesity is a disease state that is increasing in incidence and carries with it a significant health burden, including the development of diabetes mellitus and its complications. There are many proposed mechanisms for the development of obesity and diabetes mellitus and by which obesity predisposes the development of diabetes. Genetic loci and defects have been discovered that have helped to support the idea that these conditions have a hereditary component. In addition to genetic components, there are environmental factors that also seem to play a major role in the development of obesity. The ultimate cause of obesity involves ingesting more energy than is expended over time. This in turn predisposes to the development of insulin resistance and type 2 diabetes mellitus. For this reason, weight loss measures are of the utmost importance for avoiding and reversing the deleterious consequences of obesity. Thus, bariatric surgery may prove to be one of the most important therapies for both treating and preventing type 2 diabetes mellitus.

REFERENCES

1. Flegal KM, Carroll MD, Ogden CL, et al. Prevalence and trends in obesity among US adults. JAMA 2010;303(3):235–41.
2. Wolf AM, Colditz GA. Current estimates of the economic cost of obesity in the United States. Obes Res 1998;6(2):97–106.

3. Centers for Disease Control and Prevention. National diabetes fact sheet: national estimates and general information on diabetes and prediabetes in the United States, 2011. Atlanta (GA): U.S. Department of Health and Human Services, Centers for Disease Control and Prevention; 2011.

4. Gardner DG, Shoback D. Greenspan's basic & clinical endocrinology. New York: McGraw Hill; 2007. p. 661–747, 796–816.

5. Unger RH. Reinventing type 2 diabetes: pathogenesis, treatment, and prevention. JAMA 2008;299(10):1185–7.

6. AACE Diabetes Mellitus Clinical Practice Guidelines Taskforce. (2007). AACE guidelines for clinical practice for the management of diabetes mellitus. Available at: http://www.aace.com/pub/guidelines. Accessed February 15, 2011.

7. Romao I, Roth J. Genetic and environmental interactions in obesity and type 2 diabetes. J Am Diet Assoc 2008;108:824–8.

8. Belchetz P, Hammond P. Mosby's color atlas and text of diabetes and endocrinology. London: Mosby; 2003. p. 11–21, 397–407.

9. Thorens B. A toggle for type 2 diabetes? N Engl J Med 2006;354:1636.

10. Klein BE, Klein R, Moss SE, et al. Parental history of diabetes in a population-based study. Diabetes Care 1996;19:827.

11. Barnett AH, Eff C, Leslie RD, et al. Diabetes in identical twins. A study of 200 pairs. Diabetologia 1981;20:87.

12. Fajans SS, Bell GI, Polonsky KS. Molecular mechanisms and clinical pathophysiology of maturity-onset diabetes of the young. N Engl J Med 2001;345:971.

13. Abhimanyu G. HMGA1, a novel locus for type 2 diabetes mellitus. JAMA 2011; 305(9):938–9.

14. Grant SF, Thorleifsson G, Reynisdottir I, et al. Variant of transcription factor 7-like 2 (TCF7L2) gene confers risk of type 2 diabetes. Nat Genet 2006;38:320.

15. Lyssenko V, Lupi R, Marchetti P, et al. Mechanisms by which common variants in the TCF7L2 gene increase risk of type 2 diabetes. J Clin Invest 2007;117:2155.

16. Bennet WM, Beis CS, Ghatei MA, et al. Amylin tonally regulates arginine-stimulated insulin secretion in rats. Diabetologia 1994;37:436.

17. Boden G, Chen X. Effects of fat on glucose uptake and utilization in patients with non-insulin-dependent diabetes. J Clin Invest 1995;96:1261.

18. Wannamethee SG, Whincup PH, Lennon L, et al. Circulating adiponectin levels and mortality in elderly men with and without cardiovascular disease and heart failure. Arch Intern Med 2007;167:1510.

19. Mantzoros CS, Li T, Manson JE, et al. Circulating adiponectin levels are associated with better glycemic control, more favorable lipid profile, and reduced inflammation in women with type 2 diabetes. J Clin Endocrinol Metab 2005;90:4542.

20. Kadowski T, Yamauchi T, Kubota N, et al. Adiponectin and adiponectin receptors in insulin resistance, diabetes, and the metabolic syndrome. J Clin Invest 2006; 116:1784.

21. Steppen CM, Bailey ST, Bhat S, et al. The hormone resistin links obesity to diabetes. Nature 2001;409:307.

22. Kanaya AM, Wassel Fyr C, Vittinghoff E, et al. Adipocytokines and incident diabetes mellitus in older adults: the independent effect of plasminogen activator inhibitor 1. Arch Intern Med 2006;166:350.

23. Graham TE, Yang Q, Bluher M, et al. Retinol-binding protein 4 and insulin resistance in lean, obese, and diabetic subjects. N Engl J Med 2006;354:2552.

24. Hotamisligil GS, Johnson RS, Distel RJ, et al. Uncoupling of obesity from insulin resistance through a targeted mutation in aP2, the adipocyte fatty acid binding protein. Science 1996;274:1377.

25. Uysal KT, Wiesbrock SM, Marino MW, et al. Protection from obesity-induced insulin resistance in mice lacking TNF-alpha function. Nature 1997;389:610.
26. Hotamisligil GS, Shargill NS, Spiegelman BM. Adipose expression of tumor necrosis factor-alpha: direct role in obesity-linked insulin resistance. Science 1993;259:87.
27. Media centre. Obesity and overweight fact sheet. N*311. World Health Organization; 2011.
28. Eckel RH, Grundy SM, Zimmet PZ. The metabolic syndrome. Lancet 2005;365 (9468):1415–28.
29. Koh KK, Han SH, Quon MJ. Inflammatory markers and the metabolic syndrome: insights from therapeutic interventions. J Am Coll Cardiol 2005;46(11):1978–85.
30. Kohli P, Greenland P. Role of the metabolic syndrome in risk assessment for coronary heart disease. JAMA 2006;295(7):819–21.
31. Considine RV, Sinha MK, Heiman ML, et al. Serum immunoreactive leptin concentrations in normal-weight and obese humans. N Engl J Med 1996;334:292.
32. Flint A, Raben A, Astrup A, et al. Glucagon-like peptide-1 promotes satiety and suppresses energy intake in humans. J Clin Invest 1998;101:515.
33. Wren AM, Seal LJ, Cohen MA, et al. Ghrelin enhances appetite and increases food intake in humans. J Clin Endocrinol Metab 2001;86:5992.
34. Druce MR, Wren AM, Park AJ, et al. Ghrelin increases food intake in obese as well as lean subjects. Int J Obes (Lond) 2005;29:1130.
35. Foster-Schubert KE, McTiernan A, Frayo RS, et al. Human plasma ghrelin levels increase during a one-year exercise program. J Clin Endocrinol Metab 2005; 90:820.
36. Cummings D, Weigle DS, Frayo RS, et al. Plasma ghrelin levels after diet-induced weight loss or gastric bypass surgery. N Engl J Med 2002;346:1623.
37. Tymitz K, Engel A, McDonough S, et al. Changes in ghrelin levels following bariatric surgery: review of the literature. Obes Surg 2011;21:125–30.
38. Sakurai T, Amemiya A, Ishii M, et al. Orexins and orexin receptors: a family of hypothalamic neuropeptides and G protein-coupled receptors that regulate feeding behavior. Cell 1998;92:573.
39. Gerald C, Walker MW, Criscione L, et al. A receptor subtype involved in neuropeptide-Y-induced food intake. Nature 1996;382:168.
40. Bethoud HR. Multiple neural systems controlling food intake and body weight. Neurosci Biobehav Rev 2002;26:393.
41. Bray GA. Reciprocal relation between the sympathetic nervous system and food intake. Brain Res Bull 1991;27:517.
42. Tsujii S, Bray GA. A beta-3 adrenergic agonist (BRL-37,344) decreases food intake. Physiol Behav 1998;63:723.
43. Grujic D, Susulic VS, Harper ME, et al. Beta3–adrenergic receptors on white and brown adipocytes mediate beta3-selective agonist-induced effects on energy expenditure, insulin secretion, and food intake. A study using transgenic and gene knockout mice. J Biol Chem 1997;272:17686.
44. Ravussin E, Lillioja S, Knowler WC, et al. Reduced rate of energy expenditure as a risk factor for body weight gain. N Engl J Med 1988;318:467.
45. Stunkard AJ, Sorensen TI, Hanis C, et al. An adoption study of human obesity. N Engl J Med 1986;314:193–8.
46. Fontaine E, Savard R, Tremblay A, et al. Resting metabolic rate in monozygotic and dizygotic twins. Acta Genet Med Gemellol (Roma) 1985;34:41.
47. Rankinen T, Perusse L, Weisnegel SJ, et al. The human obesity gene map: the 2001 update. Obes Res 2002;10:196.

48. Chen H, Charlat O, Tartaglia LA, et al. Evidence that the diabetes gene encodes the leptin receptor: identification of a mutation in the leptin receptor gene in db/db mice. Cell 1996;84:491.

49. Campfield LA, Smith FJ, Burn P. The OB protein (leptin) pathway—a link between adipose tissue mass and central neural networks. Horm Metab Res 1996;28:619.

50. Pelleymounter MA, Cullen MJ, Baker MB, et al. Effects of the obese gene product on body weight regulation in ob/ob mice. Science 1995;269:540.

51. Montague CT, Farooqi IS, Whitehead JP, et al. Congenital leptin deficiency is associated with severe early-onset obesity in humans. Nature 1997;387:903.

52. Farooqi IS, Jebb SA, Langmack G, et al. Effects of recombinant leptin therapy in a child with congenital leptin deficiency. N Engl J Med 1999;341:879.

53. Ravussin E, Smith SR, Mitchell JA, et al. Enhanced weight loss with pramlintide/metreleptin: an integrated neurohormonal approach to obesity pharmacotherapy. Obesity (Silver Spring) 2009;17(9):1736–43.

54. Kennedy A, Gettys TW, Watson P, et al. The metabolic significance of leptin in humans: gender-based differences in relationship to adiposity, insulin sensitivity, and energy expenditure. J Clin Endocrinol Metab 1997;82:1293.

55. Jackson RS, Creemers JW, Ohagi S, et al. Obesity and impaired prohormone processing associated with mutations in the human prohormone convertase I gene. Nat Genet 1997;16:303.

56. Hill J, Peters J. Environmental contributions to the obesity pandemic. Science 1998;29:1271–374.

57. Christakis NA, Fowler JH. The spread of obesity in a large social network over 32 years. N Engl J Med 2007;357:379.

58. Patel MS, Srinivasan M. Metabolic programming: causes and consequences. J Biol Chem 2002;277:1629–32.

59. Unger RH. Minireview; weapons of lean body mass destruction: the role of ectopic lipids in the metabolic syndrome. Endocrinology 2003;144(12):5159–65.

60. McGarry JD. What if Minkowski had been ageusic? An alternative angle on diabetes. Science 1992;258(5083):766–70.

61. Boden G, Shulman GI. Free fatty acids in obesity and type 2 diabetes: defining their role in the development of insulin resistance and beta-cell dysfunction. Eur J Clin Invest 2002;32(Suppl 3):14–23.

62. Lee Y, Hirose H, Ohneda M, et al. Beta-cell lipotoxicity in the pathogenesis of non-insulin dependent diabetes mellitus of obese rats: impairment in adipocyte-beta-cell relationships. Proc Natl Acad Sci U S A 1994;91(23):10878–82.

63. The ACCORD Study Group. Long-term effects of intensive glucose lowering on cardiovascular outcomes. N Engl J Med 2011;364:818–28.

64. Dixon JB, O'Brien PE, Playfair J, et al. Adjustable gastric banding and conventional therapy for type 2 diabetes: a randomized controlled trial. JAMA 2008; 299(3):316–23.

Physiology of Weight Loss Surgery

Chan W. Park, MD, Alfonso Torquati, MD, MSCI*

KEYWORDS

- Bariatric surgery • Diabetes • Gastric bypass • Incretins
- Adipokines • Cytokines

WHY (ARE PEOPLE SO FAT?)

Several hypotheses and theories have been introduced to explain the origins of the current obesity epidemic. In 1962, a geneticist by the name of James V. Neel[1] presented his theory of how the progress of natural human evolution favored the perpetuation of obesity and diabetes promoting "thrifty genes."[1] He proposed that those individuals who had thrifty genes were better able to extract nutrients from ingested food and were more efficient in accumulating fat during times of abundance, and this resulted in an evolutionary advantage for these individuals during times of famine or food scarcity. Over time, survival of individuals with thrifty genes was favored compared with those with other genes. In light of the abundance of food in today's society and changes toward more sedentary lifestyles, this theory provides a plausible explanation for the obesity epidemic.

Opponents of this theory point to the archaeological records that refute the idea that famines were a commonly occurring phenomenon and that these events had a devastating impact on human survival.[2] Others are quick to point out that the basic principles of genetics dictate that, if thrifty genes received such favoritism throughout the course of human evolution, every person should be obese by now.[2,3] Although 70 to 100 million Americans are obese today, this number still only represents a minority (~one-third) of the population; this seems to contradict the thrifty gene theory.[3,4]

A more recent theory proposed by John Speakman[3] incorporates the observation that not all modern humans are obese, and he proposes that the obese phenotype is the result of genetic drift; it is caused by a set of "drifty genes."[3] With the elimination of predatory checks limiting the upper limit of human body weight, and perhaps accelerated by the increasing availability of food resources, humans are now in an evolutionary environment that fosters the perpetuation of fatter phenotypes. A common introduction, which most morbidly obese patients receive at their first bariatric surgery

---

Dr Alfonso Torquati is supported by National Institute of Health grant K23 DK075907.
Duke Endosurgery, Department of Surgery, Duke University, DUMC 3351, Duke University Medical Center, Durham, NC 27713, USA
* Corresponding author.
E-mail address: alfonso.torquati@duke.edu

Surg Clin N Am 91 (2011) 1149–1161
doi:10.1016/j.suc.2011.08.009
0039 6109/11/$ – see front matter © 2011 Elsevier Inc. All rights reserved.

surgical.theclinics.com

seminar, is that obesity is a result of too many calories consumed and not enough calories expended (eg, while running away from a predator).

The debate between thrifty and drifty genes continues, and the final verdict remains undelivered. It is plausible that the origins of obesity can be explained by these eloquent theories, but it is more likely that a combination of evolutionary events, socio-economic factors, and biologic stressors have resulted in the current obesity epidemic. Regardless of which evolutionary theory is correct, obesity cannot be overcome without significant changes involving both caloric intake and energy expenditure. At some point in an obese person's life, the balance between caloric intake and energy expenditure is lost, and only by reestablishing a negative balance can weight loss and resolution of obesity occur. Bariatric surgery provides this counterbalance and allows the patient to realistically achieve weight loss goals and minimize the detrimental effects of comorbid diseases.

The clinical outcomes achieved by bariatric surgery have been impressive.[5-8] However, the physiologic mechanisms and complex metabolic effects of bariatric surgery are only beginning to be understood. Ongoing research has contributed a large amount of data on the science behind obesity and its treatment, and this article reviews the current understanding of metabolic and bariatric surgery physiology.

HOW (DOES IT ALL WORK?)

One of the earliest studies reporting on the effectiveness of surgery in treating obesity-related diseases (ie, diabetes) was first published in 1955. In this study, Friedman and colleagues[9] reported observing "the amelioration of diabetes mellitus following subtotal gastrectomy." Several decades later, Pories and colleagues[10] reviewed their experience with gastric bypass surgery performed on obese patients and showed effective and durable weight loss (in a 14-year period) along with an 83% resolution of diabetes (defined as normoglycemia without medications). Further evidence for the effectiveness, long-term durability, and safety of bariatric surgery has continued to grow in the literature.[5-8,10]

Initially, the prevailing theory behind bariatric surgery was that there were 2 primary mechanisms for surgically induced weight loss: caloric restriction and/or nutrient malabsorption. Thus, bariatric operations have historically been categorized as restrictive and/or malabsorptive procedures. Restrictive procedures such as adjustable gastric banding (AGB), gastric plication, and (for the most part) sleeve gastrectomy all produce restriction of gastric capacity and limit the amount of oral intake possible in obese patients. In contrast, pure malabsorptive procedures such as jejunoileal bypass involve the surgical manipulation of the gastrointestinal tract, resulting in an alteration of the flow of nutrients and digestive enzymes through the gut. This operation results in significant malabsorption of nutrients, but has become less popular because of the unacceptably high long-term complication profile (profound malabsorption causes malnutrition, severe diarrhea, and even mortality). The benefits of both gastric restriction and intestinal malabsorption are combined in duodenal switch (DS) and Roux-en-Y gastric bypass (RYGB) procedures. Although producing the most impressive weight loss and comorbid disease resolution, the DS procedure is a more complex operation with both a higher level of difficulty and greater potential complication risk. Thus, RYGB is currently considered the gold standard bariatric surgical procedure given its favorable risk-benefit profile, and is the most commonly performed bariatric surgery today in the United States.[7,8]

Although these simple concepts of restriction and malabsorption provide a framework for categorizing bariatric operations, they do not fully explain the complex physiology of obesity and, furthermore, they grossly overlook the profound metabolic effects of bariatric surgery. In 2007, nearly 25 years after its development, the American Society for Bariatric Surgery changed its name to the American Society for Metabolic and Bariatric Surgery, reflecting a growing acceptance that bariatric surgery did more than just help patients lose weight. This acceptance was based on mounting evidence that obesity-related disease conditions often improved before any significant weight loss had taken place. Ongoing research continues to expand knowledge of bariatric surgery and its metabolic effects; as investigators continue their efforts, discovering deeper and increasingly complex interactions within the biochemical and hormonal network of human physiology, how bariatric surgery works is just beginning to be understood.

The Enteroencephalic Endocrine Axis, Obesity, and Bariatric Surgery

Since the time of Pavlov, the brain-body connection has been recognized in appetite stimulation and the physiology of eating. The process of nutrient ingestion begins even before food is consumed, and this is shown by anticipatory physiologic changes observed during the cephalic phase of ingestion, such as the release of various enteric hormones.[11] During the meal, constant interplay continues between the visceral organs and the central regulatory centers of the brain, and the simple activity of eating has been shown to activate complex neural networks and stimulate reward centers of the brain. A recent study by Ochner and colleagues[12] even showed that bariatric surgery can alter the patterns of neural activation in the mesolimbic reward centers in response to food. These changes were associated with a reduction in subjective appetite, and this highlights the importance of deciphering how bariatric surgery alters the communication pathways of the enteroencephalic endocrine axis. This axis is believed to be at the core of the physiologic regulation of human appetite, the process of nutrient intake, energy homeostasis, and human metabolism. A group of hormonal peptides facilitate the functions of this axis, and the following is a review of the key components of the enteroencephalic axis.

Ghrelin

One of the first hormones of interest for obesity and bariatric surgery is ghrelin. Also known as the hunger hormone, ghrelin is primarily produced by P/D1 cells located in the fundus of the stomach.[13] Ghrelin levels increase significantly before a meal or when a person is believed to be hungry (hence its common name), and levels quickly diminish following a meal. Although it has many physiologic effects, ghrelin's key role in obesity and bariatric surgery is in the peptide's neurotrophic effects through the enteroencephalic endocrine axis. With receptors in the arcuate nucleus and the lateral hypothalamus, ghrelin stimulates the hypothalamic release of various neuropeptides such as neuropeptide Y (NPY) and growth hormone. The result is that ghrelin facilitates an orexigenic state, or a state of heightened appetite, via activation of the appetite-regulating and metabolism-regulating NPY neurons. Conversely, a significant reduction in the level of ghrelin, such as that observed immediately following a meal, results in a person achieving a sense of satiety. Ghrelin is the only known circulating orexin, a hormone that stimulates appetite.

Numerous studies have established the role of ghrelin as a premeal, appetite-stimulating hormone, and it is thought that ghrelin provides an important survival mechanism that stimulates nutrient intake in underweight people.[14–18] However, the effects of ghrelin on human metabolism (and vice versa) may be more complicated than that. It has been shown that basal ghrelin levels may have an inverse relationship to body weight and energy balance.[19,20] Basal ghrelin levels in individuals of normal and lower weight are significantly higher compared with the obese, and this may seem counterintuitive. Why would an obese person have lower levels of a hormone that causes appetite stimulation and favors greater caloric intake? In obese individuals, ghrelin's function as an orexin may be overshadowed by the existing, positive energy balance (more calories in/available than out).[20] In a study by English and colleagues,[21] obese subjects had significantly lower levels of basal ghrelin, but eating did not cause a significant decrease in the level of circulating ghrelin.[21,22] Thus, in obese individuals, it seems that the protective function of ghrelin (against weight loss) has been turned off. In addition, the loss of a significant ghrelin level reduction following a meal may make it impossible for obese individuals to attain a sense of satiety after eating. How and why this occurs is not yet known, and further research may elucidate this physiologic phenomenon.

Basal ghrelin levels increase as body weight is lost. In studies of normal-weight and obese subjects who lost weight through nonsurgical methods (diet and exercise), ghrelin levels were shown to increase when weight was lost.[23–25] In another study, subjects who greatly restricted their own eating (ie, dieting) were found to have higher serum ghrelin levels compared with those who had less restrictive diets.[26] What is most remarkable about this finding is that ghrelin levels were increased without any real change in weight. This reflex physiologic increase in ghrelin may make it increasingly difficult for people to lose weight through diet and exercise alone. In this sense, bariatric surgery may offer what no other therapy can. Studies in patients after RYGB have reported that plasma ghrelin is low despite significant weight loss.[23,27] However, this finding has been inconsistent in the literature, with some studies reporting either no change or increased levels of ghrelin after bariatric surgery.[28–31]

The confusing picture of how bariatric surgery affects ghrelin may be caused by several factors, including differences in surgical technique, different ways to assay levels, as well as the complex and multiple physiologic functions of ghrelin.[32] The AGB procedure does not actively exclude ghrelin-producing cells within the stomach fundus, and this may account for the observations that ghrelin levels are higher after surgery.[33,34] Likewise, sleeve gastrectomy and RYGB procedures involve exclusion of most of the ghrelin-producing stomach from the flow of nutrients, and favors a lower postsurgical ghrelin level. However, the extent of fundal exclusion may vary across the surgical centers performing these operations and this may contribute to the conflicting results. Recent scientific discoveries have identified multiple products of the gene that produces ghrelin (such as obestatin and desacyl ghrelin). These peptides have been shown to both augment and contradict the effects of ghrelin at differing receptor sites throughout the body.[32] How these interactions affect the enteroendocrine functions of ghrelin are yet to be fully understood. In addition, a study by le Roux and colleagues[35] reported that ghrelin did not affect appetite or stimulate food intake in patients who received a surgical vagotomy. Thus, bariatric operations involving gastric resection (and concomitant vagotomy) may effectively inhibit the role of ghrelin on appetite stimulation and food consumption.

Neuropeptide Y

At the level of the hypothalamus and the central regulatory centers of the brain, NPY is the dominant hormonal signal regulating nutrient intake and metabolism. NPY activity is ubiquitous throughout the body, and NPY is one of the most abundant neuropeptides in the human brain. NPY serves as the primary neuropeptide affecting numerous physiologic processes such as the regulation of circadian rhythm, stress response, and human metabolism. The complex and numerous physiologic relationships affecting NPY's role in the regulation of human metabolism and obesity are just beginning to be understood.

Release of NPY is stimulated by orexigenic signals such as ghrelin and inhibited by anorexigenic signals such as leptin and peptide YY (PYY).[36] Among its many activities, NPY is a potent appetite-stimulating neuropeptide, and animal studies have confirmed the relationship between NPY and increased food intake as well as the development of obesity.[37,38] In human studies, NPY has also been shown to promote obesity and the development of metabolic syndrome.[39] This study showed that NPY promotes abdominal obesity and fat angiogenesis as a result of stress through an increased glucocorticoid (stress hormone) response. However, attempts to antagonize the orexigenic effects of NPY using novel NPY receptor antagonists have only been marginally effective.[40] In this large, multicenter, randomized controlled-study, NPY antagonism resulted in statistically significant, but clinically insignificant, weight loss (~2 kg more than control) in a 52-week period. Similarly, NPY levels following RYGB have been unimpressive.[41] In this study, measurements of post-RYGB enteroendocrine changes in both diabetic and nondiabetic patients showed no significant changes in NPY despite effective weight loss and changes in body mass index (BMI) across groups. Thus, despite its known orexigenic effects, NPY as a potential target for obesity treatment is not well established.

Peptide YY

Another enterokine that acts on NPY neurons to regulate metabolism and appetite is PYY. Similar in structure and belonging to the same class of hormones as NPY, PYY is secreted in response to the presence of nutrients within the lumen of the gut by L-cells found throughout the small and large intestines (the highest concentrations of L-cells are found in the terminal ileum and colon.).[36,42] In contrast with NPY, PYY exerts an anorexigenic stimulus on NPY neurons resulting in the termination of feeding and nutrient intake. In addition, PYY has many visceral effects such as the inhibition of gastrointestinal motility and reduction in both pancreatic and intestinal secretions. All of these effects promote a slowing of nutrient flow through the gastrointestinal tract, an effect referred to as the ileal brake, and PYY is considered to be one of the key components of this negative-feedback mechanism.[43–45] The ileal brake negative-feedback mechanism is thought to be responsible for the suppression of appetite, leading to the termination of a meal.

Studies have confirmed PYY's effectiveness in suppressing appetite and nutrient consumption.[46–48] In one study, PYY infusion was shown to reduce nutrient intake in both obese and lean subjects who received exogenous PYY.[47] Another study quantified the effects of PYY administration and showed a 30% decrease in the amount of food consumed during a buffet meal by both obese and lean subjects. In addition, this study also showed that PYY infusion caused a decrease in ghrelin levels, suggesting an interaction between appetite suppression and stimulation along the enteroendocrine axis.[48] Obese individuals have been shown to produce lower baseline levels of PYY compared with those who are lean and of normal weight, but not all reports have confirmed this finding.[46–48]

Bariatric surgery, RYGB in particular, has been shown to increase PYY levels,[49] and this observation has been made as early as 48 hours after surgery.[49–51] RYGB increases the rate of transit of nutrients to PYY-secreting areas of the intestine (ileum and colon), and this may cause the observed increase in postprandial PYY response after RYGB. Consistent with this mechanism, AGB did not increase PYY levels in obese patients,[50] whereas RYGB and sleeve gastrectomy resulted in sustained increase of PYY levels during a 12-month study period.[51] Furthermore, in meal-stimulation studies, increased postprandial PYY levels were seen in patients with RYGB, but not in patients undergoing medical weight loss.[24]

Leptin

Released primarily by adipose tissues, leptin acts at the level of the hypothalamus to counteract the orexigenic signals induced by ghrelin and NPY. Leptin activates pro-piomelanocortin containing (POMC) neurons which in turn release anorexigenic peptides such as α-melanocyte–stimulating hormone (α-MSH), and it also directly inhibits the release of NPY.[52] Leptin is not an enteric hormone per se and is more appropriately categorized as an adipokine. Nevertheless, leptin's counter-activity to ghrelin and NPY makes it a key negative peptide signal within the enteroencephalic axis. Leptin promotes anorexic behavior and is believed to be intricately involved in the production of the sense of fullness or satiety following a meal.

In contrast with ghrelin, serum leptin levels are not dependent on short-term caloric intake; leptin levels are more reflective of an individual's metabolic profile over time and are dictated by the amount of existing adipose tissue.[46] Thus, obese individuals have higher levels of circulating leptin; a counterintuitive phenomenon in light of leptin's known anorexigenic properties. However, it is thought that obese individuals become resistant to the anorexigenic effects of leptin, greatly reducing the potency of leptin's inhibitory effects on the regulatory centers controlling appetite. In addition to its activity counter to ghrelin and NPY, leptin also blocks other appetite-stimulating signals. Leptin blocks anandamide (an appetite stimulant) and stimulates the release of an appetite-antagonist (α-MSH).

Given these mechanisms, administration of exogenous leptin has been tried as a treatment of obesity. In 1999, a multicenter, randomized, controlled trial showed promising results with weight loss occurring in both lean and obese subjects in response to escalating doses of leptin.[53] However, subsequent studies using leptin for weight loss have failed to replicate this finding.[54,55] It seems that leptin may be more effective as a marker for weight loss rather than an effector, and recent reports have confirmed that leptin levels decrease as weight is lost regardless of how this is achieved.[56–58]

Several studies have shown resolution of the leptin-resistance status after bariatric surgery procedures.[30,46,56] Leptin levels decrease significantly in individuals who have had gastric bypass surgery and correlate with percent of weight loss.

Enteroinsular Axis, Diabetes, and Bariatric Surgery

One of the greatest benefits of bariatric surgery is the resolution in comorbid disease conditions such as type 2 diabetes mellitus. With more than 25 million Americans suffering from this disease and nearly $120 billion spent annually on the treatment of diabetes,[59] developing an effective treatment of diabetes is of utmost importance. Bariatric surgery has been shown to be more than just an effective treatment of diabetes; it is capable of achieving unrivaled therapeutic results. Supported by a growing body of evidence in the literature, the American Diabetes Association has endorsed bariatric surgery for the treatment of type 2 diabetes in patients with BMI greater than or equal to 35 kg/m². [60] Thus, understanding the mechanisms responsible for the high rate of diabetes resolution/remission after bariatric surgery is clinically relevant and may lead to new therapeutic targets.

As stated previously, bariatric surgery results in significant improvements in diabetes (and other comorbid conditions of obesity) before any significant weight loss has taken place, and this challenges the established notion that weight loss is the only mechanism for normalization of glucose metabolism. Studies have elucidated the effects of bariatric surgery on the enteroinsular axis; specifically on a family of peptides involved in the synthesis, secretion, and regulation of insulin: the incretins.[61–64] Incretin levels have been shown to significantly change following bariatric surgery, and consequently there is much interest in developing novel techniques for using these hormones in the treatment of diabetes.

Glucose-dependent Insulinotropic Peptide

Glucose-dependent insulinotropic peptide (GIP), also known as gastric inhibitory polypeptide, is an incretin produced by the K-cells located within the mucosa of the duodenum and jejunum. GIP has several major roles in obesity and diabetes physiology: the regulation of pancreatic β-cells, control of glucose-dependent insulin and postprandial glucagon levels, and fatty acid metabolism.[65,66] It is thought that GIP is released by the proximal intestine in response to the presence of glucose within the lumen. The foregut hypothesis of bariatric surgery physiology is based mostly on this mechanism of GIP release.[67,68] According to this theory, bariatric procedures that bypass the duodenum/proximal jejunum (eg, RYGB) result in the complete exclusion of nutrients/glucose from the proximal intestines/foregut. This exclusion results in the loss of K-cell stimulation, a resultant reduction in GIP levels, and a reduction in β-cell stimulation/insulin release. It has been postulated that this mechanism is responsible for the early resolution of diabetes.

However, studies of GIP, its role in bariatric surgery, and the resolution of diabetes have not been conclusive. Although some have shown decreased levels in patients after RYGB,[66,69] others have shown an increase or lack of change in GIP levels.[41,61,66,70] These conflicting results are open for interpretation, and it is not well understood what role GIP has in bariatric surgery physiology.

Glucagon-like Peptide-1

Glucagon-like Peptide-1 (GLP-1) is another important incretin in the physiology of obesity. GLP-1 has many physiologic functions, including the stimulation of insulin secretion by the pancreas, an increase in the insulin sensitivity of pancreatic cells (α-cells and β-cells), inhibition of glucagon secretion, and reduction of hunger and food intake through activation of central regulatory centers of the brain.[65,71] Released by L-cells in the distal gastrointestinal tract, namely the terminal ileum and colon, GLP-1 levels increase in response to the presence of nutrients in the lumen of the distal or hindgut intestines. Increasing the level of GLP-1 has been shown to induce appetite suppression in both obese and normal-weight humans, and it is also considered to be a component of the ileal brake mechanism.[71,72] Again, this mechanism for appetite suppression and the termination of food intake is a negative-feedback circuit that is triggered by the presence of nutrients in the ileum and mediated by the anorexigenic properties of GLP-1 and PYY.[46]

In addition to its contributions to the ileal brake mechanism, it has been proposed that GLP-1 is a key factor leading to the rapid resolution/remission of diabetes mellitus after bariatric surgery. In contrast with the foregut hypothesis, the hindgut hypothesis proposes that RYGB allows faster arrival of nutrients into the hindgut, which then results in a quicker increase in GLP-1 levels. GLP-1 in turn alters metabolic physiology to limit further intake of nutrients, increase insulin production, and improve insulin sensitivity.[72]

The Incretin Effect, Diabetes, and Bariatric Surgery

Based on these results, there have been attempts to stimulate incretin release through intravenous glucose infusion. However, it has been shown that intravenous administration of glucose does not have the same intensity of effect on human metabolism and the enteroinsular axis as is seen after the same dose of orally ingested glucose. This effect has been called the incretin effect and gives additional relevance to the enteric production of incretins as an important mechanism by which glycemic control and remission of diabetes is achieved after bariatric surgery.[73]

In a randomized, prospective trial comparing the effects of RYGB and sleeve gastrectomy, both procedures resulted in improved insulin resistance (as measured by Homeostatic Model Assessment [HOMA]), diminished fasting insulin levels, and an increased postprandial GLP-1 response as early as 1 week following surgery, and before any significant weight loss.[74] Another study confirmed these rapid effects of RYGB on insulin resistance and GLP-1, which resulted in 72% diabetes remission (defined as fasting glucose <7 mmol/L and 2-hour glucose <11.1 mmol/L after oral glucose tolerance test in subjects not on medications).[75] However, despite similar weight loss results in the RYGB group, this same study showed that AGB and diet restriction did not result in any early improvements in insulin resistance or changes in postprandial GLP-1 levels, and diabetes remission was observed in only 17% after AGB. Although the RYGB effects on the enteroinsular axis are consistent with current understanding, the effects of sleeve gastrectomy are not well understood and require further study. In addition, diabetes resolution after AGB is likely more the result of caloric restriction and weight loss over time. In a recent randomized, controlled trial with close, long-term follow-up, AGB resulted in much higher rates of remission (73%).[76]

In contrast, some investigators have tried to isolate and synthesize peptide signals that can replicate the effects of GIP and GLP-1, but there are unfavorable side effect profiles, variability in efficacy and bioavailability, and marginal outcome results.[73,77] Although novel medical therapies hold promise, to date there exists no known substance or medication capable of modulating multiple mechanisms and achieving weight loss results and diabetes resolution with the speed and of the magnitude that are possible through bariatric surgery. Despite this, most of the lay public, and even some practitioners, still fail to recognize the benefits possible with metabolic and bariatric surgery.

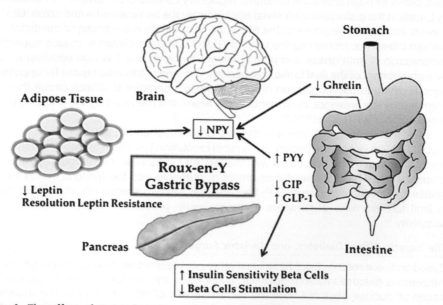

Fig. 1. The effect of gastric bypass surgery is mediated by changes in the brain, stomach, intestine, pancreas, and adipose tissue.

Furthermore, current guidelines for the medical therapy for type 2 diabetes are based on a strategy of progressively increasing the number and types of diabetes medications, based on worsening glycemic control over time. This waiting-for-failure approach has been criticized because hyperglycemia itself may have immediate and sustained negative effects on the β-cell reserve, worsening a patient's prognosis for reversal of diabetes progression. It is thought that one of the factors associated with incomplete remission of diabetes after bariatric surgery is a long history of the disease.[78] Likewise, other studies have shown that earlier glycemic control in diabetics can result in improved diabetes remission and preservation of β-cell function; ultimately resulting in a reduction of diabetes-related morbidity.[77] The American Diabetes Association recently acknowledged the merits of bariatric surgery and recognized it as a viable treatment option in class II and III obese patients meeting the necessary prerequisites.

SUMMARY

Although the root cause of the current obesity epidemic has not been discovered, it warrants considerable attention and the appropriate use of all the treatment options available. As shown in **Fig. 1**, bariatric surgery is a proven and unrivaled treatment of obesity and the management of obesity-related diseases. Gastric bypass produces profound physiologic and metabolic changes in many organs as a result of surgical anatomic manipulation, as shown by the many studies available in the literature. However, understanding of the complex physiologic interactions that regulate energy homeostasis, appetite stimulation, and of the factors that provide the impetus for human obesity is still limited. Furthermore, the effects of bariatric surgery on obesity-related diseases such as diabetes are intriguing and present a tremendous potential for maximizing the treatment of millions of suffering Americans. Additional studies investigating the current hypotheses and theories of obesity and bariatric surgery should lead to new approaches for less invasive treatments.

This article only discusses half of the weight loss equation. As mentioned earlier, weight loss can only be achieved by balancing caloric intake and energy expenditure. However, novel ways of increasing human metabolism and developing an effective method for maximizing the amount of calories expended by the obese individual have not yet been discovered. Apart from increasing exercise and physical activities (which is difficult and, in some cases, impractical to initiate), there are no other means by which an increased metabolism can be achieved. Future research might capitalize on this untapped resource for developing novel treatments for obesity.

REFERENCES

1. Neel JV. Diabetes mellitus: a "thrifty" genotype rendered detrimental by "progress"? Am J Hum Genet 1962;14:353–62.
2. Prentice AM, Hennig BJ, Fulford AJ. Evolutionary origins of the obesity epidemic: natural selection of thrifty genes or genetic drift following predation release? Int J Obes 2008;32:1607–10.
3. Speakman JB. Thrifty genes for obesity, an attractive but flawed idea, and an alternative perspective: the 'drifty gene' hypothesis. Int J Obes 2008;32:1611–7.
4. Flegal KM, Carroll MD, Ogden CL, et al. Prevalence and trends in obesity among US adults, 1999-2008. JAMA 2010;303(3):235–41.
5. Sjöström L, Narbro K, Sjöström CD, et al. Effects of bariatric surgery on mortality in Swedish obese subjects. N Engl J Med 2007;357(8):741–52.

6. Buchwald H, Avidor Y, Braunwald E, et al. Bariatric surgery: a systematic review and meta-analysis. JAMA 2004;292(14):1724–37.
7. DeMaria EJ, Pate V, Warthen M, et al. Baseline data from American Society for Metabolic and Bariatric Surgery-designated bariatric surgery centers of excellence using the bariatric outcomes longitudinal database. Surg Obes Relat Dis 2010;6(4):347–55.
8. Flum DR, Belle SH, King WC, et al. Perioperative safety in the longitudinal assessment of bariatric surgery. N Engl J Med 2009;361(5):445–54.
9. Frideman MN, Sancetta AJ, Magovern GJ. The amelioration of diabetes mellitus following subtotal gastrectomy. Surg Gynecol Obstet 1955;100(2):201–4.
10. Pories WJ, Swanson MS, MacDonald KG, et al. Who would have thought it? An operation proves to be the most effective therapy for adult-onset diabetes mellitus. Ann Surg 1995;222(3):339–50.
11. Power ML, Schulkin J. Anticipatory physiological regulation in feeding biology: cephalic phase responses. Appetite 2008;50(2):194–206.
12. Ochner CN, Kwok Y, Coceicao E, et al. Selective reduction in neural responses to high calorie foods following gastric bypass surgery. Ann Surg 2011;253(3):502–7.
13. Sakata I, Sakai T. Ghrelin cells in the gastrointestinal tract. Int J Pept 2010. DOI: 10.1155/2010/945056.
14. Cummings DE, Purnell JQ, Frayo RS, et al. A preprandial rise in plasma ghrelin levels suggests a role in meal initiation in humans. Diabetes 2001;50(8):1714–9.
15. Diniz Mde F, Azeredo Passos VM, Diniz MT. Bariatric surgery and the gut-brain communication–the state of the art three years later. Nutrition 2010;10:925–31.
16. Cummings DE, Overduin J. Gastrointestinal regulation of food intake. J Clin Investig 2007;117:13–23.
17. Hansen TK, Dall R, Hosoda H, et al. Weight loss increases circulating levels of ghrelin in human obesity. Clin Endocrinol 2002;56:203–6.
18. Wren AM, Bloom SR. Gut hormones and appetite control. Gastroenterology 2007; 132:2116–57.
19. Marzullo P, Verti B, Savia G, et al. The relationship between active ghrelin levels and human obesity involves alterations in resting energy expenditure. J Clin Endocrinol Metab 2004;89(2):936–9.
20. Shiiya T, Nakazato M, Mizuta M, et al. Plasma ghrelin levels in lean and obese humans and the effect of glucose on ghrelin secretion. J Clin Endocrinol Metab 2002;87(1):240–4.
21. English PJ, Ghatei MA, Malik IA, et al. Food fails to suppress ghrelin levels in obese humans. J Clin Endocrinol Metab 2002;87(6):2984.
22. Tritos NA, Mun E, Bertkau A, et al. Serum ghrelin levels in response to glucose load in obese subjects post-gastric bypass surgery. Obes Res 2003;11(8):919–24.
23. Cummings DE, Weigle DS, Frayo RS, et al. Plasma ghrelin levels after diet-induced weight loss or gastric bypass surgery. N Engl J Med 2002;346(21): 1623–30.
24. Oliván B, Teixeira J, Bose M, et al. Effect of weight loss by diet or gastric bypass surgery on peptide YY3-36 levels. Ann Surg 2009;249(6):948–53.
25. Kelishadi R, Hashemipour M, Mohammadifard N, et al. Short- and long-term relationships of serum ghrelin with changes in body composition and the metabolic syndrome in prepubescent obese children following two different weight loss programmes. Clin Endocrinol 2008;69(5):721–9.
26. Schur EA, Cummings DE, Callahan HS, et al. Association of cognitive restraint with ghrelin, leptin, and insulin levels in subjects who are not weight-reduced. Physiol Behav 2008;93(4–5):706–12.

27. Morínigo R, Casamitjana R, Moizé V, et al. Short-term effects of gastric bypass surgery on circulating ghrelin levels. Obes Res 2004;12:1108–16.
28. Frühbeck G, Rotellar F, Hernández-Lizoain JL, et al. Fasting plasma ghrelin concentrations 6 months after gastric bypass are not determined by weight loss or changes in insulinemia. Obes Surg 2004;14:1208–15.
29. Shak JR, Roper J, Perez-Perez GI, et al. The effect of laparoscopic gastric banding surgery on plasma levels of appetite-control, insulinotropic, and digestive hormones. Obes Surg 2008;18:1089–96.
30. Faraj M, Havel PJ, Phélis S, et al. Plasma acylation-stimulating protein, adiponectin, leptin, and ghrelin before and after weight loss induced by gastric bypass surgery in morbidly obese subjects. J Clin Endocrinol Metab 2003;88: 1594–602.
31. Holdstock C, Engström BE, Ohrvall M, et al. Ghrelin and adipose tissue regulatory peptides: effect of gastric bypass surgery in obese humans. J Clin Endocrinol Metab 2003;88:3177–83.
32. Soares JB, Leite-Moreira AF. Ghrelin, des-acyl ghrelin and obestatin: three pieces of the same puzzle. Peptides 2008;29(7):1255–70.
33. Dixon AF, Dixon JB, O'Brien PE. Laparoscopic adjustable gastric banding induces prolonged satiety: a randomized blind crossover study. J Clin Endocrinol Metab 2005;90(2):813–9.
34. Wang Y, Liu J. Plasma ghrelin modulation in gastric band operation and sleeve gastrectomy. Obes Surg 2009;19(3):357–62.
35. le Roux CW, Neary NM, Halsey TJ, et al. Ghrelin does not stimulate food intake in patients with surgical procedures involving vagotomy. J Clin Endocrinol Metab 2005;90(8):4521–4.
36. Nogueiras R, Wilson H, Perez-Tilve D, et al. The role of the gastrointestinal hormones ghrelin, peptide YY, and glucagon-like peptide-1 in the regulation of energy balance. In: Donohoue PA, editor. Energy metabolism and obesity: research and clinical applications. Totowa (NJ): Humana Press; 2008. p. 107–24.
37. Hanson ES, Dallman MF. Neuropeptide Y (NPY) may integrate responses of hypothalamic feeding systems and the hypothalamo-pituitary-adrenal axis. J Neuroendocrinol 1995;7(4):273–9.
38. Dryden S, Pickavance L, Frankish HM, et al. Increased neuropeptide Y secretion in the hypothalamic paraventricular nucleus of obese (fa/fa) Zucker rats. Brain Res 1995;690(2):185–8.
39. Kuo LE, Kitlinska JB, Tilan JU, et al. Neuropeptide Y acts directly in the periphery on fat tissue and mediates stress-induced obesity and metabolic syndrome. Nat Med 2007;13(7):803–11.
40. Erondu N, Gantz I, Musser B, et al. Neuropeptide Y5 receptor antagonism does not induce clinically meaningful weight loss in overweight and obese adults. Cell Metab 2006;4(4):275–82.
41. Whitson BA, Leslie DB, Kellogg TA, et al. Entero-endocrine changes after gastric bypass in diabetic and nondiabetic patients: a preliminary study. J Surg Res 2007;141(1):31–9.
42. Ballantyne GH. Peptide YY(1–36) and peptide YY(3-36): part I. Distribution, release and actions. Obes Surg 2006;16(5):651–8.
43. Pironi L, Stanghellini V, Miglioli M, et al. Fat-induced ileal brake in humans: a dose-dependent phenomenon correlated to the plasma levels of peptide YY. Gastroenterology 1993;105(3):733–9.
44. Jayasena CN, Bloom SR. Role of gut hormones in obesity. Endocrinol Metab Clin North Am 2008;37(3):769–88.

45. le Roux CW, Bloom SR. Peptide YY, appetite and food intake. Proc Nutr Soc 2005; 64(2):213–6.

46. Beckman LM, Beckman TR, Earthman CP. Changes in gastrointestinal hormones and leptin after Roux-en-Y gastric bypass procedure: a review. J Am Diet Assoc 2010;110(4):571–84.

47. Sloth B, Holst JJ, Flint A, et al. Effects of PYY1-36 and PYY3-36 on appetite, energy intake, energy expenditure, glucose and fat metabolism in obese and lean subjects. Am J Physiol Endocrinol Metab 2007;292(4):E1062–8.

48. Batterham RL, Cohen MA, Ellis SM, et al. Inhibition of food intake in obese subjects by peptide YY3-36. N Engl J Med 2003;349(10):941–8.

49. le Roux CW, Welbourn R, Werling M, et al. Gut hormones as mediators of appetite and weight loss after Roux-en-Y gastric bypass. Ann Surg 2007;246(5): 780–5.

50. Korner J, Inabnet W, Febres G, et al. Prospective study of gut hormone and metabolic changes after adjustable gastric banding and Roux-en-Y gastric bypass. Int J Obes 2009;33(7):786–95.

51. Karamanakos SN, Vagenas K, Kalfarentzos F, et al. Weight loss, appetite suppression, and changes in fasting and postprandial ghrelin and peptide-YY levels after Roux-en-Y gastric bypass and sleeve gastrectomy: a prospective, double blind study. Ann Surg 2008;247(3):401–17.

52. Sikaris KA. The clinical biochemistry of obesity. Clin Biochem 2004;25(3):165–81.

53. Heymsfield SB, Greenberg AS, Fujioka K, et al. Recombinant leptin for weight loss in obese and lean adults: a randomized, controlled, dose-escalation trial. JAMA 1999;282(16):1568–75.

54. Fogteloo AJ, Pijl H, Frölich M, et al. Effects of recombinant human leptin treatment as an adjunct of moderate energy restriction on body weight, resting energy expenditure and energy intake in obese humans. Diabetes Nutr Metab 2003; 16(2):109–14.

55. Zelissen PM, Stenlof K, Lean ME, et al. Effect of three treatment schedules of recombinant methionyl human leptin on body weight in obese adults: a randomized, placebo-controlled trial. Diabetes Obes Metab 2005;7(6):755–61.

56. Ram E, Vishne T, Maayan R, et al. The relationship between BMI, plasma leptin, insulin and proinsulin before and after laparoscopic adjustable gastric banding. Obes Surg 2005;15(10):1456–62.

57. Kotidis EV, Koliakos GG, Baltzopoulos VG, et al. Serum ghrelin, leptin and adiponectin levels before and after weight loss: comparison of three methods of treatment–a prospective study. Obes Surg 2006;16(11):1425–32.

58. Pardina E, Ferrer R, Baena-Fustegueras JA, et al. The relationships between IGF-1 and CRP, NO, leptin, and adiponectin during weight loss in the morbidly obese. Obes Surg 2010;20(5):623–32.

59. Centers for Disease Control and Prevention. National diabetes fact sheet: national estimates and general information on diabetes and prediabetes in the United States, 2011. Atlanta (GA): US Department of Health and Human Services, Centers for Disease Control and Prevention; 2011.

60. American Diabetes Association. Standards of medical care in diabetes – 2011. Diabetes Care 2011;34(Suppl 1):S11–61.

61. Bose M, Teixeira J, Olivan B, et al. Weight loss and incretin responsiveness improve glucose control independently after gastric bypass surgery. J Diabetes 2010;2(1):47–55.

62. Laferrère B. Effect of gastric bypass surgery on the incretins. Diabetes Metab 2009;35(6 Pt 2):513–7.

63. Kashyap SR, Daud S, Kelly KR, et al. Acute effects of gastric bypass versus gastric restrictive surgery on beta-cell function and insulinotropic hormones in severely obese patients with type 2 diabetes. Int J Obes 2010;34(3):462–71.

64. Isbell JM, Tamboli RA, Hansen EN, et al. The importance of caloric restriction in the early improvements in insulin sensitivity after Roux-en-Y gastric bypass surgery. Diabetes Care 2010;33(7):1438–42.

65. Efendic S, Portwood N. Overview of incretin hormones. Horm Metab Res 2004; 36(11–12):742–6.

66. Rao RS, Kini S. GIP and bariatric surgery. Obes Surg 2011;21(2):244–52.

67. Theodorakis MJ, Carlson O, Muller DC, et al. Elevated plasma glucose-dependent insulinotropic polypeptide associates with hyperinsulinemia in impaired glucose tolerance. Diabetes Care 2004;27(7):1692–8.

68. Hickey MS, Pories WJ, MacDonald KG Jr, et al. A new paradigm for type 2 diabetes mellitus: could it be a disease of the foregut? Ann Surg 1998;227:637–43.

69. Rubino F, Forgione A, Cummings DE, et al. The mechanism of diabetes control after gastrointestinal bypass surgery reveals a role of the proximal small intestine in the pathophysiology of type 2 diabetes. Ann Surg 2006;244:741–9.

70. Laferrère B, Heshka S, Wang K, et al. Incretin levels and effect are markedly enhanced 1 month after Roux-en-Y gastric bypass surgery in obese patients with type 2 diabetes. Diabetes Care 2007;30(7):1709–16.

71. Doyle ME, Egan JM. Glucagon-like peptide-1. Recent Prog Horm Res 2001;56: 377–99.

72. Thomas S, Schauer P. Bariatric surgery and the gut hormone response. Nutr Clin Pract 2010;25(2):175–82.

73. Barber TM, Begbie H, Levy J. The incretin pathway as a new therapeutic target for obesity. Maturitas 2010;67(3):197–202.

74. Peterli R, Wölnerhanssen B, Peters T, et al. Improvement in glucose metabolism after bariatric surgery: comparison of laparoscopic Roux-en-Y gastric bypass and laparoscopic sleeve gastrectomy: a prospective randomized trial. Ann Surg 2009;250(2):234–41.

75. Pournaras DJ, Osborne A, Hawkins SC, et al. Remission of type 2 diabetes after gastric bypass and banding: mechanisms and 2 year outcomes. Ann Surg 2010; 252(6):966–71.

76. Dixon JB, O'Brien PE, Playfair J, et al. Adjustable gastric banding and conventional therapy for type 2 diabetes: a randomized controlled trial. JAMA 2008; 299(3):316–23.

77. Piya MK, Tahrani AA, Barnett AH. Emerging treatment options for type 2 diabetes. Br J Clin Pharmacol 2010. [Epub ahead of print]. DOI: 10.1111/j.1365-2125.2010.03711.x.

78. Deitel M. Update: why diabetes does not resolve in some patients. Obes Surg 2011;21(6):794–6.

Epidemiology and Economic Impact of Obesity and Type 2 Diabetes

Hazem Shamseddeen, MD, Jorge Zelada Getty, MD,
Isam N. Hamdallah, MD, Mohamed R. Ali, MD*

KEYWORDS

- Diabetes • Obesity • Bariatric surgery • Epidemic
- Morbid obesity

The epidemic of obesity has been increasing globally in the last 30 years. Developed countries were more affected, but developing countries have increasingly contributed to this epidemic as they continue to modernize.[1] The national and global burden of obesity, with its public health and financial implications, is projected to markedly increase in the next 2 decades.[1,2]

DEFINITION OF OBESITY
Body Mass Index Criteria

The basic definition of obesity is the accumulation of abnormal or excess body fat. It is a complex, multifactorial disease that results from the interaction of genetic and environmental factors. Excess body weight is associated with increased morbidity and mortality, including increased risk of type 2 diabetes mellitus, heart disease, dyslipidemia, osteoarthritis, sleep apnea syndrome, and some cancers.[3]

The most commonly used measurement that closely correlates with body adiposity is the body mass index (BMI), defined as the weight in kilograms divided by the square of the height in meters (kg/m^2). According to the World Health Organization (WHO), overweight and obesity are defined as a BMI equal to or greater than 25 kg/m^2 and 30 kg/m^2, respectively.[4] Obesity is further classified as class I for BMI values between 30 kg/m^2 and 34.9 kg/m^2, class II between 35 kg/m^2 and 39.9 kg/m^2, and class III for a BMI 40 kg/m^2 or greater.[4] Normal BMI values are between 18.5 kg/m^2 and 24.9 kg/m^2, and a BMI less than 18.5 kg/m^2 is considered underweight.[4]

The authors have nothing to disclose.
University of California Davis Medical Center, 2221 Stockton Boulevard, Cypress Building, Sacramento, CA 95817, USA
* Corresponding author.
E-mail address: mohamed.ali@ucdmc.ucdavis.edu

Surg Clin N Am 91 (2011) 1163–1172
doi:10.1016/j.suc.2011.08.001
0039-6109/11/$ – see front matter © 2011 Elsevier Inc. All rights reserved.

Among obese individuals, health risks increase proportionately with increasing BMI.[5] The BMI criteria used to establish the classifications of obesity are based on statistical data from reference populations that reflect excess morbidity and mortality associated with increasing body fat content.[5] BMI definitions of obesity classifications are the same for both genders and for all ages of adults.

However, BMI may not be an accurate measurement of body fat when considering specific populations, because of differences in body proportions. In Asian populations, for example, it has been identified that type 2 diabetes and cardiovascular disease are prevalent among patients who do not meet the traditional definitions of overweight or obesity.[6] BMI can also overestimate the degree of adiposity in muscular patients.[7] Consequently, adiposity and associated health risks must be interpreted within the context of assessments of body composition and medical comorbidities.[7] Anthropometric measurements, such as waist circumference (WC), neck circumference (NC), and waist/hip ratio (WHR), better reflect central adiposity and are being used, with increasing frequency, to associate obesity with health risk factors.[7]

Types of Obesity (Central vs Peripheral)

Body composition differs between men and women.[8] For a given BMI, men tend to have more lean mass and central distribution of adipose tissue, whereas women exhibit a higher overall proportion of adiposity with primarily peripheral distribution.[8] The central fat distribution involves primarily the trunk and reflects a preponderance of visceral adiposity, whereas peripheral fat distribution is deposited in the limbs and hips, particularly in the lower body. The type of fat distribution has been associated with the development of obesity-related complications.[9–11] Compared with subcutaneous fat, visceral fat is more sensitive to lipolysis induced by catecholamines and less sensitive to the antilipolytic effects of insulin, which increases the levels of free fatty acids in the portal and systemic circulation.[9] The resulting metabolic abnormalities, including decreased glucose tolerance, reduced insulin sensitivity, and adverse lipid profiles, become risk factors for type 2 diabetes and cardiovascular disease.[9] The peripheral fat distribution, more common in women, is associated with improved insulin sensitivity.[8]

WC and WHR are often used as indicators of central obesity. Abdominal obesity is defined as WC greater than 88 cm or WHR greater than 0.85 in women and WC greater than 102 cm or WHR greater than 0.90 in men.[7,10] Central obesity has been shown to be a risk factor for acute myocardial infarction (AMI) in men and women.[10] Moreover, in a large study of 27,098 participants from 52 countries, the likelihood of AMI increased proportionately with WHR in both genders and in most ethnic groups.[12] Seidell[11] concluded that WC and WHR are related to increased risk of all-cause mortality, particularly in younger adults and in those with low BMI (BMI$\geq$24.9 kg/m^2). These concepts are particularly important when considering health risks caused by adiposity in patients who do not meet the BMI definitions for overweight and obesity. For example, WC and WHR have been strongly associated with risk of ischemic heart disease in the Asia Pacific region, regardless of the BMI.[13] Thus, body composition and fat distribution should factor prominently in the management of obese patients and, specifically, when considering patients for bariatric or metabolic operations.

Obesity-Associated Morbidity and Mortality

Obesity adversely affects health by causing several medical conditions. The comorbid manifestations of obesity are hypothesized to result from either hyperplasia of adipose tissue or increased metabolic activity from hypertrophic adipocytes.[14] Sleep apnea in obese patients has been attributed to an increased NC from parapharyngeal fat deposits.[15] Osteoarthritis results from the trauma to joints associated with excess body weight.[15] Other significant comorbidities associated with obesity are nonalcoholic fatty liver disease, gallbladder disease, stroke, idiopathic intracranial hypertension, several types of cancer (eg, colon, rectum, prostate, endometrium, breast), and endocrine changes in overweight women, including irregular menses, amenorrhea, and infertility.[14] Metabolic syndrome (association of type 2 diabetes mellitus, hypertension, and dyslipidemia with obesity) predisposes obese patients to cardiovascular complications.[14] The association of obesity with type 2 diabetes is strong in that overweight persons have a threefold risk of developing this comorbidity compared with individuals of normal weight, and class I obese persons are 20 times more likely to develop diabetes.[15] As expected from this significant obesity-related morbidity, several long-term epidemiologic studies have indicated that overweight and obesity are associated with increased mortality.[16]

OBESITY EPIDEMIC
Statistics in the United States

Obesity is increasing at an alarming rate in the United States.[2,17] Data from the National Health and Nutrition Examination Survey (NHANES) indicate that, in 2003 to 2004, 32.2% of US adults were obese.[17] Compared with data from 1999 to 2000, the prevalence of obesity among adult men significantly increased, from 27.5% to 31.1%, by 2003 to 2004, whereas the prevalence among adult women remained stable (33.4% vs 33.2%).[17] By 2003 to 2004, approximately 30% of non-Hispanic white adults were obese, whereas 45% of non-Hispanic black adults were obese and 36.8% of Mexican-American adults were obese.[17] In the same year, the prevalence of obesity among US adults between 20 and 39 years of age was 28.5%.[17] This rate was 36.8% for adults 40 to 59 years of age and 31.0% for individuals more than 60 years of age.[17]

Concurrently, 17.1% of children and adolescents (aged 2–19 years) had become overweight (defined as at or above the 95th percentile of the gender-specific BMI).[17] Within this group, prevalence of overweight increased significantly for women (13.8%–16%) and men (14.0%–18.2%) between 1999 to 2000 and 2003 to 2004.[17]

However, such large increases have been projected to continue in the next 2 decades. Analysis of NHANES data, collected between 1970 and 2004, predicts that 90% of US adults will become overweight or obese by 2030 and that more than 50% will become obese.[2] Among adults, black women and Mexican-American men are expected to be most affected.[2] At the same time, the prevalence of overweight and obesity in children and adolescents is expected to increase 1.6-fold to approximately 30%.[2]

Statistics Worldwide

Numerous factors contribute to the obesity pandemic. In many places worldwide, environmental factors such as food, socioeconomic status, and eating behaviors interact with genetic and physiologic characteristics and lead to metabolic changes and obesity.

In a study of 106 countries, representing 88% of the world's population, 23.2% of adults were found to be overweight (24% in men and 22.4% in women) and 9.8% were found to be obese (7.7% in men and 11.9% in women) in 2005.[1] The number of overweight people worldwide is projected to increase from 937 million in 2005 to 1.35 billion in 2030, whereas the number of obese individuals is expected to increase from 396 million to 573 million.[1]

In developed countries, the prevalence of obesity is similar for men and women.[18] However, a greater proportion of women than men is obese in the developing world.[18] In developing countries, obesity is more prevalent in urban areas because of several factors, including the shift from rural to urban lifestyles and decreased physical activity.[19] The higher prevalence of obesity in women is mainly attributed to cultural factors.[20]

Health Impact and Cost

Obesity is a major public health concern. It is associated with numerous comorbidities that range from metabolic and physiologic conditions, such as diabetes and cardiovascular disease, to psychological impairment and low quality of life. Some conditions, such as type 2 diabetes mellitus, dyslipidemia, obstructive sleep apnea, obesity hypoventilation syndrome, idiopathic intracranial hypertension, and nonalcoholic steatohepatitis, are highly associated with obesity (relative risk >5).[21] Other factors, including all-cause mortality, hypertension, myocardial infarction, stroke, cholelithiasis, polycystic ovarian syndrome, osteoarthritis, and gout, are not as strongly associated with obesity but still occur with relative risks between twofold and fivefold higher than normal.[21] Other medical issues, including cancer mortality, breast cancer, prostate cancer, colon cancer, impaired fertility, asthma, and gastroesophageal reflux, are associated with obesity at a relative risk of 1 to 2.[21] Thus, compared with the general population, obese individuals are at significantly higher risk of a multitude of medical problems, some of which can lead to significant morbidity and mortality.

Several studies have linked obesity with increased mortality.[22–24] Obese individuals are at increased risk of mortality from cardiovascular disease, diabetes, kidney disease, and obesity-related cancers.[22] In addition, obese nonsmoking women and men have been reported to lose 7.1 and 5.8 years of their life expectancy, respectively.[23] In a 16-year study of 90,000 US adults, death attributable to overweight and obesity was estimated at 4.2% to 14.2% in men and 14.3% to 19.8% in women.[24]

Obesity has become a major public health concern in the United States, and its financial impact on health care costs seems to grow every year. In an analysis of data from the Medical Expenditure Panel Surveys, the per capita medical expenditure for obese individuals was 42% higher than that for normal-weight individuals.[25] In 2008, annual medical spending related to obesity was $147 billion dollars, which accounted for 9.1% of all medical expenditure.[25] Overweight and obesity are projected to cost $860 billion to $956 billion (15.8%–17.6% of total health care costs) by 2030.[2] In addition to direct health-related costs, obesity is associated with indirect costs associated with disability, absenteeism, and loss of productivity.[26] The annual indirect cost of obesity related to absenteeism alone has been estimated at $4.3 billion .[26] Worldwide, the economic burden of obesity has been estimated at between 0.7% and 2.8% of total health expenditure.[27] This economic impact reached 9.1% for overweight and obese.[27]

TYPE 2 DIABETES MELLITUS EPIDEMIC
Statistics in the United States

Type 2 diabetes mellitus is a prevalent disease, affecting approximately 8.3% of people in the United States.[28] Of these individuals, 18.8 million have been diagnosed, whereas an additional 7 million remain undiagnosed.[28] The Centers for Disease Control (CDC) 2011 National Diabetes Fact Sheet reported that 1.9 million cases were diagnosed in 2010 and that 11.3% of adults more than the age of 25 years, and 26.9% of those more than the age of 65 years, have diabetes.[28] Although gender does not significantly affect the prevalence of diabetes (11.8% of women and 10.7% of men), ethnicity does seem to play a role.[28] This disease affects 7.1% of non-Hispanic white, 10.8% of Hispanic, and 12.8% of non-Hispanic black individuals.[28]

Statistics Worldwide

Type 2 diabetes mellitus is a worldwide epidemic, with its incidence increasing in the past few years. It is estimated that 285 million people currently have diabetes and that this figure will increase to 438 million (7.8% of the world adult population) by 2030.[29] Increases in the incidence of diabetes correlate with improvement in national socioeconomic status, as shown by sharp increases in obesity and diabetes in India and China.[29] Currently, India ranks highest in the prevalence of diabetes, with 51 million cases, followed by China, with 43 million cases, and then the United States, with 25.8 million cases.[29] It has been projected that, by the year 2030, the prevalence of diabetes will almost double.[29]

Health Impact and Cost

In the year 2004, an estimated 3.4 million people died of hyperglycemic complications.[30] The WHO projects that this mortality will double between 2005 and 2030.[30] Most direct fatalities from diabetes occur in low-income and middle-income countries.[30] Diabetes was previously ranked as the eighth leading cause of death worldwide, but now ranks fifth, following infections, cardiovascular disease, cancer, and trauma.[31]

Although mortality caused by diabetes is lower in the United States than in developing countries, it still directly accounted for 71,382 deaths and was a factor in 160,022 deaths, in 2007.[28] Thus, according to the CDC, diabetes contributed to 231,404 deaths out of almost 2.5 million total deaths.[28] These figures will likely increase, because the lifetime risk of diabetes in the United States has been predicted to reach 1 in 3 for children born in the year 2000.[32]

Along with significant health consequences, diabetes imposes a significant economic load. Several studies have examined the cost of diabetes around the world and have indicated that developed countries tend to have bigger financial burdens through direct treatment costs and indirect costs from losses in productivity.[33] In 2010, the United States was estimated to have spent $198 billion, or 52.7% of the global expenditure, on diabetes treatment.[33] This corresponds with an average annual cost of $9677 per diagnosed patient and $2864 per undiagnosed individual to treat diabetes and its associated comorbidities.[34] Indirect costs, from lost earnings and decreased productivity, reached $58 billion in the United States in 2007.[28] In India and China, these indirect costs were even higher because of early mortality related to diabetes.[29]

About 12% of the worldwide health care expenditure was spent on diabetes in 2010, corresponding with approximately 14% of total health care spending in the United States.[35] In contrast, hypertension, stroke, and myocardial infarction represented only 10% of global health care expenditure.[36] The WHO predicts that India and China will be spending 40% of their gross health care expenditure on management of diabetes by 2025, when they will be expected to have 130 million cases.[35] The global expenditure for prevention and treatment of diabetes is projected to exceed $490 billion by 2030.[29]

Pathophysiologic Connection Between Diabetes and Obesity

According to the CDC, 90% to 95% of adult US diabetics are type 2 diabetics.[28] Most of these cases are hypothesized to be secondary to insulin resistance and a hyperinsulinemic state, which increases insulin production and eventually leads to an irreversible state in which pancreatic β-cells burn out and cease to produce insulin.[37] Clinically, most of these patients can initially be managed with lifestyle modifications, but disease progression leads to a need for oral medications and, ultimately, insulin replacement. The deleterious effects of diabetes on other organs, such as the renal, cardiovascular, and ophthalmic systems, depend on the duration and management of the disease.

The development of diabetes is multifactorial. Although genetic predisposition has been shown to play a role, poor nutrition, physical inactivity, and obesity remain the most common risk factors.[30,38] There are many hormonal mediators that regulate food intake and metabolism, including several gastrointestinal, pancreatic, and adipocyte-derived peptides. Adipose tissue is not only a calorie storage organ but is an active endocrine organ, secreting factors like leptin, lipocalin 2, TNF-α, interleukin 6, and adiponectin.[39] Adiponectin is an antiinflammatory factor and an insulin sensitizer.[39] It is secreted in abundance by adipocytes in insulin-sensitive persons but is deficient in obese persons, making it a contributor to insulin resistance.[39] Leptin regulates food intake, and its absence has been shown to lead to uncontrolled food intake and obesity.[39] There is mounting evidence that these mediators link obesity to the development of diabetes and the other components of metabolic syndrome.

The association between obesity and type 2 diabetes is so strong that the new term diabesity is being used in the literature. The prevalence of obesity among patients at the initial diagnosis of diabetes has markedly increased since the 1970s.[40] It is estimated that individuals with BMI greater than 40 kg/m^2 are 7 times more likely to develop diabetes than those with BMI in the normal range.[41]

Physical activity, diet modification, and weight loss are recommended for the management of prediabetes and early diabetes, because such simple lifestyle changes can significantly delay the progression of the disease and its end-organ damage.[30] Individuals with difficulty losing weight can benefit from weight loss programs, either surgical or nonsurgical. Bariatric surgery results in clinical remission of diabetes in 64% to 83% of patients.[37] The benefit of early intervention to prevent β-cell dysfunction should be emphasized. Gastric bypass induces remission of diabetes in 95% of patients with diabetes duration less than 5 years, but in only 54% of patients with diabetes duration greater than 10 years.[42]

OPTIONS FOR MEDICAL AND SURGICAL MANAGEMENT

The health risks of obesity diminish with weight loss. Even a modest weight loss can result in a 20% reduction in all-cause mortality.[43] A weight gain of 5 to 7 kg can increase the risk of diabetes by 50%, whereas a reduction of as little as 5 kg decreases the risk by the same amount.[44] When considering obesity in the context of type 2 diabetes, management has to integrate good glycemic control with weight loss. As soon as diabetes is diagnosed, effective therapies for weight management should be implemented. By the same principle, in diabetic patients or patients with impaired glucose tolerance, the prevention of weight gain should be one of the main goals when deciding on therapy.[45]

Conventional medical therapy for diabetes includes the use of insulin, insulin sensitizers (eg, thiazolidinediones), insulin secretagogues (eg, sulfonylureas), and modulators of hepatic glucose production (metformin). Most of these medications are associated with weight gain, except for metformin, which has been associated with weight neutrality or a modest weight reduction.[45] Among newer treatment modalities are the incretin therapeutic agents, which include glucagonlike peptide-1 (GLP-1) receptor agonists (exenatide, liraglutide) and dipeptidyl peptidase-4 (DPP-4) inhibitors (sitagliptin, vildagliptin, saxagliptin). Both groups improve GLP-1 activity and, thereby, stimulate the synthesis and glucose-dependent secretion of insulin and suppress glucagon secretion. GLP-1 receptor agonists also slow gastric emptying and increase satiety, with a net effect of weight loss. They have also been associated with beneficial effects on cardiovascular risk factors. Thus, lifestyle modifications and metformin can be effective initial therapeutic choices to treat the overweight or obese patient with type 2 diabetes, and GLP-1 receptor agonists can be added to facilitate weight loss, normalize satiety, and improve postprandial glucose excursions.[16]

Weight loss therapy is recommended for patients with BMI of 30 kg/m^2 or greater and for patients with BMI between 25 kg/m^2 and 29.9 kg/m^2 or high-risk WC and 2 or more risk factors.[7] Diet should consist of low-calorie, low-fat foods with a caloric goal of 1000 to 1200 kcal/d for most women, and 1200 to 1600 kcal/d for men.[7] Physical activity increases energy expenditure, helps with weight maintenance, and reduces the risk of heart disease.[7]

Pharmacotherapy can be added if lifestyle modifications are not successful in achieving weight loss. Currently, the only medication approved for the long-term treatment of obesity is orlistat, which inhibits pancreatic lipases and, thereby, decreases fat absorption from the gastrointestinal tract.[47] A systematic review of orlistat showed that the mean weight loss at 1 year was 2.9 kg.[48] Although this minor weight loss is insufficient to make any clinical difference, it may be useful as an adjunct in patients waiting for bariatric surgery.[49]

Nonoperative management of obesity with diet, exercise, behavioral modification, and medications rarely achieves adequate durable weight loss.[50] However, bariatric surgery is effective at achieving weight loss and improving or resolving comorbidities. In a prospective, randomized trial, bariatric surgery achieved considerably better weight loss and improvement in comorbidities than medical therapy at 10 year follow-up.[51] A meta-analysis by Buchwald and colleagues[52] in 2004 reported a mean excess weight loss of 61% with bariatric surgery and substantial improvement or complete resolution of diabetes mellitus, hypertension, dyslipidemia, and obstructive sleep apnea. This study also found a low operative 30-day mortality of 0.5% for patients who underwent gastric bypass.[52] In addition, bariatric surgery has been shown to decrease overall mortality in obese individuals in the long-term, on the order of 40%.[53,54] This effect was most pronounced in mortality related to diabetes mellitus, heart disease, and cancer.[54]

SUMMARY

Obesity is a burgeoning health care crisis in the United States and around the world. This disease is closely associated with numerous medical problems, including diabetes mellitus. Weight reduction is the cornerstone of therapy for obesity and diabetes. Current nonsurgical weight loss therapies consist of lifestyle modifications and medications and have been shown to be largely ineffective. Bariatric surgery has repeatedly been shown to be safe and highly efficacious in achieving and maintaining meaningful weight loss, as well as treating the medical comorbidities of obesity. As such, early intervention must be considered in obese, diabetic patients, and bariatric surgery should play a prominent role in the treatment algorithm.

REFERENCES

1. Kelly T, Yang W, Chen CS, et al. Global burden of obesity in 2005 and projections to 2030. Int J Obes (Lond) 2008;32:1431–7.

2. Wang Y, Beydoun MA, Liang L, et al. Will all Americans become overweight or obese? Estimating the progression and cost of the US obesity epidemic. Obesity (Silver Spring) 2008;16:2323–30.

3. Daniels J. Obesity: America's epidemic. Am J Nurs 2006;106:40–9 [quiz: 9–50].

4. Anonymous. Obesity: preventing and managing the global epidemic. Report of a WHO consultation. World Health Organ Tech Rep Ser 2000;894:i–xii, 1–253.

5. WHO/IASO/IOTF. The Asia-Pacific perspective: redefining obesity and its treatment. Melbourne (Australia): Health Communications Australia; 2000.

6. Anonymous. Appropriate body-mass index for Asian populations and its implications for policy and intervention strategies. Lancet 2004;363:157–63.

7. NIH-NHLBI. North American Association for the Study of Obesity. The practical guide: identification, evaluation, and treatment of overweight and obesity in adults. Bethesda (MD): National Institutes of Health; 2000.

8. Geer EB, Shen W. Gender differences in insulin resistance, body composition, and energy balance. Gend Med 2009;6(Suppl 1):60–75.

9. Huxley R, Mendis S, Zheleznyakov E, et al. Body mass index, waist circumference and waist:hip ratio as predictors of cardiovascular risk–a review of the literature. Eur J Clin Nutr 2010;64:16–22.

10. Oliveira A, Rodriguez-Artalejo F, Severo M, et al. Indices of central and peripheral body fat: association with non-fatal acute myocardial infarction. Int J Obes (Lond) 2010;34:733–41.

11. Seidell JC. Waist circumference and waist/hip ratio in relation to all-cause mortality, cancer and sleep apnea. Eur J Clin Nutr 2010;64:35–41.

12. Yusuf S, Hawken S, Ounpuu S, et al. Obesity and the risk of myocardial infarction in 27,000 participants from 52 countries: a case-control study. Lancet 2005;366: 1640–9.

13. Anonymous. Central obesity and risk of cardiovascular disease in the Asia Pacific Region. Asia Pac J Clin Nutr 2006;15:287–92.

14. Bray GA. Medical consequences of obesity. J Clin Endocrinol Metab 2004;89: 2583–9.

15. Field AE, Coakley EH, Must A, et al. Impact of overweight on the risk of developing common chronic diseases during a 10-year period. Arch Intern Med 2001;161:1581–6.

16. Adams KF, Schatzkin A, Harris TB, et al. Overweight, obesity, and mortality in a large prospective cohort of persons 50 to 71 years old. N Engl J Med 2006; 355:763–78.

17. Ogden CL, Carroll MD, Curtin LR, et al. Prevalence of overweight and obesity in the United States, 1999-2004. JAMA 2006;295:1549–55.

18. Low S, Chin MC, Deurenberg-Yap M. Review on epidemic of obesity. Ann Acad Med Singapore 2009;38:57–9.

19. International Obesity Task Force. The global challenge of obesity and the International Obesity Task Force. International Union of Nutritional Sciences; 2002. Available at: http://www.iuns.org/features/obesity/obesity.htm. Accessed March 15, 2011.

20. Lawlor DA, Chaturvedi N. Treatment and prevention of obesity–are there critical periods for intervention? Int J Epidemiol 2006;35:3–9.

21. Dixon JB. The effect of obesity on health outcomes. Mol Cell Endocrinol 2010; 316:104–8.

22. Flegal KM, Graubard BI, Williamson DF, et al. Cause-specific excess deaths associated with underweight, overweight, and obesity. JAMA 2007;298:2028–37.

23. Peeters A, Barendregt JJ, Willekens F, et al. Obesity in adulthood and its consequences for life expectancy: a life-table analysis. Ann Intern Med 2003;138:24–32.
24. Calle EE, Rodriguez C, Walker-Thurmond K, et al. Overweight, obesity, and mortality from cancer in a prospectively studied cohort of U.S. adults. N Engl J Med 2003;348:1625–38.
25. Finkelstein EA, Trogdon JG, Cohen JW, et al. Annual medical spending attributable to obesity: payer-and service-specific estimates. Health Aff (Millwood) 2009;28:w822–31.
26. Cawley J, Rizzo JA, Haas K. Occupation-specific absenteeism costs associated with obesity and morbid obesity. J Occup Environ Med 2007;49:1317–24.
27. Withrow D, Alter DA. The economic burden of obesity worldwide: a systematic review of the direct costs of obesity. Obes Rev 2011;12:131–41.
28. CDC. National diabetes fact sheet: national estimates and general information on diabetes and prediabetes in the United States, 2011. Atlanta (GA): US Department of Health and Human Services, Centers for Disease Control and Prevention; 2011.
29. IDF. IDF diabetes atlas. 4th edition. Brussels (Belgium): International Diabetes Federation; 2009.
30. World Health Organization. Diabetes fact sheet no 213. WHO Media Center; 2011. Available at: http://www.who.int/mediacentre/factsheets/fs312/en. Accessed March 15, 2011.
31. Roglic G, Unwin N, Bennett PH, et al. The burden of mortality attributable to diabetes: realistic estimates for the year 2000. Diabetes Care 2005;28:2130–5.
32. Narayan KM, Boyle JP, Thompson TJ, et al. Lifetime risk for diabetes mellitus in the United States. JAMA 2003;290:1884–90.
33. Zhang P, Zhang X, Brown J, et al. Global healthcare expenditure on diabetes for 2010 and 2030. Diabetes Res Clin Pract 2010;87:293–301.
34. Dall TM, Zhang Y, Chen YJ, et al. The economic burden of diabetes. Health Aff (Millwood) 2010;29:297–303.
35. Farag YM, Gaballa MR. Diabesity: an overview of a rising epidemic. Nephrol Dial Transplant 2011;26:28–35.
36. Gaziano TA, Bitton A, Anand S, et al. The global cost of nonoptimal blood pressure. J Hypertens 2009;27:1472–7.
37. Dixon JB. Obesity and diabetes: the impact of bariatric surgery on type-2 diabetes. World J Surg 2009;33(10):2014–21.
38. Li S, Zhao JH, Luan J, et al. Genetic predisposition to obesity leads to increased risk of type 2 diabetes. Diabetologia 2011;54:776–82.
39. Ouchi N, Parker JL, Lugus JJ, et al. Adipokines in inflammation and metabolic disease. Nat Rev Immunol 2011;11:85–97.
40. Leibson CL, Williamson DF, Melton LJ 3rd, et al. Temporal trends in BMI among adults with diabetes. Diabetes Care 2001;24:1584–9.
41. Mokdad AH, Ford ES, Bowman BA, et al. Prevalence of obesity, diabetes, and obesity-related health risk factors, 2001. JAMA 2003;289:76–9.
42. Schauer PR, Burguera B, Ikramuddin S, et al. Effect of laparoscopic Roux-en Y gastric bypass on type 2 diabetes mellitus. Ann Surg 2003;238:467–84 [discussion: 84–5].
43. Williamson DF, Pamuk E, Thun M, et al. Prospective study of intentional weight loss and mortality in never-smoking overweight US white women aged 40–64 years. Am J Epidemiol 1995;141:1128–41.
44. Colditz GA, Willett WC, Rotnitzky A, et al. Weight gain as a risk factor for clinical diabetes mellitus in women. Ann Intern Med 1995;122:481–6.

45. Colagiuri S. Diabesity: therapeutic options. Diabetes Obes Metab 2010;12: 463–73.
46. Siram AT, Yanagisawa R, Skamagas M. Weight management in type 2 diabetes mellitus. Mt Sinai J Med 2010;77:533–48.
47. Ioannides-Demos LL, Piccenna L, McNeil JJ. Pharmacotherapies for obesity: past, current, and future therapies. J Obes 2011;2011:179674.
48. Padwal RS, Majumdar SR. Drug treatments for obesity: orlistat, sibutramine, and rimonabant. Lancet 2007;369:71–7.
49. Monkhouse SJ, Morgan JD, Bates SE, et al. An overview of the management of morbid obesity. Postgrad Med J 2009;85:678–81.
50. Goodrick GK, Poston WS 2nd, Foreyt JP. Methods for voluntary weight loss and control: update 1996. Nutrition 1996;12:672–6.
51. Sjostrom L, Lindroos AK, Peltonen M, et al. Lifestyle, diabetes, and cardiovascular risk factors 10 years after bariatric surgery. N Engl J Med 2004;351: 2683–93.
52. Buchwald H, Avidor Y, Braunwald E, et al. Bariatric surgery: a systematic review and meta-analysis. JAMA 2004;292:1724–37.
53. Sjostrom L, Narbro K, Sjostrom CD, et al. Effects of bariatric surgery on mortality in Swedish obese subjects. N Engl J Med 2007;357:741–52.
54. Adams TD, Gress RE, Smith SC, et al. Long-term mortality after gastric bypass surgery. N Engl J Med 2007;357:753–61.

The Economic Costs of Obesity and the Impact of Bariatric Surgery

Nathan G. Richards, MD, Alec C. Beekley, MD,
David S. Tichansky, MD*

KEYWORDS

• Obesity • Economic costs • Health care • Bariatric surgery

Any discussion of economic costs of a disease and associated treatment is inherently complex. The disease has direct costs to the health care system for required hospitalizations, medications, and procedures, and indirect costs to the health care system in lost opportunities to treat other patients and diseases. The disease also has direct, non–health care costs in lost economic productivity and income in patients with the disease, workforce losses from early mortality and disability, and the cost of recruitment and training of replacement personnel. Any treatment of the disease costs the health care system directly, and treatments successful in improving longevity may increase health care expenditures over time (patients who live longer may incur more health care costs in their lifetimes). Most surgical treatments also result in temporary workforce losses while patients are getting the procedure and recovering. When assessing the cost-effectiveness of a given disease treatment, the cost of the treatment must be weighed against the cost to the health care system if the patient does not get the treatment. Although economic cost cannot be the only criteria by which the health care system administers or withholds treatment, the upwardly spiraling costs of health care in the United States have made these kinds of analyses a priority.

Obesity is associated with many other diseases. Powerful links have been established between obesity and a host of illnesses or conditions including adult-onset diabetes/insulin resistance, hypertension, heart disease, obstructive sleep apnea, gastroesophageal reflux disease, nonalcoholic fatty liver disease, nonalcoholic steatohepatosis, degenerative joint disease, obesity hypoventilation syndrome, pseudotumor cerebri, depression, and even certain cancers. Hence, correction of obesity and the diseases that are caused or exacerbated by obesity has the potential to improve quality of life and longevity, reduce long-term health care costs, and reduce

Department of Surgery, Thomas Jefferson University, 1100 Walnut Street, 5th floor, Philadelphia, PA 19107, USA
* Corresponding author.
E-mail address: david.tichansky@jefferson.edu

Surg Clin N Am 91 (2011) 1173–1180
doi:10.1016/j.suc.2011.08.010
0039-6109/11/$ – see front matter © 2011 Elsevier Inc. All rights reserved.

global economic losses from lost productivity, workforce losses, absenteeism, and the costs of replacement workers.

THE ECONOMIC IMPACT OF OBESITY

When examining the economic impact of obesity and weight-loss surgery, in addition to the savings in personal health care cost after bariatric surgery, there is also the impact that obesity has on lost work productivity and absenteeism. Another concern for the workforce economy is early mortality in US workers. In theory, many employees required training to do their jobs, at many different levels of costs to employers. Their loss, through absenteeism, early retirement, or early mortality requires the recruitment and training of replacement employees, which also severely affects the national workforce and its associated economy.

The first impact of obesity on the workforce is absenteeism. Ewing and colleagues[1] recently examined the economic impact of obesity on a small region in Texas. They found that morbidly obese employees missed 11 times more days of productivity because of illness or injury (33 days vs 3 days per year) than the average US worker. Assuming people work 250 days per year, morbidly obese employees have 217 days of productivity per year versus 247 for the average US worker. Thus, the average obese worker was only 87.8% as productive as an average US worker.

However, Finkelstein and colleagues[2] found that men with a body mass index (BMI) between 35 and 40 kg/m^2 only miss about 2 more work days per year because of the illness or injury than do healthy-weight men, and overweight men who have low-grade obesity (BMI between 30 and 35 kg/m^2) did not miss significantly more days than healthy-weight men. In women, Finkelstein and colleagues[2] found that the number of additional work days missed per year was a half day for overweight women, 1.8 days for obese women, 3 days for grade II obesity, and 5 days for grade III obesity, so, although these numbers imply that absenteeism is greater in obese workers, it may not be as great as previously described by Ewing and colleagues.[1]

However, Finkelstein and colleagues[2] went on to try to quantify this absenteeism in dollars. Their conclusions were that the range of cost attributed to overweight and obesity was from $175 per year for an overweight man to $2485 per year for grade II obese woman. Thirty percent of these costs were from increased absenteeism. In addition, only 3% of the employees had a higher-grade obesity (grade III), but they accounted for 21% of the costs associated with obesity. Cawley and colleagues[3] summarized their data by estimating that absenteeism secondary to obesity costs $4.3 billion annually in the United States.

Both Cawley and colleagues[3] and Ewing and colleagues[1] put forth a concept that obese workers may be less productive even though they are present at work. The term presenteeism has been coined. Gates and colleagues[4] studied this concept of obesity in presenteeism and the impact of BMI on workplace productivity. Reviewing the work patterns of 341 manual laborers in manufacturing through a work limitations questionnaire found that workers with a BMI greater than or equal to 35 kg/m^2 experience the greatest health-related work limitations, specifically regarding time needed to complete tasks and the ability to perform physically demanding jobs. These limitations were quantified as a 4.2% loss in productivity from health-related causes, which was greater than the loss for all other employees. This equated to $506 annually in losses per worker. He put forth the concept of a threshold effect, with people with a BMI greater than 35 kg/m^2 becoming significantly less productive than mildly obese workers. This productivity loss endured in spite of the absenteeism this group not being significantly different.

Ricci and colleagues[5] studied lost productive time associated with excess weight in the whole US workforce. By using results of a health interview conducted via a telephone survey, they compared so-called lost productive time in normal-weight, overweight, and obese workers. Obese workers were more likely to report lost productive time because of obesity at 42% versus 36% in normal-weight workers. Only 34% of overweight workers reported lost productive time. There was no significant difference in lost productive time in overweight versus normal-weight individuals. Workers who reported lost productive time quantified equal amounts of lost productive time, which was 4.2 hours per week. The reasons for the lost productive time included influenza, musculoskeletal pain, headache, fatigue, or digestive issues. It was estimated that this lost productive time caused by obesity amounts to approximately $42 billion per year in the United States, approximately $1627 on average per obese worker per year. However, two-thirds of that cost was in reduced work performance and not true absenteeism, which makes the loss more difficult to pinpoint. The numbers for overweight workers are even greater at $55 billion per year. This cost is not related to overweight workers having more lost productivity per worker, but to the greater number of overweight workers nationally. When judging these results, it is important to realize that most of these employees were between 40 and 65 years old. Sixty-nine percent of these workers were educated beyond high school, 81% worked full time, and 67% worked in a white-collar job. Thus, this lost productivity or low work performance was not necessarily in people doing manual-labor jobs; which intuitively may be more susceptible to losses from injury or physically not feeling well.

Frezza and Wachtel[6] and Ewing and colleagues[1] classified loss of output income as between $1660 and $2389 per household. Most of these previous studies only discussed pure work. When adding in the approximately $60 billion in losses caused by diabetes-related absenteeism,[6] lost labor productivity, and unemployment, the financial losses to the United States business and the labor workforce directly attributable to obesity and its related diseases are huge.

As previously stated, the financial impact of weight-loss surgery in health care costs are significant largely because of the reduction of the cost of treating comorbid conditions. So does bariatric surgery have a positive impact, for example, on absenteeism, presenteeism, and productivity? Can the observed improvement in comorbid conditions also reduce absenteeism and result in more work productivity? Hawkins and colleagues[7] noted that, although obese subjects had 83% less productivity and lower earnings than normal-weight people, patients who had laparoscopic Roux-en-Y gastric bypass and laparoscopic adjustable gastric banding had significant improvement. In 59 patients, there was a 32% increase in the number of people who were in paid work since surgery, and mean weekly hours increased from 30.1 to 35.8 hours. Almost all 59 reported a decrease in physical limitations or emotional limitations on their ability to do work. In addition, the same patients claimed state benefits at a rate of approximately 3 to 4 times higher before than after surgery.

Brounts and colleagues[8] studied productivity from a more utilitarian angle. If employees cannot do their jobs for any reason, their replacements need to be recruited and trained at significant cost to the employer. They studied the outcomes of soldiers on active duty undergoing gastric bypass and found that the expected outcomes of bariatric surgery also prevailed in a military population. However, the military can base productivity on 2 solid measures: promotability and deployability into war zones. Brounts and colleagues[8] found that 5 of 27 patients who underwent gastric bypass and had previously been nonpromotable because of weight were reclassified as promotable and 24 of the 27 patients were either able to maintain or achieve deployable status after surgery. Perryman and colleagues[9] reported the effect of the gastric banding procedures and their benefits in people in the Texas Employees Retirement System. From a pure health and cost recovery model, the direct health costs of the laparoscopic gastric banding procedure were recovered in 23 to 24 months. From a societal perspective, Texas could have business gains of $195 million in expenditure, $94 million in gross product, and 1354 person years of employment if patients in the Texas Employment Retirement System were to undergo a successful laparoscopic adjustable gastric banding procedure.

The overall conclusion of studies examining bariatric surgery and improved work productivity is that most workplace losses from obesity dissipate following bariatric surgery. Thus, the benefits of bariatric surgery in workplace losses, although not well quantified in many studies, can be summarized as follows: of the billions of dollars that are lost each year because of obesity, most could be reclaimed if the obesity and morbid obesity rates were controlled with weight-loss surgery.

THE ECONOMIC IMPACT OF OBESITY SURGERY

The current medical literature supports the premise that bariatric surgery can extend life as well as quality-adjusted life years by leading to improvement or complete resolution of type II diabetes, hypertension, and heart disease.[10–12] The well-known Swedish Obese Subjects (SOS) study, for example, showed that obese patients undergoing bariatric surgery had an unadjusted, overall 23.7% reduction in mortality in a 10-year period compared with nonsurgical obese patients. When mortalities adjusted for gender, age, and risk factors were compared, this reduction in mortality increased to 30.7%. This improvement in longevity seems to be caused by the improvement in most cardiovascular risk states.[11,12] Although the long-term data are not yet available to determine whether surviving patients cost more or less to the health care system during the remainder of their lifetimes, from the shorter-term studies available, it seems that these costs will be less.

Cremieux and colleagues,[13] in 2008, published a study of the impact of bariatric surgery on overall health care costs. Between 2000 and 2005, a large increase in the rate of morbid obesity in the United States was noted. In this time period, the obesity rate increased by 24%. The morbid obesity rate (BMI$\geq$40 kg/m^2) increased by 50% and the rate of patients with a BMI greater than 50 kg/m^2 increased by 75%. "This trend in morbid obesity results in increased health care use and costs, as health care costs for the morbidly obese are 81% above those for the non-obese population and 47% above the costs for the non-morbidly obese population."[13]

The cost increases referenced later are predominantly composed of costs associated with the treatment of the components of metabolic syndrome: diabetes, hypertension, hyperlipidemia, and heart disease. As shown in this and other articles, bariatric surgery has been repeatedly shown to either ameliorate or eradicate these entities from patients who have undergone such surgical techniques.

Assuming the known benefits of bariatric surgery, Cremieux and colleagues[13] undertook a study to determine the difference in costs in patients who no longer had these diseases. The investigators analyzed the cost-effectiveness of bariatric surgery by comparing costs gathered from patients starting at 6 months before bariatric surgery with costs generated in, and measured from, patients throughout the continuous involvement in their study. Their results showed that the mean investment for bariatric surgery in their cohort, laparoscopic or open, varied from $17,000 to $26,000. After controlling for observable patient characteristics, they estimated that costs for patients having bariatric surgery who underwent laparoscopic surgery were recouped within 2 years. Costs for patients who underwent open bariatric surgery were recouped within 4 years. Subsequent articles specifically analyzed costs associated with diabetes mellitus, hypertension, and heart disease.

In 2010, Makary and colleagues[14] published their findings evaluating diabetes medication use and annual median health care costs in patients with type 2 diabetes mellitus who had undergone bariatric surgery. They retrospectively reviewed 2235 adult patients with type 2 diabetes and commercially available health insurance in the United States between 2002 and 2005. They specifically studied (1) the use of diabetes medications at specified time intervals before and after bariatric surgery, and (2) total median health care costs per year. They showed that bariatric surgery reduced the use of diabetes medications as well as total health care costs in patients with type 2 diabetes mellitus. In his study cohort, Makary and colleagues[14] found that, at 6 months, 75% of the 2235 patients who had undergone bariatric surgery had eliminated diabetes medication therapy. At 1 year, 81%, and, by 2 years, 85% of patients who had remained in follow-up had stopped taking medications for their diabetes. From a cost savings perspective, standardized annual median cost per person from 2 years to 1 year before surgery was $6375 and from 1 year before surgery, the annual cost was $10,502. After bariatric surgery, the annual median costs of health care use went from $6882 in the first postoperative year to $4197 between years 1 and 2, to $1878 between postoperative years 2 and 3.

Type 2 diabetes mellitus has had such an excellent response to bariatric operations that it has sparked interest in bariatric surgery as a primary treatment of type 2 diabetes mellitus. Obesity has been linked to inflammatory and metabolic pathway derangements leading to insulin resistance and impaired pancreatic β-cell function resulting in type 2 diabetes. Bariatric operations have been shown to result in a 50% to 85% remission rate for type 2 diabetes, particularly if the operation is performed early in the onset of the disease. Bariatric procedures that functionally result in food anatomically bypassing the C-loop of the duodenum and the head of the pancreas seem to result in an almost immediate, improvement in glycemic control that is not associated with weight loss, but through hormonal mechanisms not yet clearly elucidated. Moreover, type 2 diabetes has been shown to respond to all currently offered bariatric procedures, probably through mechanisms associated with weight loss and diet.[15]

Control of type 2 diabetes may be one of the most important economic effects of bariatric surgery, because improved glycemic control as measured by hemoglobin A1C has been shown to reduce short-term health care costs and is anticipated to reduce long-term health care costs.[16] The landmark SOS study further buttresses these data. Narbro and colleagues,[17] in 2002, found that the average annual cost for all medications in obese individuals was approximately $140, whereas, in the reference nonobese population, the annual cost of medications was only $80. This statistically significant difference underscores the significant pharmaceutical costs associated with obesity. An analysis of patient costs in the obese group who underwent bariatric surgery versus those who did not revealed, for diabetes medication, that the surgically treated group decreased their costs by an average of $9 per year. Obese patients who underwent bariatric surgery also saw their costs for medications associated with heart disease and hypertension decrease annually by $19. Performed over 6 years, Narbro and colleagues[17] concluded that surgical obesity treatment can decrease costs associated with diabetes, heart disease, and hypertension.

In 2004, Sjostrom and colleagues[18] showed that, at 10 years after bariatric surgery, rates of resolution of diabetes, hypertriglyceridemia, low high-density lipoprotein, and hypertension continued to improve in obese patients who had undergone bariatric surgery, and the average weight loss in these patients decreased by 16.1% from their presurgical weights. Conversely, in the reference (nonoperative) group of obese patients, weight had increased by 1.6% at 10 years and the rates of these diseases continued to worsen. Although the costs associated with diabetes, hypertension, and hypertriglyceridemia were not analyzed in this work, the intuitive inference is that, because the disease processes were ameliorated by the weight loss associated with bariatric operation, the need for medications decreased, as did the amount of money that needed to be spent in their treatment.

Athyros and colleagues[19] reviewed 20 years' (1990–2010) worth of studies that were searchable on bariatric surgery in MEDLINE, Current Contents, and the Cochrane Library. Their findings further revealed the effectiveness of bariatric surgery in resolving major comorbidities associated with morbid obesity, including type 2 diabetes mellitus, hypertension, dyslipidemia, metabolic syndrome, nonalcoholic fatty liver disease, nephropathy, left ventricular hypertrophy, and obstructive sleep apnea. Separately, Clifton[20] reviewed the large, recent canon of bariatric literature to further elucidate the specific effects of bariatric surgery on these diseases. He found that, although randomized controlled trials are necessary to further support the current literature, "bariatric surgery has powerful and usually persistent effects on type 2 diabetes mellitus, dyslipidemia, and hypertension."[20] Other studies have shown resolution or improvements in pseudotumor cerebri,[21] coronary artery disease, reduced cancer incidence in women,[22] and gastroesophageal reflux disease.[23]

Supported by data presented by Makary and colleagues,[14] Cremieux and colleagues,[13] and Narbro and colleagues,[17] these reviews and meta-analyses identify the considerable effect that bariatric surgery has on significantly decreasing health care costs associated with common, often mortal, comorbidities that frequently accompany morbid obesity, including type 2 diabetes mellitus, hypertension, dyslipidemia, and heart disease.

SUMMARY

The current obesity epidemic clearly has far-reaching implications for both the economic future and health care future in the United States. As recent debates about the country's budgetary issues highlight, the fate of the health care system and the economy as a whole are inextricably linked. Health care expenditures accounted for 17.6% of gross domestic product in 2009.[24] This is expected to grow; most budgetary proposals currently being debated only slow this growth. Treatments that repeatedly show reduction in health care costs over time should be approved and made available to as many patients as possible. It is our opinion that bariatric surgery meets this criterion. However, statistics show that bariatric surgery likely cannot provide the impact necessary for reduction in health care and economic costs on a national scale. In 2006, less than 0.4% of the more than 22 million Americans eligible for bariatric surgery received an operation.[25] A rough analysis shows that, with roughly 22 million obese Americans, it would take 5500 bariatric surgeons doing 400 cases a year each for 10 years to attempt to surgically treat every obese American. These numbers are not achievable with the country's current surgical and health care resources.

The conclusion from this analysis is that the obesity epidemic must begin to be addressed by long-term, concerted policy efforts at the local, state, and national levels. Such efforts could include gradual infrastructure change and incentives designed to encourage healthy commuting (eg, biking or walking), reformation and regulation of our nation's food supply, education, and continued research into novel, nonsurgical treatments for obesity. As experts on obesity, bariatric surgeons must be prepared to guide and inform these efforts.

REFERENCES

1. Ewing BT, Thompson MA, Wachtel MS, et al. A cost-benefit analysis of bariatric surgery on the South Plains region of Texas. Obes Surg 2011;21(5):644–9.
2. Finkelstein E, Fiebelkorn C, Wang G. The costs of obesity among full-time employees. Am J Health Promot 2005;20(1):45–51.
3. Cawley J, Rizzo JA, Haas K. Occupation-specific absenteeism costs associated with obesity and morbid obesity. J Occup Environ Med 2007;49(12):1317–24.
4. Gates DM, Succop P, Brehm BJ, et al. Obesity and presenteeism: the impact of body mass index on workplace productivity. J Occup Environ Med 2008;50(1): 39–45.
5. Ricci JA, Chee E. Lost productive time associated with excess weight in the U.S. workforce. J Occup Environ Med 2005;47(12):1227–34.
6. Frezza EE, Wachtel MS. The economic impact of morbid obesity. Surg Endosc 2009;23(4):677–9.
7. Hawkins SC, Osborne A, Finlay IG, et al. Paid work increases and state benefit claims decrease after bariatric surgery. Obes Surg 2007;17(4):434–7.
8. Brounts LR, Lesperance K, Lehmann R, et al. Resectional gastric bypass outcomes in active duty soldiers: a retrospective review. Surg Obes Relat Dis 2009;5(6):657–61.
9. Perryman MR, Gleghorn V. Obesity-related costs and the economic impact of laparoscopic adjustable gastric banding procedures: benefits in the Texas Employees Retirement System. J Med Econ 2010;13(2):339–50.
10. Christou NV. Impact of obesity and bariatric surgery on survival. World J Surg 2009;33(10):2022–7.
11. Sjostrom L. Bariatric surgery and reduction in morbidity and mortality: experiences from the SOS study. Int J Obes (Lond) 2008;32(Suppl 7):S93–7.
12. Sjostrom L, Narbro K, Sjostrom CD, et al. Effects of bariatric surgery on mortality in Swedish obese subjects. N Engl J Med 2007;357(8):741–52.
13. Cremieux PY, Buchwald H, Shikora SA, et al. A study on the economic impact of bariatric surgery. Am J Manag Care 2008;14(9):589–96.
14. Makary MA, Clarke JM, Shore AD, et al. Medication utilization and annual health care costs in patients with type 2 diabetes mellitus before and after bariatric surgery. Arch Surg 2010;145(8):726–31.
15. Dixon JB. Obesity and diabetes: the impact of bariatric surgery on type-2 diabetes. World J Surg 2009;33(10):2014–21.
16. Aagren M, Luo W. Association between glycemic control and short-term health-care costs among commercially insured diabetes patients in the United States. J Med Econ 2011;14(1):108–14.
17. Narbro K, Agren G, Jonsson E, et al. Pharmaceutical costs in obese individuals: comparison with a randomly selected population sample and long-term changes after conventional and surgical treatment: the SOS intervention study. Arch Intern Med 2002;162(18):2061–9.
18. Sjostrom L, Lindroos AK, Peltonen M, et al. Lifestyle, diabetes, and cardiovascular risk factors 10 years after bariatric surgery. N Engl J Med 2004;351(26): 2683–93.
19. Athyros VG, Tziomalos K, Karagiannis A, et al. Cardiovascular benefits of bariatric surgery in morbidly obese patients. Obes Rev 2011;12(7):515–24.

20. Clifton PM. Bariatric surgery: results in obesity and effects on metabolic parameters. Curr Opin Lipidol 2011;22(1):1–5.
21. Fraser C, Plant GT. The syndrome of pseudotumour cerebri and idiopathic intracranial hypertension. Curr Opin Neurol 2011;24(1):12–7.
22. Sjostrom L, Gummesson A, Sjostrom CD, et al. Effects of bariatric surgery on cancer incidence in obese patients in Sweden (Swedish Obese Subjects Study): a prospective, controlled intervention trial. Lancet Oncol 2009;10(7):653–62.
23. Al Harakeh AB, Burkhamer KJ, Kallies KJ, et al. Natural history and metabolic consequences of morbid obesity for patients denied coverage for bariatric surgery. Surg Obes Relat Dis 2010;6(6):591–6.
24. Available at: https://www.cms.gov/NationalHealthExpendData/25_NHE_Fact_Sheet. asp. Accessed April 28, 2011.
25. Martin M, Beekley A, Kjorstad R, et al. Socioeconomic disparities in eligibility and access to bariatric surgery: a national population-based analysis. Surg Obes Relat Dis 2010;6(1):8–15.

The History and Evolution of Bariatric Surgical Procedures

Matthew T. Baker, MD

KEYWORDS

• Bariatric surgery • Outcomes • Obesity

Although the origins of surgery to treat obesity can be traced back to the 1950s, its practice remained in obscurity until 2 things happened. First, obesity became recognized as a disease state with life-threatening comorbidities such as diabetes, hypertension, sleep apnea, dyslipidemia, and venous stasis, resulting in a higher risk for premature death.[1,2] Second, obesity became an epidemic. Recent data show that up to 35% of Americans are now considered obese, whereas that number was only 12.8% in 1962.[3] Given these developments, a renewed interest in surgical procedures to treat obesity led to a large increase in the number of operations performed annually in the past decade. In an attempt to find the best weight loss operation, many procedures have been tried, with varying results and outcomes. This article reviews the history of bariatric surgical procedures and discusses why some survived to the present day and others became less popular.

All bariatric procedures can be categorized as restrictive, malabsorptive, or a combination of the two. Restrictive procedures are designed to decrease the amount of caloric intake by reducing the volume of food able to be consumed. Malabsorptive procedures bypass a large portion of the nutrient absorptive circuit, thereby reducing the amount of caloric absorption. Other procedures combine restriction and malabsorption in varying amounts.

MALABSORPTIVE PROCEDURES
Jejunoileal Bypass

Given the fact that all nonsurgical attempts at weight reduction have involved limiting or reducing caloric intake, it is interesting that the first surgical attempts involved malabsorption, not restriction. Dr Viktor Henrikson[4] of Sweden is credited with being the first to perform surgery for inducing weight loss and improving comorbidities. His 1952 article describes a case report in which he resected a 105-cm segment of small

The author has nothing to disclose.
Department of General and Vascular Surgery, Gundersen Lutheran Health System, 1900 South Avenue C05-001, La Crosse, WI 5460, USA
E-mail address: mtbaker@gundluth.org

bowel in a 32-year-old woman suffering from obesity, constipation, slowed metabolism, and the inability to complete a weight loss program successfully. The idea apparently came to him after becoming aware of a couple of reported cases in which "favorable side-effects concerning weight and intestinal function occurred" after small bowel resection. He does not mention why he chose the length of 105 cm, or which segment of bowel was removed, but it apparently was not enough to induce significant weight loss because, at 14 months after her operation, the patient not only had failed to lose weight, but had gained 2 kg. Despite this numerical failure, the patient was "content, subjectively felt healthier and more energetic. Her intestines were functioning without problem and her metabolism was somewhat higher than before the operation."

The first attempts at surgical weight loss in the United States were similar in concept, but different in design. In 1954, Kremen and colleagues,[5] from the University of Minnesota, published the results of their elaborate experiments on dogs followed by a jejunoileal bypass (JIB) in a human subject on April 9, 1954. The procedure involved joining the proximal small intestine to the distal ileum, thereby bypassing a large segment of small bowel, instead of resecting it as described by Henrikson.[4] Around the same time, Dr Richard Varco, also of the University of Minnesota, independently performed a JIB, but the case was unpublished and the patient record was lost.[6] Variations of the JIB procedure were introduced during the next 2 decades. In the early 1960s, Payne and colleagues[7] published a case series involving 10 patients in whom a segment of proximal jejunum 38 to 51 cm long was anastomosed to the transverse colon. The jejunocolic shunt procedure (**Fig. 1**), as it was termed, resulted in considerable weight loss with comorbidity resolution, but the associated debilitating diarrhea, dehydration, and severe electrolyte imbalances led to either complete reversal of the procedure or conversion to a JIB. This latter procedure involved anastomosing the proximal 36 cm of jejunum to the distal 10 cm of ileum in an end-to-side fashion (**Fig. 2**). Payne and colleagues[7] eventually advised against the jejunocolic

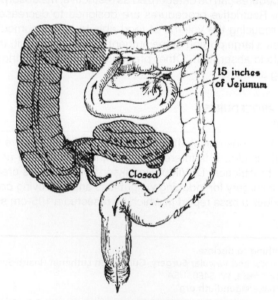

Fig. 1. Initial intestinal bypass operation with jejunocolic anastomosis. (*From* Payne JH, Dewind LT, Commons RR. Metabolic observations in patients with jejunocolic shunts. Am J Surg 1963;106:274; with permission.)

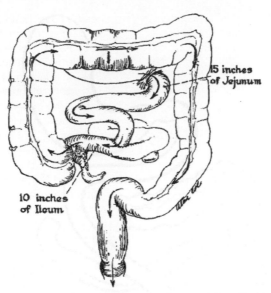

Fig. 2. Intestinal continuity only partially restored; note jejunoileal anastomosis. (*From* Payne JH, Dewind LT, Commons RR. Metabolic observations in patients with jejunocolic shunts. Am J Surg 1963;106:279; with permission.)

shunt and recommended the JIB procedure. However, it was eventually noted that approximately 10% of patients having JIB either did not experience satisfactory weight loss or developed significant weight regain. This finding was caused by reflux of nutrients back up the defunctionalized limb of small bowel, allowing absorption of the refluxed material, and led to other JIB variations in which an end-to-end anastomosis was performed and the defunctionalized, or bypassed, limb was drained into the cecum, transverse colon, or sigmoid colon (**Fig. 3**).[8]

Despite the popularity and weight loss success of the JIB procedure in the late 1960s and early 1970s, it was also associated with serious complications. The so-called blind loop syndrome was believed to be caused by bacterial overgrowth in the defunctionalized limb. The syndrome was characterized by abdominal bloating, migratory arthralgias, and, eventually, liver problems. The severity of liver dysfunction ranged from mild, in about 25% of patients, to full-blown cirrhosis in up to 5%, and liver failure in 1% to 2%.[9,10] Significant diarrhea became synonymous with the jejunoileal bypass. The associated anal burning, electrolyte abnormalities, and dehydration compromised quality of life and led to frequent physician visits and hospitalizations. Other malabsorptive sequelae included protein depletion, calcium and vitamin D deficiencies, nephrolithiasis, cholelithiasis, and vitamin B_{12} deficiency. Only about one-third of patients having JIB had a benign course. By the mid-1970s, other less morbid bariatric procedures were being developed and the jejunoileal bypass became less popular.[11]

COMBINED MALABSORPTIVE AND RESTRICTIVE PROCEDURES
Biliopancreatic Diversion

Because of the morbidity associated with the defunctionalized limb in the jejunoileal procedures, Scopinaro and colleagues[12] of Genoa, Italy developed the biliopancreatic diversion (BPD) procedure in the mid-1970s. The procedure involved a partial distal

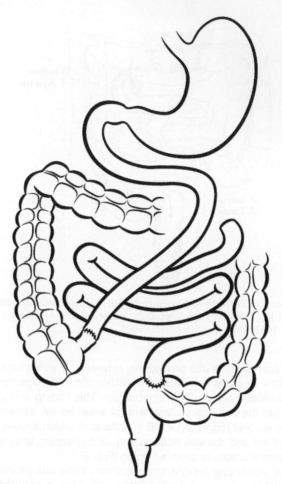

Fig. 3. Jejunoileal bypass, end-to-end.

gastrectomy with closure of the duodenal stump. The jejunum was divided 250 cm proximal to the ileocecal valve. The distal limb (Roux limb) was then anastomosed to the proximal stomach. The proximal limb (biliopancreatic limb) was anastomosed to the ileum 50 cm proximal to the ileocecal valve (**Fig. 4**). The result was a Roux-en-Y version of the JIB. Although the biliopancreatic limb was not part of the alimentary channel, conveyance of bile and gastropancreatic juices prevented bacterial overgrowth and thus eliminated the blind loop syndrome of the JIB. The resulting 200-cm Roux limb and 50-cm common channel allowed for rapid transit of food and minimal contact time with digestive enzymes, thereby greatly reducing caloric and nutrient absorption. The partial gastrectomy introduced a restrictive component to the procedure that was believed to enhance the overall initial weight loss achieved. The long-term maintenance of weight loss was attributed to the jejunoileal bypass portion of the procedure.

The BPD proved to be effective. In 1998, Scopinaro and colleagues[13] reported their long-term outcomes in 2241 patients in a 21-year period. The excess weight loss achieved after 1 year averaged 75% and most patients were able to maintain most

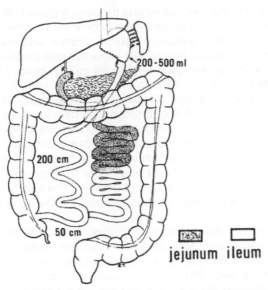

jejunum ileum

Fig. 4. Ad hoc stomach BPD. Alimentary limb, from gastroenterostomy to enteroenterostomy (EEA); biliopancreatic limb, from duodenum to EEA; common limb, from EEA to ileocecal valve. (*From* Scopinaro N, Gianetta E, Adami GF, et al. Biliopancreatic diversion for obesity at eighteen years. Surgery 1996;119:262; with permission.)

of this throughout the follow-up period. These results are the best, in terms of initial and maintained weight loss, reported in the bariatric surgical literature to date. The effect on glycemic control in patients with diabetes was equally impressive, with a 98% cure at 10 years. The effect of BPD on hypertension and hyperlipidemia was also favorable. However, the long-term side effects were significant. The main complications were diarrhea, foul-smelling stools, flatulence, anemia, stomal ulceration, protein malabsorption, dumping syndrome, peripheral neuropathy, Wernicke encephalopathy, and bone demineralization secondary to poor calcium and vitamin D absorption.[14] The incidence of most of these side effects were greatly reduced with close lifelong follow-up, early detection, intervention, and even prevention. There was a particular problem with protein malnutrition (PM), which was characterized by hypoalbuminemia, anemia, edema, asthenia, and alopecia. The cause was multifactorial, including insufficient intake from gastric restriction and insufficient absorption from deficient alimentary limb length. Attempts to increase weight loss led to drastic reductions in gastric pouch size. Although the weight loss was excellent, it was associated with a 30% incidence of PM. Treatment typically involved 2 to 3 weeks of parenteral feeding. PM was rare, but did occasionally recur. Larger gastric volumes were associated with less PM but also less weight loss. To maximize weight loss and minimize PM, alimentary limb lengths were increased from between 200 and 250 cm to between 300 and 350 cm. This increase led to further reduction of PM without significantly compromising weight loss. Scopinaro[15] eventually adopted a tailored approach to the BPD and altered gastric pouch size and alimentary limb length according to specific patient characteristics and risk factors.

BPD with Duodenal Switch

To reduce some of the morbidity associated with the BPD, Hess and Marceau developed a variation of that procedure in the late 1980s.[16,17] By preserving the pylorus, gastric emptying control was maintained and the dumping syndrome was eliminated. Preservation of the proximal duodenum helped to neutralize gastric acid and therefore minimize the risk of stomal ulcerations. Gastric restriction was maintained as in the BPD, which not only decreased parietal cell mass but also preserved the restrictive component of the operation. However, to keep the pylorus intact, the partial gastrectomy was converted to a 70% to 80% greater curve gastrectomy (sleeve configuration). The entire small bowel was measured from the ligament of Treitz to the ileocecal valve. Forty percent of this distance was calculated and measured from the ileocecal valve in a retrograde fashion. The jejunum was divided at this distance and the distal (Roux) limb was brought up and anastomosed to the proximal duodenum. The long biliopancreatic limb was anastomosed to the ileum, 75 to 100 cm proximal to the ileocecal valve, creating a longer common channel than the classically described 50-cm common channel of the BPD. The resulting alimentary limb, which includes the Roux limb and common channel, usually became 250 to 300 cm (**Fig. 5**).

Hess and colleagues[17] developed the procedure while addressing the problem of weight regain in patients with prior failed restrictive operations. In their attempts to revise the failed procedures, they adopted the BPD as the revisional procedure of choice. However, frustrated with dense adhesions in the upper abdomen, the associated difficulty of creating the gastrojejunostomy on a scarred, previously stapled

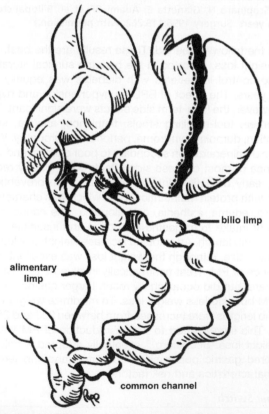

Fig. 5. BPD with DS. (*From* Hess DS, Hess DW. Biliopancreatic diversion with a duodenal switch. Obes Surg 1998;8:269; with permission.)

stomach, along with the trouble with marginal ulcerations, they began to look for alternative solutions. They came across an article by DeMeester and colleagues[18] about a duodenal switch (DS) procedure for duodenogastric reflux, and adapted it to their use. With time, they noticed the success of the procedure in their revisional patients and soon began using the procedure as a primary operation for both morbidly obese and supermorbidly obese patients. In 1998, Hess and Hess[17] published their experience with the BPD/DS procedure in 440 patients with follow-up data available for some patients up to 9 years. They reported weight loss outcomes similar to those of the BPD procedure. As expected, comorbidity resolution was also similar. The main differences between the 2 procedures were found in the lack of marginal ulcers and dumping syndrome in patients who had BDP/DS. Because of the slightly longer common channel, there was also less liver failure, renal failure, and severe electrolyte abnormalities. However, revisional procedures were required to lengthen the common channel for PM and excess weight loss in 8 patients and for excess diarrhea in 2 patients. The common channel was shortened in 7 patients for poor weight loss.

Gastric Bypass

In search of a weight loss operation without the detrimental side effects of the JIB, Dr Edward E. Mason, of the University of Iowa developed the gastric bypass. As opposed to the previously mentioned operations, this procedure introduced gastric restriction as the main force driving weight loss. The concept was based on observations in patients who had undergone partial gastrectomy with Billroth II gastrojejunostomy for peptic ulcer disease. These patients were noted to lose weight after surgery and had difficulty regaining weight long term. The first gastric bypass was performed by Mason and Ito[19] on May 10, 1966, on a 50-year-old woman with a body mass index (BMI) of 43 kg/m^2. She had undergone multiple failed ventral hernia repairs and the gastric bypass was performed in hopes of helping her achieve a more manageable, less morbid weight. Nine months later, she was 27 kg lighter and her hernia was successfully repaired.[19] The procedure consisted of dividing the stomach horizontally and connecting a loop gastrojejunostomy to the proximal gastric pouch (**Fig. 6**). Small pouch size to force smaller portions and small diameter anastomosis to delay gastric emptying and enhance satiety was emphasized.

As the popularity of the JIB waned, more surgeons began to perform the gastric bypass, each adding different modifications to improve weight loss, avoid weight regain, or to lessen the morbidity, mortality, or detrimental side effects of the procedure. Initially, the pouch size was not measured or calibrated. In 1977, Alder and Terry[20] published a study that correlated pouch size with observed long-term weight loss. Implementing the law of Laplace, they argued that the larger the pouch, the more the wall tension, which would lead to more dilatation. Based on their findings, they concluded that an adequate size for the gastric pouch was less than 30mL. In the same year, Alden[21] published a study in which, instead of dividing the stomach in pouch creation, he proposed just stapling a partition without division to decrease the incidence of gastric leaks. However, the frequent failure of staple lines led to restoration of stomach and pouch continuity and subsequent weight regain. The technique was eventually abandoned.

Also in 1977, Griffen and colleagues[11] introduced the Roux-en-Y configuration to replace the loop gastrojejunostomy (**Fig. 7**). This modification improved the technique in 3 ways: it lessened tension on the jejunal loop, eliminated bile reflux into the pouch, and added a malabsorptive component to the operation. With the Mason bypass, bringing up a loop of jejunum to reach the proximal stomach was often difficult to do without tension. Subsequent leaks led to the escape of gastric, duodenal, biliary,

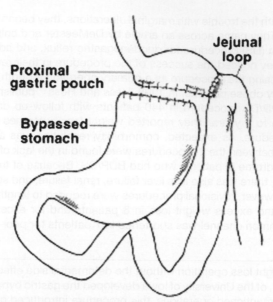

Fig. 6. Mason loop gastric bypass. (*From* Deitel M. A Synopsis of the development of bariatric operations. Obes Surg 2007;17:708; with permission.)

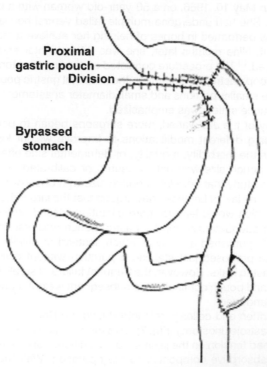

Fig. 7. Griffen Roux-en-Y gastric bypass. (*From* Deitel M. A synopsis of the development of bariatric operations. Obes Surg 2007;17:708; with permission.)

and pancreatic secretions, which was morbid and often fatal. Less tension with the Roux-en-Y decreased anastomotic leak risk. Moreover, if a leak did occur at this anastomosis, the escaping fluid was mainly saliva and patients were more likely to survive.[22]

In 1983, Torres and colleagues[23] introduced another modification. Creating an anastomosis to the upper greater curve of the stomach was technically challenging because of exposure problems in the obese patient. Furthermore, mobilizing the upper fundus for pouch creation often left the lateral segment, to which the jejunum was anastomosed, potentially ischemic. In addition, many cases of pouch dilatation and weight regain were reported. To overcome these factors, Torres and colleagues[23] created a pouch based on the lesser curve of the upper stomach, in which blood supply could be better preserved, the wall was more muscular and less prone to distention, and exposure was less cumbersome (**Fig. 8**). The late 1980s brought additional modifications to prevent dilatation of the pouch and its outlet. Salmon[24] added a banded gastroplasty and Fobi[25] used a silastic ring. Other surgeons began experimenting with Roux limb length and found that additional weight loss could be achieved if the Roux limb was longer than 150 cm, compared with the traditional limb lengths of less than 100 cm. This finding was mainly significant in superobese patients (BMI>50 kg/m^2).[26]

Although the gastric bypass offered advantages compared with the JIB and BPD, with less diarrhea, PM, and liver disease, it came at the expense of poorer weight loss and weight regain.[11] In addition, the issues with dumping syndrome and marginal ulcers, not encountered with the JIB, could be problematic. Also, like the BPD, bypassing the distal stomach and duodenum leads to calcium, iron, and B$_{12}$ malabsorption, and lifelong supplementation and monitoring is crucial to prevent bone demineralization and anemia.

PURELY RESTRICTIVE PROCEDURES
Gastroplasty

In search of a bariatric operation without the morbidity of intestinal or gastric bypass, several surgeons began developing gastroplasty procedures in the 1970s and 1980s. Gastroplasty procedures altered gastric anatomy to restrict caloric intake and induce

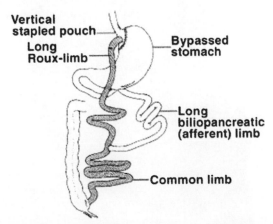

Fig. 8. The Torres and colleagues[23] variation with stapled lesser curvature pouch. (*From* Deitel M. A synopsis of the development of bariatric operations. Obes Surg 2007;17:708; with permission.)

early satiety, but avoided intestinal bypass and the associated long-term morbidity. The first attempts by Printen and Mason[27] were performed in 1971. This procedure consisted of horizontal division of the upper stomach, creating a small upper pouch connecting to the larger lower pouch through a small channel along the greater curvature of the stomach (**Fig. 9**). The unsatisfactory weight loss and/or weight regain was believed to be secondary to staple line dehiscence and/or dilatation of the pouch and connecting channel.

In the late 1970s, Gomez[28,29] advocated modifications to avoid these problems. He added a second staple line application to the partition to avoid staple line dehiscence, and reinforced the channel with an external mersilene mesh collar to avoid channel dilatation. This latter modification was associated with excessive fibrosis and gastric obstruction, so he abandoned the mesh for a running polypropylene seromuscular suture ring. However, the suture ring was complicated by suture erosion into the stomach and subsequent stomal dilatation.[29] About the same time, Pace and colleagues[30] and Carey and Martin[31] described gastric partitioning but, in contrast with the procedures described earlier, the 1-cm stoma was created midway between the lesser and greater curvatures by removing 3 of the middle staples from a TA-90 stapling device (**Fig. 10**). Despite attempts to reinforce staple lines and stomas, such as those by Gomez,[28,29] failures continued. Moreover, none of these modifications addressed pouch dilatation. To address this shortcoming, Long and Collins[32] in 1978 began using an oblique staple line from the fundus, just lateral to the angle of His, to a stoma based on the lesser curvature of the stomach. This technique was based on the idea that the lesser curvature has thicker muscle and would therefore be less prone to dilatation. The stoma was reinforced with polypropylene suture to prevent dilatation (**Fig. 11**). Recognizing that polypropylene suture reinforcement of stomas frequently led to suture erosion and subsequent stomal dilatation, Laws[33] introduced a silastic ring threaded over a suture and around the stoma to prevent this problem.

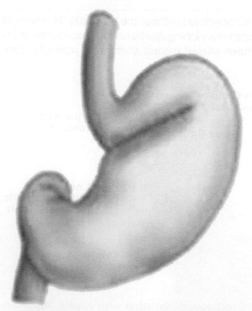

Fig. 9. Horizontal gastroplasty (Mason). (*From* Saber AA, Elgamal MH, McLeod MK. Bariatric surgery: the past, present, and future. Obes Surg 2008;18:124; with permission.)

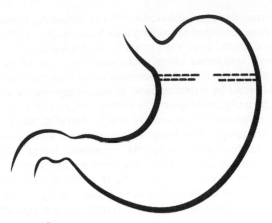

Fig. 10. Horizontal gastroplasty.

Subscribing to the theory that lesser curvature–based pouches are more resistant to dilatation, as did Long and Collins,[32] Mason[34] developed the vertical banded gastroplasty (VBG) procedure and began performing it in 1980. Disillusioned by the increased operative risks and undesirable side effects of the gastric bypass, Mason[34] was in search of a better bariatric procedure. His strict criteria included "effectiveness, safety, freedom from undesirable side effects, and reversibility." He believed that gastric restriction, if performed appropriately, could meet these ideal criteria by

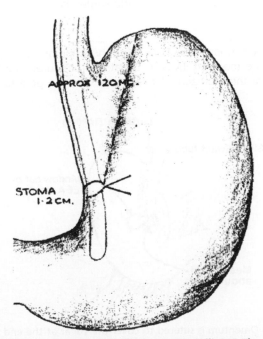

Fig. 11. Closure of defect in stomach wall. (*From* Long M, Collins JP. The technique and early results of high gastric reduction for obesity. Aust N Z J Surg 1980;50(2):147; with permission.)

"eliminating the stomach's reservoir function without disturbing digestion and absorption."[34] The procedure consisted of creating a vertical pouch oriented along the proximal lesser curve separated from the fundus by a stapled partition. The size of the pouch was precisely calibrated using a standardized hydrostatic pressure measurement. The ideal pouch size was determined to be less than 50 mL. The outlet of the pouch was reinforced by a narrow band of polypropylene mesh passed through a window created by a circular stapler. The stoma was also carefully calibrated using a bougie to assure a diameter of between 10 and 12 mm (**Fig. 12**). The VBG proved to be less technically challenging than the gastric bypass and eliminated the problems of dumping, ulcers, and anemia. Its popularity increased during the next decade as short-term outcomes proved to be favorable, with excess weight loss at 1 year of 60% or more. By 5 years, however, only 50% of patients were maintaining a 50% excess weight loss and this decreased to 40% of patients by 10 years.[35] The failures were in part caused by staple line dehiscence in up to 48% of patients, depending on the technique used.[36] This problem allowed ingested food to reenter the main body of the stomach, thereby negating effective restriction of the proximal gastric pouch. Mason and colleagues[35] reported only a 10% dehiscence rate, and many of these were only partial breakdowns allowing maintenance of some weight loss success. Although less common, stomal stenosis from excessive scarring from the mesh wrap requiring revision was also occasionally seen. Direct comparisons with the gastric bypass showed the VBG to be associated with less sustained weight loss over time and was less successful at controlling type 2 diabetes.[37,38] With the development of new technologies and laparoscopic techniques, many surgeons began performing laparoscopic VBGs and gastric bypasses. Although favorable reports of comparable long-term outcomes were published,[39] reports of high revision rates and conversions of VBG to gastric bypass became more prevalent.[40,41] VBG popularity subsequently waned and it is used less and less by bariatric surgeons.

Gastric Band

Gastric banding, which does not involve any transection or stapling of the stomach, was developed to be the least invasive bariatric procedure. Like the VBG, drastic volume reduction of the stomach inlet reservoir was the goal to limit food intake

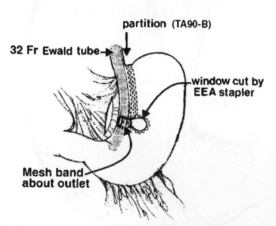

Fig. 12. Mason VBG. Omentum is sutured to cover the collar at the end of the procedure. (*From* Deitel M. A synopsis of the development of bariatric operations. Obes Surg 2007;17:709; with permission.)

without altering the continuity of the gastrointestinal tract. In 1978, Wilkinson and Peloso[42] of New Mexico were the first to place a nonadjustable band in a human. The band consisted of a 2-cm wide strip of Marlex mesh around the upper part of the patient's stomach (**Fig. 13**). About this same time, Molina and Oria[43] of Houston performed similar operations using a nonadjustable Dacron graft to encircle the upper stomach. Other surgeons, like Kolle[44] of Norway[44] and Naslund and colleagues[45] of Sweden, also used mesh to perform their versions of the nonadjustable band procedures in the early 1980s, and this was soon followed by the use of silicone as a safer alternative to nonadjustable gastric banding.[46,47]

These early gastric bands and grafts were unsuccessful. It was nearly impossible to create an ideal stoma diameter during surgery or to revise it later. Slippage was common and the stomach would prolapse either anteriorly or posteriorly up through the band, especially with the silicone variety. Band erosions and strictures led to intractable vomiting, severe food intolerances, and esophageal dilatation. In time, the proximal pouches would gradually dilate and lead to weight regain.[48] However, important developments were occurring during this period. Austrian surgeon Szinicz and colleagues[49] described experiments in rabbits in which the upper stomach was encircled with a ring of silicone, lined with a balloon on its inner surface. This balloon was attached to a subcutaneous port that could be accessed (**Fig. 14**). By adding, or removing saline, the balloon volume could be adjusted, thereby adjusting the stoma size.[49] Other researchers were quick to develop and bring this concept into clinical practice. Hallberg and Forsell[50] of Sweden described their experience with an inflatable gastric band in 1985, and Dr Lubomyr Kuzmak,[47] a Ukrainian surgeon working

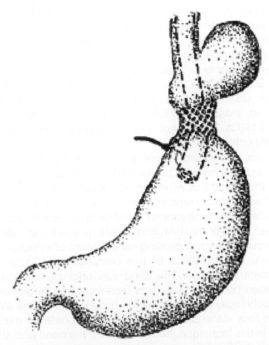

Fig. 13. Placement of a nonadjustable band with Marlex mesh (Wilkinson and Peloso[42]). (*From* Steffen R. The history and role of gastric banding. Surg Obes Relat Dis 2008;4(Suppl 3):S8; with permission.)

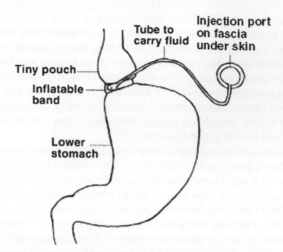

Tube to carry fluid

Injection port on fascia under skin

Tiny pouch

Inflatable band

Lower stomach

Fig. 14. Adjustable gastric band with small pouch. (*From* Deitel M. A synopsis of the development of bariatric operations. Obes Surg 2007;17:710; with permission.)

in the United States, published his experience in 1986. Kuzmak[47] showed improved weight loss and reduced complications when comparing the inflatable band with the nonadjustable version.

It soon became evident that the adjustable bands were superior to their nonadjustable counterparts. The stoma could be sized appropriately to maximize the effect for patients individually. The bands created and developed by Forsell and Kuzmak underwent numerous modifications and were eventually commercialized. With the advent of laparoscopic placement, this led to an increase in banding procedures, first in Europe and Australia, then later in the United States. Forsell's band became known as the Swedish Adjustable Gastric Band and was approved for use in Europe in 1996, although it had been available in Sweden since 1987. It was eventually approved for use in the United States in late 2007 as the Realize Band (Ethicon Endo-Surgery, Inc, Cincinnati, OH, USA). Kuzmak's band came to be known as the LAP-BAND system (Allergen, Inc, Irvine, CA, USA) and was accepted for use in Europe and Australia in the mid-1990s, but did not receive approval from the US Food and Drug Administration (FDA) until 2001.[48]

Like all the bariatric procedures mentioned earlier, outcomes and complication rates improved as experience with the banding procedures grew. Early studies, all performed outside the United States, reported favorable results.[51–55] However, similar outcomes were not seen in early reports from US centers.[56] This was likely because of the relative inexperience with advanced laparoscopic techniques and variability in surgical procedures.[57] One of the main complications was band slippage and upward gastric prolapse through the band causing either gastric obstruction or proximal gastric pouch dilatation. The incidence of this complication was greatly reduced by altering the placement technique. The band was originally introduced through the lesser sac and placed perigastrically. This technique has largely been replaced by the pars flaccida technique, which places the band higher on the stomach, resulting in a smaller pouch less vulnerable to dilatation. The posterior gastric attachments are also preserved in this technique, further securing the band posteriorly. In addition, gastrogastric imbricating sutures around the band anteriorly provide additional support and resistance to slippage.[58] Other observed complications include band erosion, esophageal dilatation, and problems related to the reservoir and tubing.

There are many studies documenting outcomes in thousands of patients having adjustable gastric bands with long-term follow-up.[59] Although technically safer and less challenging, with favorable weight loss and comorbidity reduction, it has not achieved the outcomes seen with the other bariatric procedures. Excess weight loss percentage, although variable among studies, averages around 50%, but in general takes 2 to 3 years to achieve, compared with 12 to 18 months with other bariatric procedures. Closer follow-up for adjustments is also required for optimal results.[60] Reoperation rates also vary and have improved with time, but approach 5% per year.[48] Many of the reoperations include band removal, replacement, or conversion to a different bariatric procedure.

Sleeve Gastrectomy

Another purely restrictive procedure involving only the stomach is sleeve gastrectomy. However, compared with other gastroplasty procedures in which partitioning, or dividing, is involved, this procedure resects the excluded, or divided, part of the stomach, thereby eliminating reversibility, one of the proposed advantages of gastroplasty. The procedure involves a vertical gastrectomy that excises the most compliant, or distensible, part of the stomach, the fundus and lateral 80% of the body, leaving a narrow, sleevelike gastric tube that preserves the antrum and an intact pylorus (**Fig. 15**). The procedure was originally described by Marceau and colleagues[61] in the early 1990s as the restrictive component of the BPD/DS. However, its true origins as a standalone procedure began in the late 1980s as the magenstrasse and mill procedure.

Disappointed with the results of the VBG procedure and the morbidity of the gastric bypass, Johnston and colleagues[62] of Leeds, United Kingdom, sought to develop a simpler procedure that would avoid the use of implanted foreign material such as bands and reservoirs. The new type of gastroplasty they developed was to create a narrow tube along the lesser curvature of stomach, longer than that of the VBG. A circularly stapled hole in the stomach was created that differed from that of the VBG in that it was located more distally, just beyond the incisura angularis. The outlet into the antrum was not wrapped in mesh to avoid erosion or stenosis, as seen in the

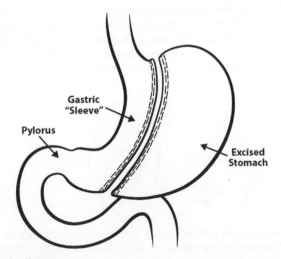

Pylorus

Gastric "Sleeve"

Excised Stomach

Fig. 15. Sleeve gastrectomy.

VBG. The tube was then created by stapling just lateral and parallel to the lesser curve from the doughnut hole up to the angle of His around a prepositioned bougie (**Fig. 16**). The magenstrasse, or "street of the stomach", conveyed the restricted volume of food from the esophagus to the antral "mill", where normal antral grinding of solid food would take place. Normal gastric emptying was then regulated by an intact and functioning pylorus. At first, a 40-French bougie was used, but, because of unsatisfactory weight loss, the size was reduced incrementally, and they found that a 32-French bougie resulted in a 63% excess weight loss at 3 years.

Modifications were made to the original procedure in subsequent years to simplify the technique, improve weight loss maintenance, and to facilitate adaptation to the laparoscopic approach. To overcome the challenges of creating the circular hole, this step was omitted by starting the staple line on the greater curve, 5 to 6 cm proximal to the pylorus, stapling up to and then along the bougie. This method also addressed the rare, but troubling, complication of gastric fistula formation from the staple line on the greater curved side of the stomach, as well as weight regain from food refluxing up into the lateral stomach reservoir. This modification required removal of the resected part of the stomach and division of the short gastric vessels, which became less risky with the advent of laparoscopic techniques, instrumentation, and improved visualization. After implementing these changes, new outcomes showed an increased leak rate, almost always high on the staple line near the gastroesophageal junction. Because a 32-French bougie is smaller in diameter than the lumen of the esophagus, it was believed that encroachment of the staple line onto the esophagus compromised staple line integrity. To overcome this shortfall, surgeons began swinging the last staple load application to the left, thereby leaving a small triangular pouch of stomach near the esophagus. This modification resulted in a large decrease in leaks.[63]

With the shift from open surgery to laparoscopy in bariatric surgery, the sleeve gastrectomy has also been used as part of a staging approach in the massively obese patient, preceding either a DS or gastric bypass. These complex procedures in such large patients often pose significant technical challenges for laparoscopic surgeons. Because the sleeve gastrectomy is technically less challenging to perform, surgeons began performing this procedure, waiting a year or two for adequate weight loss, then returning to the operating room for the definitive procedure within a more friendly environment. Many of these patients lost enough weight with the sleeve that the secondary procedure was often not pursued or thought to be unnecessary.[64] The sleeve gastrectomy as a standalone procedure has become more popular in the last decade. It is technically less demanding than the gastric bypass or DS, is associated with minimal morbidity, avoids the use of foreign material like the VBG or gastric band, and has

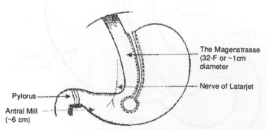

Fig. 16. The magenstrasse and mill procedure. (*From* Johnston D, Dachtler J, Sue-Ling HM, et al. The magenstrasse and mill operation for morbid obesity. Obes Surg 2003;13(1):11; with permission.)

fewer long-term problems such as dumping, marginal ulcers, internal hernias, and malabsorptive deficiencies. Complications associated with the sleeve procedure include staple line leaks and strictures. This latter complication usually occurs at the incisura angularis and can be avoided with added attention to detail when constructing the sleeve at this area. Staple line leaks can be troubling because the gastric tube is a high-pressure cylinder, making it resistant to spontaneous healing. Long-term weight loss data are lacking, but intermediate-term follow-up data up to 5 years show an overall 55% excess weight loss, with a range from 33% to 85%. Weight regain, or insufficient weight loss, has led to conversion of the sleeve to either a gastric bypass or DS.[65]

LAPAROSCOPY IN BARIATRIC SURGERY

The introduction, development, and refinement of laparoscopic techniques have been the biggest contributor to the increase in the number of bariatric procedures performed in the last decade. The associated shorter length of stay, quicker recovery, less pain, and large reduction in wound-related problems such as infections and incisional hernias, with similar results in other outcomes, has led to increased patient demand.[66]

The first laparoscopic procedures for obesity were performed in the early 1990s. Broadbent and colleagues[67] first successfully placed a nonadjustable gastric band in a patient on September 10, 1992, in Australia, and published their preliminary results in 1993. After initial animal experiments in 1992, Belachew and colleagues[68] placed the first laparoscopic adjustable band in a human on September 1, 1993, in Belgium. The first laparoscopic VBG was performed by Hess and Hess[69,70] on July 29, 1993, in Bowling Green, Ohio. However, only 2 laparoscopic VBGs were performed before changing to the DS procedure they were developing. Just 3 months later, Wittgrove and Clark[71] performed the first laparoscopic Roux-en-Y gastric bypass procedure in October, 1993, and published their results on 500 patients in 2000. Gagner performed the first laparoscopic DS procedure in 1999.[72]

Early outcome comparisons between laparoscopic procedures and their open counterparts showed that a learning curve existed to achieve similar results.[73,74] Young surgeons eager to overcome this learning curve and to learn the advanced, minimally invasive techniques required to perform these procedures began enrolling in newly developed fellowship training programs. With time, mortality, anastomotic leak rates, operative times, and other outcomes have improved to equal, or surpass, those associated with the open era.[75,76] Currently, more laparoscopic bariatric procedures than open procedures are performed annually.

SUMMARY

The search for the ideal weight loss operation began more than 50 years ago when obesity was rare, but its detrimental health effects were coming to light. Surgical pioneers, recognizing the growing need to help these patients, developed innovative, but unproven procedures that initially created malabsorption, then restricted volume intake, and eventually combined both techniques. Variations, alterations, and modifications of these original procedures, combined with intense efforts to follow and document outcomes, have led to the evolution of bariatric surgery as it is known today. Hundreds of thousands of patients have benefited from their work. No single procedure is right for every patient and no single patient is right for every procedure. Patient factors such as preference, risk tolerance, co-morbid conditions, and surgical history all play a role in determining which procedure is suitable. More recent research has focused on the hormonal and metabolic effects of these procedures. These discoveries at the cellular level will help develop possible mechanisms of weight loss and comorbidity reduction beyond the traditional explanation of reduced food consumption and malabsorption. As more lifelong data become available, further modifications and recommendations will surface. Until then, what Dr Edward E. Mason said in 2004 is still true today: The best lifelong surgical treatment of severe obesity remains to be developed.[77]

REFERENCES

1. Sjostrom L, Narbro K, Sjostrom D, et al. Effects of bariatric surgery on mortality in Swedish obese subjects. N Engl J Med 2007;357(8):741–52.
2. Adams T, Gress M, Smith S, et al. Long-term mortality after gastric bypass surgery. N Engl J Med 2007;357(8):753–61.
3. Flegal K, Carroll M, Ogden C, et al. Prevalence and trends in obesity among US adults. JAMA 2010;303(3):235–41.
4. Henrikson V. [Kan tunnfarmsresektion forsvaras som terapi mot fettsot? Nordisk Medicin 1952;47:744]. Can small bowel resection be defended for therapy for obesity? Obes Surg 1994;4:54–5.
5. Kremen A, Linner J, Nelson C. An experimental evaluation of the nutritional importance of proximal and distal small intestine. Ann Surg 1954;140:439–44.
6. Buchwald H, Rucker R. The rise and fall of jejunoileal bypass. In: Nelson RL, Nyhus LM, editors. Surgery of the small intestine. Norwalk (CT): Appleton Century Crofts; 1987. p. 529–41.
7. Payne J, DeWind L, Commons R. Metabolic observations in patients with jejuno-colic shunts. Am J Surg 1963;106:273–89.
8. Scott H Jr, Sandstead J, Brill A, et al. Experience with a new technic of intestinal bypass in the treatment of morbid obesity. Ann Surg 1971;70(1):62–70.
9. Brown R, O'Leary J, Woodward E. Hepatic effects of jejunoileal bypass for morbid obesity. Am J Surg 1974;127:53–8.
10. Deitel M, Shahi B, Ahand P, et al. Long-term outcome in a series of jejunoileal bypass patients. Obes Surg 1993;3:247–52.
11. Griffen W Jr, Young VL, Stevenson CC. A prospective comparison of gastric and jejunoileal bypass procedures for morbid obesity. Ann Surg 1977;186(4):500–9.
12. Scopinaro N, Gianetta E, Civalleri D, et al. Bilio-pancreatic by-pass for obesity: II. Initial experience in man. Br J Surg 1979;66:619–20.
13. Scopinaro N, Adami G, Marinari G, et al. Biliopancreatic diversion. World J Surg 1998;22:936–46.
14. Scopinaro N, Gianetti E, Adami G, et al. Biliopancreatic diversion for obesity at eighteen years. Surgery 1996;119:261–8.
15. Scopinaro N. Biliopancreatic diversion: mechanisms of action and long-term results. Obes Surg 2006;16(6):683–9.
16. Lagace M, Marceau P, Marceau S, et al. Biliopancreatic diversion with a new type of gastrectomy: some previous conclusions revisited. Obes Surg 1995;5:411–8.
17. Hess DS, Hess DW. Biliopancreatic diversion with a duodenal switch. Obes Surg 1998;8:267–82.
18. DeMeester T, Fuchs K, Ball C, et al. Experimental and clinical results with proximal end-to-end duodenojejunostomy for the pathologic duodenogastric reflux. Ann Surg 1987;206:414–24.
19. Mason EE, Ito C. Gastric bypass in obesity. Surg Clin North Am 1967;47(6):1345–51.

20. Alder RL, Terry BE. Measurement and standardization of the gastric pouch in gastric bypass. Surg Gynecol Obstet 1977;144(5):762–3.
21. Alden JF. Gastric and jejunoileal bypass. A comparison in the treatment of morbid obesity. Arch Surg 1977;112(7):799–806.
22. Deitel M. A synopsis of the development of bariatric operations. Obes Surg 2007; 17:707–10.
23. Torres JC, Oca CF, Garrison RN. Roux-en-Y gastrojejunostomy from the lesser curvature. South Med J 1983;76:1217–21.
24. Salmon PA. Gastroplasty with distal gastric bypass: a new and more successful weight loss operation for the morbidly obese. Can J Surg 1988;31(2):111–3.
25. Fobi M. Why the operation I prefer is silastic ring vertical gastric bypass. Obes Surg 1991;1(4):423–6.
26. Brolin RE. Long limb Roux-en-Y gastric bypass revisited. Surg Clin North Am 2005;85(4):807–17.
27. Printen KJ, Mason EE. Gastric surgery or relief of morbid obesity. Arch Surg 1973; 106:428–31.
28. Gomez CA. Gastroplasty in the surgical treatment of morbid obesity. Am J Clin Nutr 1980;33:406–15.
29. Gomez CA. Gastroplasty in morbid obesity: a progress report. World J Surg 1981;5(6):823–8.
30. Pace WG, Martin EW Jr, Tetirick T, et al. Gastric partitioning for morbid obesity. Ann Surg 1979;190(3):392–400.
31. Carey LC, Martin EW Jr. Treatment of morbid obesity by gastric partitioning. World J Surg 1981;5:829–31.
32. Long M, Collins JP. The technique and early results of high gastric reduction for obesity. Aust N Z J Surg 1980;50(2):146–9.
33. Laws HL. Standardized gastroplasty orifice. Am J Surg 1981;141(3):393–4.
34. Mason EE. Vertical banded gastroplasty for obesity. Arch Surg 1982;117:701–6.
35. Mason EE, Maher JW, Scott DH, et al. Ten years of vertical banded gastroplasty for severe obesity. Probl Gen Surg 1992;9(2):280–9.
36. Balsiger BM, Poggio JL, Mai J, et al. Ten and more years after vertical banded gastroplasty as primary operation for morbid obesity. J Gastrointest Surg 2000; 4:598–605.
37. Capella JF, Capella RF. The weight reduction operation of choice: vertical banded gastroplasty or gastric bypass? Am J Surg 1996;171:74–9.
38. Pories WJ, Swanson MS, MacDonald KG, et al. Who would have thought it? An operation proves to be the most effective therapy for adult-onset diabetes mellitus. Ann Surg 1995;222:339–52.
39. Scozzari G, Toppino M, Famiglietti F, et al. 10-year follow-up of laparoscopic vertical banded gastroplasty: good results in selected patients. Ann Surg 2010; 252:831–9.
40. Iannelli A, Amato D, Addeo P, et al. Laparoscopic conversion of vertical banded gastroplasty (Mason MacLean) into Roux-en-Y gastric bypass. Obes Surg 2008; 18:43–6.
41. Marsk R, Jonas E, Gartzios H, et al. High revision rates after laparoscopic vertical banded gastroplasty. Surg Obes Relat Dis 2009;5:94–8.
42. Wilkinson LH, Peloso OA. Gastric (reservoir) reduction for morbid obesity. Arch Surg 1981;116:602–5.
43. Molina M, Oria HE. Gastric segmentation: a new, safe, effective, simple, readily revised and fully reversible surgical procedure for the correction of morbid obesity [abstract 15]. In: 6th Bariatric Surgery Colloquium. Iowa City (IA), June 2–3, 1983.

44. Kolle K. Gastric banding [abstract]. In: OMGI 7th Congress, vol. 145. Stockholm (Sweden): 1982. p. 37.

45. Naslund I, Granstrom L, Stockeld D, et al. Marlex mesh gastric banding: a 7–12 year follow-up. Obes Surg 1994;4:269–73.

46. Frydenberg HB. Modification of gastric banding using a fundal suture. Obes Surg 1991;1:314–7.

47. Kuzmak LI. Silicone gastric banding: a simple and effective operation for morbid obesity. Contemp Surg 1986;28:13–8.

48. Steffen R. The history and role of gastric banding. Surg Obes Relat Dis 2008;4: S7–13.

49. Szinicz G, Mueller L, Erhard W, et al. "Reversible gastric banding" in surgical treatment of morbid obesity – results of animal experiments. Res Exp Med (Berl) 1989;189:55–60.

50. Hallberg D, Forsell O. Ballongband vid behandling av massiv oberwikt. Svinsk Kiriurgi 1985;344:106–8 [in Swedish].

51. Belachew M, Legrand M, Vincent V, et al. Laparoscopic adjustable banding. World J Surg 1998;22:955–63.

52. Fielding GA, Rhodes M, Nathanson LK. Laparoscopic gastric banding for morbid obesity: surgical outcomes in 335 cases. Surg Endosc 1999;13:550–4.

53. Weiner R, Wagner D, Bockhorn H. Laparoscopic gastric banding for morbid obesity. J Laparoendosc Adv Surg Tech A 1999;9:23–30.

54. Allen JW, Coleman MG, Fielding GA. Lesson learned from laparoscopic gastric banding for morbid obesity. Am J Surg 2001;182:10–4.

55. O'Brien PE, Dixon JB, Brown W, et al. The laparoscopic adjustable gastric band (Lap-Band): a prospective study of medium-term effects on weight, health and quality of life. Obes Surg 2002;84:42S–5S.

56. DeMaria EJ, Sugerman HG, Meador JG, et al. High failure rate after laparoscopic adjustable silicone gastric banding for the treatment of morbid obesity. Ann Surg 2001;233:809–18.

57. Ren CJ, Horgan S, Ponce J. US experience with the LAP-BAND system. Am J Surg 2002;184:46S–50S.

58. Fielding GA, Ren CJ. Laparoscopic adjustable gastric band. Surg Clin North Am 2005;85:129–40.

59. Buchwald H, Avidor Y, Braunwald E, et al. Bariatric surgery: a systematic review and meta-analysis. JAMA 2004;292:1724–37.

60. Shen R, Dugay G, Rajaram K, et al. Impact of patient follow-up on weight loss after bariatric surgery. Obes Surg 2004;14:514–9.

61. Marceau P, Biron S, Bourque RA, et al. Biliopancreatic diversion with a new type of gastrectomy. Obes Surg 1993;3(1):29–35.

62. Johnston D, Dachtler J, Sue-Ling HM, et al. The magenstrasse and Mill operation for morbid obesity. Obes Surg 2003;13(1):10–6.

63. McMahon MJ. Laparoscopic sleeve gastrectomy: from magenstrasse and mill to sleeve. [supplement A]. In: Proceedings supplement from the international consensus summit on sleeve gastrectomy. New York (NY): Bariatric Times; 2007. p. 3–4.

64. Silecchia G, Boru C. Effectiveness of laparoscopic sleeve gastrectomy (first stage of biliopancreatic diversion with duodenal switch) on comorbidities in super-obese high-risk patients. Obes Surg 2006;16(9):1138–44.

65. ASMBS clinical issues committee. Updated position statement on sleeve gastrectomy as a bariatric procedure. Surg Obes Relat Dis 2010;6(1):1–5.

66. Westling A, Gustavsson S. Laparoscopic vs. open Roux-en-Y gastric bypass: a prospective, randomized trial. Obes Surg 2001;11:284–92.

67. Broadbent R, Tracy M, Harrington P. Laparoscopic gastric banding: a preliminary report. Obes Surg 1993;3:63–7.
68. Belachew M, Legrand M, Jacquet N. Laparoscopic placement of adjustable silicone gastric banding in the treatment of morbid obesity: an animal model experimental study: a video film: a preliminary report [abstract 5]. Obes Surg 1993;3:140.
69. Hess DS. Letter to the editor: first laparoscopic bariatric surgery. Obes Surg 2008;18:1656.
70. Hess DW, Hess DS. Laparoscopic vertical banded gastroplasty with complete transection of the staple-line. Obes Surg 1994;4:44–6.
71. Wittgrove AC, Clark GW. Laparoscopic gastric bypass, Roux-en-Y 500 patients: technique and results, with 3–60 month follow-up. Obes Surg 2000;10:233–9.
72. Ren CJ, Patterson E, Gagner M. Early results of laparoscopic biliopancreatic diversion with duodenal switch: a case series of 40 consecutive patients. Obes Surg 2000;10:514–23.
73. See C, Carter PL, Elliott D, et al. An institutional experience with laparoscopic gastric bypass complications seen in the first year compared with open gastric bypass complications during the same period. Am J Surg 2002;183:533–8.
74. Schauer P, Ikramuddin S, Hamad G, et al. The learning curve for laparoscopic Roux-en-Y gastric bypass is 100 cases. Surg Endosc 2003;17:212–5.
75. Nguyen NT, Goldman C, Rosenquist CJ, et al. Laparoscopic versus open gastric bypass: a randomized study of outcomes, quality of life and costs. Ann Surg 2001;234:279–91.
76. Lujan JA, Frutos MD, Hernandez Q, et al. Laparoscopic versus open gastric bypass in the treatment of morbid obesity: a randomized prospective study. Ann Surg 2004;239(4):433–40.
77. Mason EE. History of obesity surgery. 2004 ASBS Consensus Conference. Surg Obes Relat Dis 2005;1:123–5.

Surgical Treatment for Morbid Obesity: The Laparoscopic Roux-en-Y Gastric Bypass

Myron S. Powell, MD, Adolfo Z. Fernandez Jr, MD*

KEYWORDS

• Obesity • Gastric bypass • Roux-en-Y • Laparoscopy

Obesity, defined as a body mass index (BMI) of 30 (ie, body weight of 30 kg divided by height in meters squared [30 kg/m²]) or greater, is the excess accumulation of body fat that adversely effects health and decreases life expectancy.[1,2] A body weight that exceeds the ideal body weight by more than 100 lb (45.4 kg) or a BMI greater than 35 has been termed morbid obesity. Historically obesity was widely perceived as a symbol of wealth and fertility, and still is in some parts of the world.[2] Viewed as one of the most serious public health problems of the twenty-first century, it is now the leading cause of preventable death in the United States, with increasing prevalence both in adults and children.[3]

During the past 20 years there has been a dramatic increase in obesity in the United States. In 2009, only Colorado and the District of Columbia had a prevalence of obesity less than 20%.[4] Thirty-three states had a prevalence equal to or greater than 25%; 9 of these states (Alabama, Arkansas, Kentucky, Louisiana, Mississippi, Missouri, Oklahoma, Tennessee, and West Virginia) had a prevalence of obesity equal to or greater than 30%.[4] Medical weight reduction programs have not been able to yield substantial long-lasting success in comparison with surgical intervention.[5]

BRIEF HISTORY OF THE EVOLUTION OF THE LAPAROSCOPIC ROUX-EN-Y GASTRIC BYPASS PROCEDURE

The history of surgery for obesity dates back to the 1950s but because of the growing obesity epidemic, the most rapid advances have occurred in the last several decades.

Department of General Surgery, Wake Forest University School Of Medicine, Winston-Salem, NC 27157, USA
* Corresponding author.
E-mail address: afernand@wfu.edu

Surg Clin N Am 91 (2011) 1203–1224
doi:10.1016/j.suc.2011.08.013
0039-6109/11/$ – see front matter © 2011 Published by Elsevier Inc.

A.J. Kremen is credited with the first bariatric operation in the United States, in 1954. He introduced the jejunoileal bypass procedure for weight loss. This procedure induced a state of malabsorption by bypassing most of the intestines while keeping the stomach intact, and was successful for weight loss. However, the morbidity of the procedure was high, having complications such as severe electrolyte imbalances, dehydration, bypass enteritis from bacterial overgrowth of the bypassed intestine, diarrhea, cirrhosis, interstitial nephritis, and various vitamin and mineral deficiencies. The mortality rate was high, and many patients have required reversal of the procedure.[6,7] In the 1980s the jejunoileal bypass was abandoned and is no longer a recommended bariatric surgical procedure. Many experimental operations were tested on morbidly obese patients throughout the 1950s and 1960s. Surgery involving the stomach became the more prevalent choice for the surgical treatment of morbid obesity.[6,7]

The development of the gastric bypass procedure for the treatment of morbid obesity has been credited to Dr Edward E. Mason.[8] In 1966 Mason and Ito applied the concepts of partial gastrectomy to obese females for weight reduction, because of the observation that female patients undergoing partial gastrectomy for ulcer disease remained underweight and had difficulty gaining weight. Mason and Ito[8] introduced the first case series of gastric restrictive procedures. The procedure, referred to as gastric bypass, involved horizontally transecting the stomach.[8] The pouch was composed of cardia and fundus, and was completely divided from the distal part of the stomach.[8] As with its predecessor, the Billroth II, their procedure incorporated a retrocolic "loop" with a hand-sewn gastrojejunostomy (**Fig. 1**).[9]

The gastric outlet was measured and restricted to maximize weight loss. Mason and Ito modified the procedure and reported the specifics of the gastrojejunostomy as related to weight loss. Further refinements were made, such as calibrating the volume of the gastric pouch and changing the diameter of the gastrojejunostomy.[9] The best

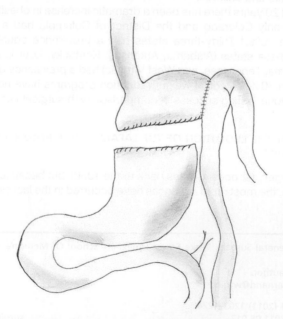

Fig. 1. Mason gastric bypass with loop gastrojejunostomy, 1966.

results were demonstrated with a calibrated 50-mL gastric pouch and a 12-mm stoma.[9] After receiving criticism from surgeons worldwide because of an increased risk of the development of a marginal ulcer as a consequence of the gastric restriction and anastomosis, Mason and colleagues[10] published a study reporting that the upper part of the stomach produces relatively little acid and that marginal ulceration would be unlikely. Later, in 1977, Alden[11] introduced a modification of the gastric bypass that did not involve complete transection of the stomach and separation of the gastric pouch from the distal stomach. Instead, surgical staplers were used to create a partition across the upper portion of the stomach to reduce the intake of food and create the feeling of satiety, with a small amount of food.[11] Surgeons continued to modify the initial attempts of Mason and Ito in gastric restrictive procedures, which ultimately contributed to the evolution of the current laparoscopic Roux-en-Y (RNY) gastric bypass procedure.

In 1977, Griffen and colleagues[12] modified the early gastric bypass procedure by replacing the loop with the RNY gastrojejunostomy, which reduced bile reflux and became the accepted technique for the anastomosis (**Fig. 2**). Several years later the jejunoileal bypass was dismissed as an acceptable procedure for weight loss, due to the increased evidence of serious complications including cirrhosis, interstitial nephritis, and renal and liver failure.[13] Fewer surgeons attempted to develop more technically challenging gastric bypass procedures, evidenced by the increased use of stapled gastroplasty techniques.[14] The 1980s presented an opportunity for bariatric surgery as more centers became committed to improving the gastric bypass procedure.[13] Improvements introduced by Torres and colleagues[15] included the use of a vertical gastric pouch along the lesser curvature, which served as a prototype for

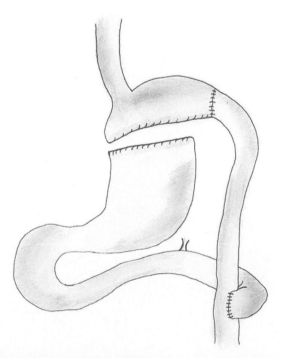

Fig. 2. Griffen Roux-en-Y gastric bypass, 1977.

the lesser curve vertical pouches currently used in today's gastric bypass (**Fig. 3**). The distal RNY was also introduced, describing various lengths of efferent and common limbs.[13] Other variations introduced by Fobi and colleagues[16] in 1998 and Capella and Capella[17] in 1996 included the use of a silastic ring at the gastric pouch to prevent dilatation of the gastric stoma. Although the concept behind the ring was intuitive, many surgeons did not accept the use of these devices because of the added risk of erosion.[13]

In 1991, the National Institutes of Health (NIH) Consensus determined that the RNY and the vertical banded gastroplasty provided a significant benefit to patients with morbid obesity, and were indicated for patients with a BMI greater than 35 and obesity-related comorbidities or for all patients with a BMI greater than 40.[13] However, long-term evaluation of patients who had undergone vertical banded gastroplasty has shown that frequent postoperative changes in dietary habits, including ingestion of high-calorie soft foods and liquids, leads to weight regain.[18] These long-term results have largely caused this operation to be abandoned. Nowadays the RNY has emerged and become the gold standard of surgical treatment for clinically severe or morbid obesity because of sustained long-term weight loss, with acceptable short-term and long-term complication rates.

Laparoscopy has had a tremendous impact on surgery by reducing perioperative complications. Morbidly obese patients can be high-risk surgical candidates who are more vulnerable to cardiopulmonary and wound-related complications, and stand to benefit from a less invasive approach.[19–22] Although the open RNY procedure has been performed with a relatively low morbidity and mortality rate, the wound-related

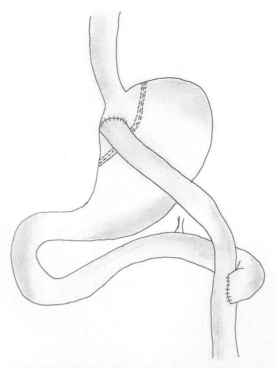

Fig. 3. Torres Roux-en-Y gastric bypass with lesser curvature pouch, 1980.

complications have been challenging. The laparoscopic Roux-en-Y gastric bypass (LRNY) has reduced the number of wound complications seen in open bariatric surgical procedures.[23] The development of laparoscopic surgical staplers changed bariatric surgery in the 1990s. The first case series to perform an LRNY was published in 1994 by Wittgrove and Clark.[24]

CURRENT TECHNIQUES OF THE LAPAROSCOPIC ROUX-EN-Y GASTRIC BYPASS

Despite the technically demanding nature of the LRNY procedure, it has swiftly gained popularity over the open technique since its inception in 1994 and has become the procedure of choice for clinically severe obesity. The totally LRNY procedure requires the operating surgeon to have an advanced laparoscopic skill set. The long learning curve and inexperience with advanced laparoscopic techniques can be a major hitch to this procedure. An alternative to the totally laparoscopic approach is the hand-assisted LRNY. Hand-assisted laparoscopy typically has been used in colorectal surgery and less frequently in bariatric procedures. Several published studies containing small series of patients in which hand-assisted techniques are used in laparoscopic gastric banding[23] and laparoscopic vertical banded gastroplasty show the benefits of hand-assisted laparoscopy in bariatrics.[25,26]

An article in 2000 by Sundbom and Gustavsson[27] highlighted the advantages of the hand-assisted technique over the total LRNY approach, as follows: (1) the avoidance of the blind abdominal puncture (Veress or trocar-assisted optical view entry, as the surgeon's left hand inside the abdomen can guide the introduction of the first trocar); (2) the ability of the surgeon's hand to directly palpate intra-abdominal structures, allowing for better anatomic orientation; (3) the surgeon's hand being used for dissection of tissue as an alternative to conventional laparoscopic instruments such as hook cautery, dissecting instruments, and ultrasonic dissectors; (4) the surgeon's hand being used for proper exposure of the surgical field without the use of mechanical retractors. In 2003, a follow-up randomized clinical trial of hand-assisted laparoscopic versus open RNY for the treatment of morbid obesity found that patients did not appear to derive any significant benefit from a hand-assisted LRNY technique in comparison with open surgery,[28] as the results did not demonstrate the proposed advantages of laparoscopy over open surgery of early mobilization, reduction in postoperative pain, and shorter hospital stay.[28] Although the bariatric surgeon who is trying to learn LRNY techniques may benefit early on from a hand-assisted approach, nonrandomized comparative studies have recently shown that hand assistance was more expensive than open surgery and did not improve patient outcome.[29]

When compared with the open technique the LRNY has been validated in multiple studies over the span of a decade, being shown to have comparable weight loss, safety, cost effectiveness, and decreased morbidity.[23,30,31] The LRNY has been shown to decrease wound complications, decrease operative blood loss, shorten hospital stay, improve postsurgical quality of life, and decrease the incidence of postoperative pulmonary complications.[32–34] However, there is no consensus on one uniform way that the LRNY is performed. There are variations on whether the Roux limb is passed in an antecolic antegastric, antecolic retrogastric, or retrocolic retrogastric fashion to form the gastrojejunostomy. Multiple techniques of creating the gastrojejunostomy have been described. Described by Wittgrove and colleagues in 1994,[24] the transoral circular-stapled technique is the most commonly used method for creating the gastrojejunostomy. Other techniques used by surgeons to create the gastrojejunostomy include the linear-stapled technique, the hand-sewn technique, and the transgastric circular-stapled technique.

Laparoscopic Roux-en-Y Transoral Circular-Stapled Technique

After appropriate patient selection, the patient is brought to the operating room and placed supine on the operating room table. A time-out is taken to verify the patient's identity, procedure, and procedure location. Appropriate preoperative antibiotics are given, deep venous thrombosis (DVT) prophylaxis is given, and sequential compression devices are placed to incision. A Foley catheter is optionally placed. The abdomen is prepped and draped in the usual sterile fashion. At this point in the procedure, many different variations are seen based on surgeon preference and training. Examples of this include how the abdominal cavity is accessed, size of ports, location of ports, and location of the operating surgeon and assistants based on use of split-leg extenders (Skytron, Grand Rapids, MI, USA). The manner in which the authors perform this procedure at their institution is detailed here.

A 1:1 mixture of 0.25% marcaine and 1% lidocaine with epinephrine is used to pre-infiltrate all incision sites. The first incision is made at the left anterior axillary line just subcostally. A 5-mm Optiview port (Ethicon Endosurgery, Cincinnati, OH) with a 0° laparoscope inserted is used to enter the abdomen under direct vision. The abdomen is insufflated with carbon dioxide gas to a pressure of 12–18 mm Hg. Once adequate insufflation has been obtained, a 5-mm 45° angled scope is inserted into the abdomen. Exploratory laparoscopy is then performed. The visualized portions of the stomach, spleen, colon, small intestine, liver, and gallbladder are all assessed. At this point, a 5-mm port is placed above and to the left of the umbilicus. Additional 5-mm and 15-mm ports are placed in the right upper quadrant (**Fig. 4**). Using abdominal graspers, the omentum is retracted cephalad and the ligament of Treitz is identified. The small bowel is measured 50 cm distal to the ligament of Treitz and the small bowel is transected with a laparoscopic linear stapler (Echelon 60 mm length, 2.5 mm thickness; Ethicon Endosurgery). Then 100 cm of small bowel is measured distal to

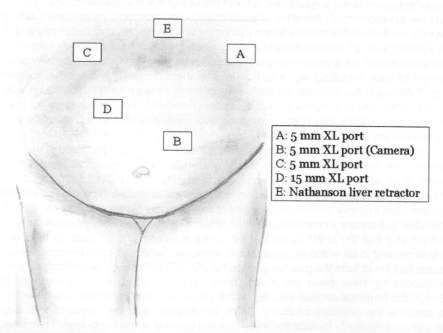

A: 5 mm XL port
B: 5 mm XL port (Camera)
C: 5 mm XL port
D: 15 mm XL port
E: Nathanson liver retractor

Fig. 4. Port site placement for the LRNY.

this and a side-to-side functional end-to-side jejunojejunostomy is created. Using an ultrasonic dissector, an enterotomy is made in the Roux limb as well as in the distal portion of the biliopancreatic limb. The linear stapler is used again to create the enteroenterostomy by placing each end of the stapler in the corresponding enterotomies. Once the stapler is fired, the common opening is closed using a running 2-0 Surgidac suture with an endoscopic suturing device (EndoStitch, 10 mm; Covidien, Mansfield, MA). A triple-staple technique may also be used to create this anastomosis. To perform this technique, enterotomies are made as previously described using the ultrasonic dissector. A linear stapler is used to create a long enteroenterostomy. The common enterotomy is then closed transversely with the linear stapler. The mesenteric defect between the anastomosis is closed using a running 2-0 Surgidac suture with an endoscopic suturing device (EndoStitch, 10 mm). The omentum is split just to the left of midline to allow for a tension-free path of the Roux limb up to the pouch to create an antecolic, antegastric gastrojejunostomy.

The Nathanson liver retractor (Cook Medical, Bloomington, IN) is inserted through a subxiphoid stab wound to retract the left lateral lobe of the liver (see **Fig. 4**). The gastrohepatic ligament is opened in an avascular plane. A linear stapler with bovine pericardial reinforcement strips (Peri-strips; Synovis Surgical Innovations, St. Paul, MN) is fired into the lesser curve of the stomach 5 cm distal to the gastroesophageal junction. Prior to this point all tubes are removed from the stomach. A linear stapler (Echelon 60 mm length, 3.8 mm thickness) is fired perpendicularly into the lesser curve of the stomach at this same point. The transection is completed up to the angle of His using an articulating linear stapler with bovine pericardial reinforcement strips (Peri-strips). A gastrotomy is created into the distal end of the pouch through the unreinforced staple line. The OrVil (EEA OrVil 21 mm Device; Covidien) tube is pulled out through this gastrotomy and the 15-mm port site. Once the stem of the anvil is visualized, the strings holding the tube are cut and the tube is removed, leaving the anvil in place. A Lembert suture is placed on either side of the anvil stem to purse-string the stomach.

Next, the Roux limb is identified. It is brought up to the upper abdomen. Care is taken to make sure that the mesentery is not twisted. An enterotomy is made in the proximal Roux limb. The EEA stapler is introduced through the 15-mm port site. It is deeply intubated into the Roux limb and brought up to the pouch. The anvil and the stapler are married and fired. The stapler is removed and inspected for two complete donuts of tissue. The anastomosis is visualized through the opening in the Roux limb, and active sites of bleeding are assessed. The proximal portion of the Roux limb is excised using a linear stapler. The mesentery is divided with the ultrasonic dissector. Lembert sutures are used to reinforce the corners of the gastrojejunostomy. A bowel clamp is placed proximally on the Roux limb, and an intraoperative gastroscopy is performed to visualize portions of the esophagus, pouch, anastomosis, and Roux limb for evidence of bleeding. The upper abdomen is filled with water to submerge the gastric pouch and anastomosis simultaneously for an air leak test. The air and the gastroscope are withdrawn once the anastomosis has been adequately accessed. The irrigation fluid is suctioned from the abdomen, and a Jackson Pratt drain is placed in the left upper quadrant. The drain is pulled out through the 5-mm left upper quadrant port site and secured to the skin using a 3-0 nylon suture. The Roux remnant is placed in a laparoscopic specimen retrieval bag (Endopouch, 10 mm; Ethicon Endosurgery) and pulled out through the 15-mm port site. The Nathanson liver retractor and upper abdominal ports are removed under direct vision. Bleeding from the port sites is assessed. The abdomen is desufflated. A 0-Vicryl suture is used to close the 15-mm port site fascial defect. The skin incisions are closed with 4-0 Monocryl suture and the skin covered with Dermabond.

Laparoscopic Roux-en-Y Linear-Stapled Technique

The LRNY linear-stapled technique is performed in a similar fashion to the previously described transoral stapled technique, with the exception of the creation of the gastrojejunostomy. The jejunojejunostomy and gastric pouch are created in a similar fashion. In this technique a 2-layer anastomosis is then created between the pouch and the Roux limb. The outer layer is a running 2-0 Surgidac suture using the endoscopic suturing device. The inner layer is a partial firing of a linear stapler (Echelon 60 mm length, 3.5 mm thickness). The gastroscope is passed through the common enterotomy. The common enterotomy is closed over the top of the gastroscope using a running 2-0 Polysorb suture. A second layering of 2-0 Surgidac is then performed over the anastomosis in a Lembert fashion. Once both layers are complete, a bowel clamp is placed proximally on the Roux limb and an intraoperative gastroscopy is performed. The esophagus, pouch, and proximal Roux limb are visualized. An underwater air leak test is performed at this point. The air and the gastroscope are withdrawn. The irrigation fluid is suctioned from the abdomen. The anastomosis is circumferentially wrapped with omentum, and held in place using 2-0 Surgidac suture.

ANALYZING THE CURRENT TECHNIQUES OF THE LAPAROSCOPIC ROUX-EN-Y GASTRIC BYPASS

It is widely apparent that the art or technique of creation of the gastrojejunostomy is one of the most challenging steps during the LRNY. As a result, multiple different techniques for creating the gastrojejunostomy have been used by bariatric surgeons to facilitate this step, as previously discussed. Countless studies and series have reported that the main complications using a circular stapler for the gastrojejunostomy are anastomotic leaks and strictures.[35] Historical data for the open RNY for morbid obesity indicate that the hand-sewn technique has lower stricture and leak rates in comparison with the circular-stapled technique.[36] The LRNY data mimic the historical data with the open RNY with regard to the techniques in creating the gastrojejunostomy and the stomal stenosis rates (**Table 1**). Leak rates have been reported from 0% to 3% in multiple large LRNY series using the various techniques for creating the gastrojejunostomy. A 0% leak rate after 1000 LRNY procedures using either

Table 1
Comparison of published data for the incidence of gastrojejunostomy stenosis

Authors, Year	No. of Patients	Technique	Stenosis Number (Percentage)
Wittgrove et al,[31] 2000	500	CS	8 (1.6%)
Matthews et al,[37] 2000	48	CS	13 (27.1%)
Champion et al,[38] 1999	63	LS	4 (6.3%)
Schauer et al,[23] 2000	275	LS	13 (4.7%)
Higa et al,[39] 2001	1500	HS	73 (4.9%)
Wittgrove et al,[40] 2002	1000	CS	40 (4.0%)
DeMaria et al,[41] 2002	281	LS	18 (6.6%)
Gonzalez et al,[42] 2003	108 (87/13/8)	HS/CS/LS	3 (3%)/4 (31%)/0 (0%)
Carrodeguas et al,[43] 2006	1291	LS	94 (7.3%)
Leyba et al,[44] 2008	80 (40/40)	CS/LS	7 (17.5%)/1 (2.5%)
Kravetz et al,[45] 2011	222 (123/99)	HS/LS	5 (4.1%)/10 (10.1%)

Abbreviations: CS, circular stapled; HS, hand sewn; LS, linear stapled.

hand-sewn or circular-stapled techniques for the gastrojejunostomy has been reported.[39,46]

As we approach a second decade in the era of LRNY, the circular-stapled anastomosis technique originally described by Wittgrove and Clark[24] is still the most commonly used technique for creation of the gastrojejunostomy. As modern technology continues to evolve so does the surgical technology, affording better devices to assist in difficult problems faced with older devices. The original and early use of the circular stapler by surgeons was with a 21-mm circular stapler to create the gastrojejunostomy. Since then the 25-mm circular stapler has been developed. Some surgeons have adopted use of the 25-mm stapler secondary to decreased rates of stomal stenosis at the gastrojejunostomy. Despite skepticism from some surgeons to change their approach from the 21-mm to the 25-mm circular stapler in creating the gastrojejunostomy, published data would suggest that the use of 25-mm circular stapler shows a decrease in stomal stenosis rates when compared with those of the 21-mm circular stapler, with no effect on long-term weight loss (**Table 2**). Higher potential for esophageal injury[23,32] contributes to the skepticism in passing a larger-diameter transoral anvil, but this has not been demonstrated. Some reports have shown this potential in passing a 21-mm anvil transorally. However, Wittgrove and Clark published a series of more than 1400 patients using the pull-wire technique of passing a 21-mm anvil for a circular-stapled anastomosis. This technique was evaluated with intraoperative upper endoscopy and water-soluble upper gastrointestinal series (UGI) on postoperative day 1, with no demonstration of esophageal injuries.[53]

A transgastric technique of anvil placement to avoid the transoral route has been described, and has been reported to decrease the incidence of wound infections and operative times.[54,55] Although the circular-stapled technique remains the popular choice among surgeons for creating the gastrojejunostomy, complications specifically reported for the circular-stapled technique include stapler malfunction and increased wound infection rate at the extended abdominal port site where the contaminated stapler is withdrawn from the abdomen.[23]

COMPLICATIONS OF LAPAROSCOPIC ROUX-EN-Y GASTRIC BYPASS SURGERY

As obesity continues to increase nationwide, so does the number of bariatric surgical procedures performed. Data from the American Society for Metabolic and Bariatric Surgery (ASMBS) estimates that the number of procedures increased from about 16,000 in the early 1990s to more than 103,000 in 2003. The ASMBS estimates that 220,000 people in the United States had bariatric surgery in 2008. Since the inception

Table 2
Comparison of published data for the incidence of gastrojejunostomy stenosis with 21-mm and 25-mm circular stapler

Authors, Year	No. of Patients	Circular Stapler Size (mm)	Stenosis Number (Percentage)
Nguyen et al,[47] 2003	185 (114/71)	25/21	10 (8.8%)/19 (26.8%)
Gould et al,[48] 2006	226 (81/145)	25/21	5 (6.2%)/23 (15.9%)
Fisher et al,[49] 2007	200 (100/100)	25/21	7 (7%)/17 (17%)
Suggs et al,[50] 2007	438 (374/64)	25/21	11 (2.9%)/6 (9.4%)
Alasfar et al,[51] 2009	126	21	29 (23%)
Dolce et al,[52] 2009	159	21	15 (9.4%)

of LRNY in 1993, it has now become the preferred method and procedure of choice for morbid obesity over its open counterpart. This adoption is mostly attributable to the decreased complication profile with respect to wound infection and incisional hernia rates. Other published data demonstrated further advantages of the laparoscopic approach with regard to less postoperative pain, decreased operative blood loss, shorter in patient hospital stay, lower pulmonary complications, and an overall better quality of life.[32–34] All surgical procedures include a list of potential complications, and the LRNY procedure is no exception.

Intestinal Leaks

Intestinal leaks can be fatal, and are likely related to the learning curve associated with advanced surgical techniques required to perform the procedure. Wittgrove and Clark reported 11 leaks in their first 500 patients; 9 (3.0%) leaks occurred in the first 300 cases, with only 2 (1.0%) leaks in the final 200 cases.[56] Leaks can occur at the gastro-jejunostomy, jejunojejunostomy, the bypassed stomach staple line, or the gastric pouch staple line. Leak rates as high as 6.9% have been reported.[42] Abdominal pain and peritonitis are not readily found in this group of patients. Clinical findings are nonspecific and can also represent an acute myocardial infarction or pulmonary embolus. It is imperative that if a high index of suspicion exists of an intestinal leak then the appropriate tests be expeditiously performed to guide to the appropriate therapy. Failure to act quickly could result in the rapid demise of the patient. Diagnosing intestinal leaks are usually made clinically, by UGI or computed tomography (CT). Greater than 50% of leaks can be missed by the UGI but CT is more reliable.[56] Subjective symptoms of a leak include the patient's feeling of "impending doom," left shoulder pain, back pain, pelvic pressure or pain, tenesmus, or worsening abdominal pain. Objective signs are often late and include tachycardia, fever, tachypnea, oliguria, fluid sequestration, hypotension, hypoxia, or shock. Treatment often depends on the clinical situation present. If the leak is well contained and the patient is hemodynamically stable, the patient can be treated conservatively with nothing by mouth, percutaneous drainage, intravenous antibiotics, and intravenous nutrition. If the leak is not well contained and the patient is hemodynamically stable, laparoscopic exploration is warranted. If the patient is hemodynamically compromised, open exploration should be performed. During exploration, whether open or laparoscopic, there are 3 principles that must be addressed at the time of exploration: repair of the leak, drain placement, and placement of a gastrostomy tube in the bypassed stomach.

Pulmonary Embolism

Multiple series of LRNY procedures have shown that the rates of pulmonary embolism (PE) are less than 1%.[57] Despite the low incidence of PE, all precautions should be undertaken for the prevention of a fatal PE. Obesity itself is a risk factor for the development of DVT and PE. The combination of increased intra-abdominal pressure and a baseline hypercoagulable state places the patient at high risk of DVT and PE. Prevention of DVT includes the use of preoperative heparin or low molecular weight heparin, as well as intraoperative sequential compression devices.

Death

The risk of death associated with the LRNY is reported in most series to be less than 1%. Historical data reported from the open RNY experience shows that the two most significant postoperative events that cause mortality are intestinal leak and PE. For this reason a high index of suspicion must be maintained to prevent this from occurring.

Cholelithiasis

Rapid weight loss is associated with the formation of gallstones as a result of the increased concentration of cholesterol in the bile. The concentrated bile leads to the formation of sludge with cholesterol crystals that serve as the nidus for gallstone formation. The best treatment is prevention. Sugerman and colleagues[58] showed that 32% of patients form gallstones after the open RNY. The risk of gallstone formation can be reduced with the addition of prophylactic ursodiol for the first 6 months postoperatively, thus reducing the risk to just 2%.[58]

Stomal Stenosis

Much debate has taken place regarding the complication of stomal stenosis and its causes. Stomal stenosis, or stricture, is usually at the constructed gastrojejunostomy and not the jejunojejunostomy. As previously discussed, there are multiple techniques used by surgeons to create the gastrojejunostomy, which include a hand-sewn technique, linear-stapled technique, and circular-stapled technique. Gonzalez and colleagues[42] published an analysis of the 3 techniques and showed that the hand-sewn technique resulted in a lower postoperative stricture rate. There are subtle differences within the same technique that can also contribute to increased incidence of stomal stenosis, such as the size of circular stapler used (21 mm or 25 mm). Stricture at the gastrojejunostomy site has been reported to occur at as high a rate as 6.6%. The reason for which stomal stenosis occurs is not well understood. Symptoms include dysphagia, nausea/vomiting, or odynophagia. Diagnosis and treatment are usually well tolerated by patients, and consists of upper endoscopy with balloon dilatation. Endoscopic balloon dilatation is usually successful after the first attempt, although multiple dilatations may be necessary to relieve the symptoms associated with stomal stenosis or stricture.

Internal Hernia

Internal hernia is another potential complication after the LRNY procedure, and is reported in less than 2% of cases.[41] The RNY has 3 potential sites of small intestine herniation: at the jejunojejunostomy, at the area between the Roux limb mesentery and the transverse colon mesentery (Petersen defect), and at the transverse colon mesentery. The mesocolic defect is created only if the Roux limb is brought retrocolic. This diagnosis can be very difficult to make. The symptoms associated with an internal hernia are vague and most commonly include periumbilical or left-sided crampy abdominal pain. Multiple episodes may occur with only transient symptoms. Patients may also present with a small-bowel obstruction. The diagnostic tests of choice include a UGI series or a CT of the abdomen with oral and intravenous contrast. Unfortunately, both of these tests will likely be normal if performed after symptoms have subsided. Treatment is laparoscopic reduction and closure of the hernia defect. Rarely is open exploration needed unless there is necrotic bowel or loss of domain due to dilated small-bowel loops.

Marginal Ulcers

Marginal ulcers can occur early or late, and are located on the jejunal side of the gastrojejunostomy anastomosis. The rate of ulceration is less than 2%.[41] Diagnosis is based on strong clinical suspicion and an upper endoscopy. Treatment is antacid therapy using proton-pump inhibitors. *Helicobacter pylori* infection should also be identified and treated. Use of tobacco and nonsteroidal anti-inflammatory drugs also contributes to ulcer formation, and should be discontinued. If treatment should fail, a UGI should be performed to rule out a gastrogastric fistula with regurgitation of acid from the excluded stomach. If a gastrogastric fistula is discovered, surgical ablation of the gastrogastric fistula may be required.

Bypassed Stomach Dilatation

Acute dilatation of the bypassed stomach can occur as a result of obstruction at the jejunojejunostomy, or may occur spontaneously. Interruption of the nerves of Laterjet resulting in a loss of vagal innervation can also result in dilatation. This complication can still be seen in patients despite the preservation of these nerves. Diagnosis can be made either clinically or radiographically. Signs and symptoms include hiccups, bloating, tympani, tachycardia, and cardiopulmonary compromise. A plain abdominal radiograph may show a large gastric bubble or air-fluid level. If the stomach is fluid-filled without air, the radiograph may not be helpful. Treatment involves needle decompression of the excluded stomach under fluoroscopy. If the problem recurs, percutaneous placement of a gastrostomy tube may be necessary. If these fail or the patient becomes hemodynamically unstable, placement of a gastrostomy tube in the operating room will be necessary.

Wound Complications

One of the advantages of the laparoscopic approach is the significant decrease in wound complications, including hernias and surgical site infections, in comparison with the open RNY. The rate of trocar site hernia is less than 1%, and wound infection rates are less than 8%.[42,59] Diagnosis is made in most instances by physical examination. If the problem arises before any significant weight loss, a CT scan of the abdomen will be required, as the patient's body habitus may obscure the diagnosis. Treatment of simple wound infections or cellulitis includes antibiotic therapy, and incision and drainage of any fluid collections. Asymptomatic hernias may be postponed until the patient's weight has stabilized to increase the success of the repair. Obviously if the hernia is incarcerated, strangulated, or symptomatic, immediate repair is necessary.

Inadequate Weight Loss

Inadequate weight loss may be a problem after gastric bypass surgery. Wittgrove and Clark[56] reported that 15% of their patients failed to lose more than 50% of their excess weight after the LRNY. These data correlate well with what is known from the open literature. The solution to this problem is not easy and potentially adds more risk for the patient. Two mechanical causes of inadequate weight loss are gastrogastric fistula and dilated stoma. Diagnosis of these can be made with a UGI series or esophagogastroduodenoscopy. Another cause of inadequate weight loss is noncompliance with dietary recommendations. Patients can "eat through" an RNY if they have a daily intake composed of high fat and carbohydrate foods or drinks. Treatment for a gastrogastric fistula is surgical. In most cases the reexploration can be performed laparoscopically because of the minimal adhesions left from the initial LRNY. Surgical treatment for a dilated stoma has been met with a high failure rate and a higher risk of leak for the patient. The noncompliant patient with inadequate weight loss should be treated with dietetic interventions to help the patient attain more weight loss. The added risk of a second procedure for these patients is not justified if the patient's compliance is the issue. For those compliant patients who are dissatisfied with their weight loss, conversion to a malabsorptive procedure should only be done if serious comorbidities remain, as the risk of malnutrition is high.

Dumping Syndrome

Gastric dumping is seen in 70% to 76% of RNY patients.[60,61] These patients report symptoms of abdominal pain and cramping, nausea, diarrhea, lightheadedness, flushing, tachycardia, and syncope. These side effects are seen as a beneficial side effect of surgical alteration of the gastrointestinal physiology by some patients, by contributing to decreasing the consumption of energy-dense foods and beverages and ultimately encouraging weight loss.[61–63] Recently, the etiology of dumping syndrome has been elucidated. It was once thought to be caused by the hyperosmolarity of intestinal contents accompanied by increased fluid in the intestinal lumen resulting in intestinal distention, decreased intravascular volume, and hypotension.[64] Recent data suggest that the release of gut peptides, as a result of food bypassing the stomach and entering the small intestines, is responsible for dumping symptoms due to the fact that the symptoms can be countered with a somatostatin analogue.[65] Dumping symptoms decrease with severity and frequency with time, and most symptoms are well controlled by dietary and nutritional changes.[63] Dietary modifications found to improve symptoms include eating small frequent meals and avoiding ingestion of foods with concentrated simple sugars, while increasing intake of foods containing complex carbohydrates high in fiber and protein.[66] Fifty milligrams of octreotide 30 minutes before meals may also decrease symptoms if dietary changes are ineffective.[66] Reactive hypoglycemia may cause late dumping, and can be managed with nutritional guidance and alterations or by simply eating small snacks.

Hyperinsulinemic Hypoglycemia

The phenomenon of severe hyperinsulinemic hypoglycemia after RNY is extremely rare. Also termed nesidioblastosis, this condition is characterized by inappropriately elevated insulin concentrations and neuroglycopenia.[67,68] Service and colleagues[68,69] described nesidioblastosis, a pathologic hyperplasia of pancreatic β cells, as a noninsulinoma pancreatogenous hypoglycemia, which is far less common than insulinoma as a cause of hyperinsulinemic hypoglycemia. This rare condition of postprandial neuroglycopenic, hyperinsulinemic, hypoglycemia, and pancreatic nesidioblastosis has been described only in small series of patients.[67,68]

The mechanisms underlying this disorder are unclear. One theory is that an intestinal hormone glucagon-like peptide 1 (GLP-1) mediates expansion of pancreatic β cells.[70] Others would argue that postprandial hypoglycemia after malabsorptive bariatric surgery is attributable to a combination of gastric dumping and inappropriately increased insulin secretion, either as a failure to adaptively decrease insulin secretion after malabsorptive bariatric surgery or as an acquired phenomenon.[71]

Several different treatment strategies are available, ranging from conservative medical therapies and diet modification to those of radical surgical treatments.[71–73] If debilitating nesidioblastosis occurs, it will likely require another major operation. The result of that second operation could be permanent insulin-dependent diabetes if the entire pancreas is removed or failure to control the attacks of hypoglycemia if some pancreas is left in place. Recommendations for pancreatic resection for nesidioblastosis require approximately 80% to 90% of pancreatic tissue to be removed.[74] As previously stated, pancreatic resection comes with its own host of problems. Despite the reported morbidity of 20% to 40% and mortality of 1% to 5%, and the risk of developing lifelong diabetes mellitus after pancreatic resection for nesidioblastosis, it can be life saving.[75,76] Z'graggen and colleagues[77] concluded in a small study of 12 patients that the majority of patients with severe postprandial hypoglycemia after gastric bypass, who are unresponsive to diet modifications, can be controlled by simple laparoscopic restoration of gastric restriction with surgical placement of a silastic ring as a first-line surgical treatment before consideration for pancreatic resection.

NUTRITIONAL COMPLICATIONS OF THE ROUX-EN-Y GASTRIC BYPASS

Although routinely performed, the LRNY necessitates the knowledge of potential long-term nutritional metabolic complications and their treatments. The RNY combines the two mechanisms of restriction and malabsorption which, in turn, promote effective long-term weight loss and improvement of obesity-associated medical conditions. This intervention is fraught with alterations of digestive physiology, leading to nutritional and metabolic complications.

Routine laboratory studies looking for vitamin and mineral deficiencies in the postoperative gastric bypass patient should be performed and monitored on a regular basis. The deficits most frequently observed after the RNY are deficiencies concerning proteins, iron, calcium, vitamin B12, and vitamin D.[78–81] Iron deficiency is common after RNY and presents primarily as microcytic anemia.[82] Various studies have shown an incidence ranging from 20% to 49% of patients.[61,83–88] The reduced intake and common intolerance of iron-rich foods such as red meat may contribute to the deficiency. Coupled with the alterations seen in the changes of digestive physiology of the bypassed stomach contributing to the malabsorption of dietary iron, this makes the etiology of iron deficiency in these patients multifactorial.[89–93] Oral iron supplementation given as ferrous sulfate, 300 mg 3 times daily, is usually adequate treatment when anemia is identified.[82] Iron supplements are sometimes poorly tolerated because of constipation and dyspepsia, which may fail to correct the underlying anemia. In rare instances patients may require intravenous iron infusions for correction.[94,95] While these patients require lifelong multivitamin supplementation, iron supplementation is also recommended for all RNY patients.[96] Commercially available daily standard multivitamins with iron are not adequate for this population of patients secondary to the small amount of elemental iron contained within. Two randomized double-blind studies have demonstrated that supplementing with 320 mg of ferrous sulfate twice daily prevented iron deficiency anemia.[94,97]

Playing a vital role in neurologic function and DNA synthesis, vitamin B12 absorption begins in the stomach where pepsin and hydrochloric acid cleave it from dietary intake. Normal vitamin metabolism is altered secondary to the surgical alterations of the gastrointestinal anatomy in the RNY. In the duodenum vitamin B12 normally binds to intrinsic factor released from the stomach, and is absorbed in the terminal ileum. Vitamin B12 deficiency occurs in 26% to 70% of gastric bypass patients.[83–85] Even though clinically symptomatic B12 deficiency is rare, the ability to maintain adequate serum levels without supplementation is difficult.[98,99] While multiple forms of supplementation are available including sublingual and nasal sprays, some clinicians recommend intramuscular injections. However, several studies have shown that a 300- to 500-μg dose of oral vitamin B12 supplementation may be sufficient if tolerated.[98,99]

Folic acid deficiency rarely causes anemia following the RNY. Essential for reactions of carbon transfer and playing an important role in DNA synthesis, folic acid must not be ignored as a potential cause of anemia in the RNY patient. The study of 1067 patients by Mallory and Macgregor[99] demonstrated that only 1% of RNY patients developed folate deficiency. Folic acid deficiency has been reported to affect as many as 9% to 18% of RNY patients at different points in follow-up.[83–85] Although folate can be absorbed throughout the entire length of the small intestine, folate absorption occurs primarily in the upper one-third of the small intestine.[85] The principal cause of folate deficiency appears to be a decreased consumption from dietary sources, which are easily corrected with vitamin supplementation.[88,100] Most daily multivitamin tablets contain between 400 and 500 µg of folate. Folate deficiency should be avoided with a daily multivitamin, although additional folate supplementation (1 mg/d) should correct deficiencies and is essential for women who become pregnant after RNY, preventing neural tube defects in infants.[101–103]

Fat-soluble vitamin deficiencies may also occur after RNY, but more commonly occur after the biliopancreatic diversion procedure secondary to the delayed interaction of dietary fats with bile salts and pancreatic enzymes from the duodenum. Vitamin D and calcium deficiencies are less likely because they are absorbed preferentially in the jejunum and ileum. Complications related to this deficiency are clinically seen as osteomalacia, and have been reported in several studies after RNY procedures.[104,105] Moderate to severe vitamin D deficiency can cause significant muscle aches and fatigue, and is common in the overall population. Daily supplementation of 400 IU of vitamin D and 1500 mg of elemental calcium is adequate for replacement. Vitamin A deficiency has also been seen after RNY procedures, clinically recognized as night blindness. Halverson[82] reported vitamin A deficiency in as many as 10% of gastric bypass patients. Oral supplemental therapy is occasionally needed for correction.

Thiamine or vitamin B1 is found in a wide variety of foods at low concentrations, and was the first of the water-soluble vitamins to be described.[106] It is not often evaluated; nevertheless, deficiency in this vitamin can occur after malabsorptive procedures such as the RNY as a result of bypass of the jejunum, where thiamine is primarily absorbed. Vitamin B1 deficiency can also be seen as a result of impaired nutritional intake or frequent emesis.[107,108] Early recognition is essential to initiate appropriate supplementation and to avoid potential complications resulting in neurologic deficits. Neurologic deficits have been reported as soon as 1 to 3 months after surgery.[89–93,109–114] Patients with active neurologic symptoms should be started on parenteral supplementation for 1 to 2 weeks with thiamine (100 mg/d).[114,115] An oral preparation of (10 mg/d)

Table 3
Nutritional deficiencies with treatment strategies

Nutritional Deficiency	Primary Treatment	Secondary Treatment
Vitamin B1 (thiamine)	Parenteral thiamine (100 mg/d) for 7–14 d	Oral preparation of thiamine (10 mg/d)
Vitamin B12 (cobalamin)	Oral crystalline B12, 350 µg/d	1000–2000 µg/2–3 mo intramuscular
Folic acid	Oral folate, 400 mg/d (included in multivitamin)	Oral folate, 1000 mg/d
Vitamin A	Oral vitamin A, 5000–10,000 IU/d	Oral vitamin A, 50,000 IU/d
Iron	Ferrous sulfate 300 mg 2–3 times/d, taken with vitamin C	Parenteral iron administration
Protein malnutrition	Enteral protein supplements	Enteral or parenteral nutrition; reversal of surgical procedure
Calcium/vitamin D	Calcium citrate, 1200–2000 mg, oral vitamin D, 50,000 IU/d	Calcitriol oral vitamin D, 1000 IU/d

Data from Heber D, Greenway F, Kaplan L, et al. Endocrine and nutritional management of the postbariatric surgery patient: an Endocrine Society Clinical Practice Guideline. J Clin Endocrinol Metab 2010;95(11):4823–43.

can be used following parenteral supplementation until neurologic symptoms resolve.[116–118] Severe thiamine deficiency typically occurs in patients after bariatric surgery, who develop intractable vomiting due to stomal stenosis. It is important that unrelenting vomiting be evaluated and resolved aggressively to prevent this complication.

The anatomic changes imposed by bariatric or malabsorptive surgery increase the risk for various vitamin and mineral deficiencies that occur as soon as the first year after surgery.[59,97,119–124] Malabsorptive procedures can be associated with micronutrient and macronutrient deficiencies, and require lifelong supplementation and monitoring.[125,126] Patients with existing osteoporosis and heavy menstruation who undergo bariatric surgery are at increased risk, and prophylactic supplementation should be considered.[119,127–129] Proper screening and supplementation of deficiencies with a multivitamin-mineral, iron, vitamin B12, or calcium with vitamin D is routinely conducted. Best-practice guidelines recently published recommend a daily multivitamin and calcium supplementation with added vitamin D for all weight-loss surgery patients.[130] **Table 3** highlights the list of common nutritional deficiencies and treatment plans seen in the RNY patient.

SUMMARY

Morbid obesity has become a pandemic problem of this century, and has accelerated to the forefront of leading causes of preventable death. The trend for bariatric surgery has followed this trend because it has proved to be a valid treatment strategy for reduction and elimination of obesity-related diseases and long-term sustainable weight loss. Over the past 60 years bariatric surgery has embraced surgical innovation, which has refined techniques to offer multiple unique and effective surgical treatment options. As in most fields of surgery, the minimally invasive or laparoscopic techniques have replaced the open procedures. Despite the need for advanced technical skills to achieve success and assure adequate patient safety, bariatric surgery has been no exception to a new generation of minimally invasive surgical techniques. Published data of case series, improvements in surgical technology, surgical training, and surgeon preference are all factors that play a critical role in the small intricacies and variations of the procedure. The largest variable in technical aspects of the LRNY is the creation and size of the gastrojejunostomy. These factors contribute to the lack of a single universal way in which the LRNY is performed. Regardless of the variations in technique, over the past 20 years the LRNY has remained the gold standard for the surgical treatment of clinically severe or morbid obesity, with relatively low morbidity and mortality.

REFERENCES

1. Calle EE, Thun MJ, Petrelli JM, et al. Body mass index and mortality in a prospective cohort of U.S. adults. N Engl J Med 1999;341:1097–105.
2. Haslam DW, James WP. "Obesity". Lancet 2005;366(9492):1197–209.
3. Flegal KM, Graubard BI, Williamson DF, et al. "Obesity". JAMA 2005;293(15): 1861–7.
4. Centers for Disease Control and Prevention (CDC). Vital signs: state-specific obesity prevalence among adults—United States, 2009. MMWR Morb Mortal Wkly Rep 2010;59(30):951–5.
5. Pories WJ, Swanson MS, MacDonald KG, et al. Who would have thought it? An operation proves to be the most effective therapy for adult-onset diabetes mellitus. Ann Surg 1995;222:339–50.

6. Kremen AJ, Linner JH, Nelson CH, et al. An experimental evaluation of the nutritional importance of proximal and distal small intestine. Ann Surg 1954;140: 439–48.
7. Griffen WO Jr, Bivins BA, Bell RM, et al. The decline and fall of jejunoileal bypass. Surg Gynecol Obstet 1983;157:301–8.
8. Mason EE, Ito C. Gastric bypass in obesity. Surg Clin North Am 1967;47: 1345–51.
9. Mason EE, Printen KJ, Hartford CE, et al. Optimizing results of gastric bypass. Ann Surg 1975;182:405–14.
10. Mason EE, Munns JR, Printen KJ, et al. Effect of gastric bypass on gastric secretion. Am J Surg 1976;131:162–8.
11. Alden JF. Gastric and jejunoileal bypass. Arch Surg 1977;112:799–806.
12. Griffen WO, Young VL, Stevenson CC. A prospective comparison of gastric and jejunoileal bypass procedures for morbid obesity. Ann Surg 1977;186:500–9.
13. McGrath V, Needleman BJ, Melvin WS. Evolution of the laparoscopic gastric bypass. J Laparoendosc Adv Surg Tech A 2003;13(4):221–7.
14. Brolin RE. Gastric bypass. Surg Clin North Am 2001;81:1077–95.
15. Torres JC, Oca CF, Garrison RN. Gastric bypass Roux-en-Y gastrojejunostomy from the lesser curvature. South Med J 1983;76:1217.
16. Fobi MA, Lee H, Holness R, et al. Gastric bypass operation for obesity. World J Surg 1998;22:925–35.
17. Capella JF, Capella RF. The weight reduction operation of choice: vertical banded gastroplasty or gastric bypass. Am J Surg 1996;171:74–9.
18. Brolin RE, Robertson LB, Kenler HA, et al. Weight loss and dietary intake after vertical banded gastroplasty and Roux-en-Y gastric bypass. Ann Surg 1994; 220:782–90.
19. Williams LF Jr, Chapman WC, Bonau RA, et al. Comparison of laparoscopic cholecystectomy with open cholecystectomy in a single center. Am J Surg 1993;165:459–65.
20. Buanes T, Mjaland O. Complications in laparoscopic and open cholecystectomy: a prospective comparative trial. Surg Laparosc Endosc 1996;6:266–72.
21. Schauer PR, Luna J, Ghiatas AA, et al. Pulmonary function after laparoscopic cholecystectomy. Surgery 1993;114:389–99.
22. Schauer PR, Sirinek KR. The laparoscopic approach reduces the endocrine response to elective cholecystectomy. Am Surg 1995;61:106–11.
23. Schauer PR, Ikramuddin S, Gourash W, et al. Outcomes after laparoscopic Roux-en-Y gastric bypass for morbid obesity. Ann Surg 2000;232:515–29.
24. Wittgrove AC, Clark GW, Tremblay LJ. Laparoscopic gastric bypass, Roux-en-Y: preliminary report of five cases. Obes Surg 1994;4:353–7.
25. Vasallo C, Negri L, Della Valle A, et al. Divided vertical banded gastroplasty either for correction or as a first choice operation. Obes Surg 1999;9:177–9.
26. Watson DI, Game PA. Hand-assisted laparoscopic vertical banded gastroplasty. Initial report. Surg Endosc 1997;11:1218–20.
27. Sundbom M, Gustavsson S. Hand-assisted laparoscopic Roux-en-Y gastric bypass: aspects of surgical technique and early results. Obes Surg 2000;10: 420–7.
28. Sundbom M, Gustavsson S. Randomized clinical trial of hand-assisted laparoscopic versus open Roux-en-Y gastric bypass for the treatment of morbid obesity. Br J Surg 2004;91:418–23.
29. DeMaria EJ, Schweitzer MA, Kellum JM, et al. Hand-assisted laparoscopic gastric bypass does not improve outcome and increases costs when compared

to open gastric bypass for the surgical treatment of obesity. Surg Endosc 2002; 16:1452–5.

30. Higa KD, Boone KB, Ho T, et al. Laparoscopic Roux-en-Y gastric bypass for morbid obesity; technique and preliminary results of our first 400 patients. Arch Surg 2000;135:1029–34.

31. Wittgrove AC, Clark GW, Schubert KR. Laparoscopic gastric bypass, Roux-en-Y: the results in 500 patients with 5-year follow-up. Obes Surg 2000;10:233–9.

32. Nguyen NT, Goldman C, Rosenquist CJ, et al. Laparoscopic versus open gastric bypass: a randomized study of outcomes, quality of life, and costs. Ann Surg 2001;234:279–91.

33. Nguyen NT, Lee SL, Goldman C, et al. Comparison of pulmonary function and post-operative pain after laparoscopic versus open gastric bypass: a randomized trial. J Am Coll Surg 2001;192:469–77.

34. Westling A, Gustavsson S. Laparoscopic vs open Roux-en-Y gastric bypass: a prospective, randomized trial. Obes Surg 2001;11:284–92.

35. Wong J. Esophagogastric anastomosis performed with a stapler: the occurrence of leakage and stricture. Surgery 1987;101:408–15.

36. Kellum JM, DeMaria EJ, Sugerman HJ. The surgical treatment of morbid obesity. Curr Probl Surg 1998;35:791–858.

37. Matthews BD, Sing RF, DeLegge MH, et al. Initial results with a stapled gastrojejunostomy for the laparoscopic isolated roux-en-Y gastric bypass. Am J Surg 2000;179(6):476–81.

38. Champion JK, Hunt T, DeLisle N. Laparoscopic vertical banded gastroplasty and Roux-en-Y gastric bypass in morbid obesity. Obes Surg 1999;9:123–44.

39. Higa K, Ho T, Boone K. Laparoscopic Roux-en-Y gastric bypass; technique and 3-year follow-up. J Laparoendosc Adv Surg Tech A 2001;11:377–82.

40. Wittgrove AC, Endres JE, Davis M, et al. Perioperative complications in a single surgeon's experience with 1,000 consecutive laparoscopic Roux-en-Y gastric bypass operations for morbid obesity [abstract L4]. Obes Surg 2002;12:457–8.

41. DeMaria EJ, Sugerman HJ, Kellum JM, et al. Results of 281 consecutive total laparoscopic Roux-en-Y gastric bypass in morbid obesity. Ann Surg 2002;235:640–7.

42. Gonzalez R, Lin E, Venkatesh KR, et al. Gastrojejunostomy during laparoscopic gastric bypass: analysis of 3 techniques. Arch Surg 2003;138:181–4.

43. Carrodeguas L, Szomstein S, Zundel N, et al. Gastrojejunal anastomotic strictures following laparoscopic Roux-en-Y gastric bypass surgery: analysis of 1291 patients. Surg Obes Relat Dis 2006;2(2):92–7.

44. Leyba JL, Llopis SN, Isaac J, et al. Laparoscopic gastric bypass for morbid obesity-a randomized controlled trial comparing two gastrojejunal anastomosis techniques. JSLS 2008;12(4):385–8.

45. Kravetz AJ, Reddy S, Murtaza G, et al. A comparative study of handsewn versus stapled gastrojejunal anastomosis in laparoscopic Roux-en-Y gastric bypass. Surg Endosc 2011;25(4):1287–92.

46. Carrasquilla C, English WJ, Esposito P, et al. Total stapled, total intra-abdominal (TSTI) laparoscopic Roux-en-Y gastric bypass: one leak in 1,000 cases. Obes Surg 2004;14:613–7.

47. Nguyen NT, Stevens CM, Wolfe BM. Incidence and outcome of anastomotic stricture after laparoscopic gastric bypass. J Gastrointest Surg 2003;7(8): 997–1003 [discussion: 1003].

48. Gould JC, Garren M, Boll V, et al. The impact of circular stapler diameter on the incidence of gastrojejunostomy stenosis and weight loss following laparoscopic Roux-en-Y gastric bypass. Surg Endosc 2006;20(7):1017–20.

49. Fisher BL, Atkinson JD, Cottam D. Incidence of gastroenterostomy stenosis in laparoscopic Roux-en-Y gastric bypass using 21- or 25-mm circular stapler: a randomized prospective blinded study. Surg Obes Relat Dis 2007;3(2):176–9.

50. Suggs WJ, Kouli W, Lupovici M, et al. Complications at gastrojejunostomy after laparoscopic Roux-en-Y gastric bypass: comparison between 21- and 25-mm circular staplers. Surg Obes Relat Dis 2007;3(5):508–14.

51. Alasfar F, Sabnis AA, Liu RC, et al. Stricture rate after laparoscopic Roux-en-Y gastric bypass with a 21-mm circular stapler: the Cleveland Clinic experience. Med Princ Pract 2009;18(5):364 7.

52. Dolce CJ, Dunnican WJ, Kushnir L, et al. Gastrojejunal strictures after Roux-en-Y gastric bypass with a 21-mm circular stapler. JSLS 2009;13(3):306–11.

53. Wittgrove AC, Clark GW. Combined laparoscopic/endoscopic anvil placement for the performance of the gastroenterostomy. Obes Surg 2001;11(5):565–9.

54. Scott DJ, Provost DA, Jones DB. Laparoscopic Roux-en-Y gastric bypass: transoral or transgastric anvil placement? Obes Surg 2000;10:361–5.

55. Teixeira JA, Borao FJ, Thomas TA, et al. An alternative technique for creating the gastrojejunostomy in laparoscopic Roux-en-Y gastric bypass: experience with 28 consecutive patients. Obes Surg 2000;10:240–4.

56. Wittgrove AC, Clark GW. Laparoscopic gastric bypass, Roux-en-Y—500 patients: technique and results, with 3-60 month follow-up. Obes Surg 2000; 10:233–9.

57. Sugerman HJ, Sugerman EL, Wolfe L, et al. Risks/benefits of gastric bypass in morbidly obese patients with severe venous stasis disease. Gastroenterology 2000;118:A1051.

58. Sugerman HJ, Brewer WH, Shiffman ML, et al. A multicenter, placebo-controlled, randomized, double-blind, prospective trial of prophylactic ursodiol for the prevention of gallstone formation following gastric-bypass-induced rapid weight loss. Am J Surg 1995;169:91–7.

59. Monteforte MJ, Turkelson CM. Bariatric surgery for morbid obesity. Obes Surg 2000;10:391–401.

60. Hsu LK, Mulliken B, McDonagh B, et al. Binge eating disorder in extreme obesity. Int J Obes Relat Metab Disord 2002;26:1398–403.

61. Balsiger BM, Kennedy FP, Abu-Lebdeh HS, et al. Prospective evaluation of Roux-en Y gastric bypass as primary operation for medically complicated obesity. Mayo Clin Proc 2000;75:673–80.

62. Collene AL, Hertzler S. Metabolic outcomes of gastric bypass. Nutr Clin Pract 2003;18:136–40.

63. Mallory GN, Macgregor AM, Rand CS. The influence of dumping on weight loss after gastric restrictive surgery for morbid obesity. Obes Surg 1996;6:474–8.

64. Heber D, Greenway F, Kaplan L, et al. Endocrine and nutritional management of the post-bariatric surgery patient: an endocrine society clinical practice guide-line. J Clin Endocrinol Metab 2010;95(11):4823–43.

65. Ukleja A. Dumping syndrome: pathophysiology and treatment. Nutr Clin Pract 2005;20:517–25.

66. Carvajal SH, Mulvihill SJ. Postgastrectomy syndromes: dumping and diarrhea. Gastroenterol Clin North Am 1994;23:261–79.

67. Service GJ, Thompson GB, Service FJ, et al. Hyperinsulinemic hypoglycemia with nesidioblastosis after gastric-bypass surgery. N Engl J Med 2005;353:249–54.

68. Patti ME, McMahon G, Mun EC, et al. Severe hypoglycemia post-gastric bypass requiring partial pancreatectomy: evidence for inappropriate insulin secretion and pancreatic islet hyperplasia. Diabetologia 2005;48:2236–40.

69. Service FJ. Classification of hypoglycemic disorders. Endocrinol Metab Clin North Am 1999;28:501–17.

70. Buchwald H, Avidor Y, Braunwald E, et al. Bariatric surgery: a systematic review and metaanalysis. JAMA 2004;292:1724–37.

71. Kellogg TA, Bantle JP, Leslie DB, et al. Postgastric bypass hyperinsulinemic hypoglycemia syndrome: characterization and response to a modified diet. Surg Obes Relat Dis 2008;4:492–9.

72. McLaughlin T, Peck M, Holst J, et al. Reversible hyperinsulinemic hypoglycemia after gastric bypass: a consequence of altered nutrient delivery. J Clin Endocrinol Metab 2010;95(4):1851–5.

73. Clancy TE, Moore FD Jr, Zinner MJ. Post-gastric bypass hyperinsulinism with nesidioblastosis: subtotal or total pancreatectomy may be needed to prevent recurrent hypoglycemia. J Gastrointest Surg 2006;10(8):1116–9.

74. Witteles RM, Straus IF, Sugg SL, et al. Adult-onset nesidioblastosis causing hypoglycemia: an important clinical entity and continuing treatment dilemma. Arch Surg 2001;136(6):656–63.

75. Kleeff J, Diener MK, Z'graggen K, et al. Distal pancreatectomy: risk factors for surgical failure in 302 consecutive cases. Ann Surg 2007;245(4):573–82.

76. Buchler MW, Wagner M, Schmied BM, et al. Changes in morbidity after pancreatic resection: toward the end of completion pancreatectomy. Arch Surg 2003; 138(12):1310–4 [discussion: 5].

77. Z'graggen K, Guweidhi A, Steffen R, et al. Severe recurrent hypoglycemia after gastric bypass surgery. Obes Surg 2008;18(8):981–8.

78. Mott T. How effective is gastric bypass for weight loss? J Fam Pract 2004;53(11): 914–7.

79. Crowley LV, Seay J, Mullin G. Late effects of gastric bypass for morbid obesity. Am J Gastroenterol 1984;79:850–60.

80. Mason ME, Jalagani H, Vinik AI. Metabolic complications of bariatric surgery: diagnosis and management issues. Gastroenterol Clin North Am 2005;34:25–33.

81. Livingston EH. Complications of bariatric surgery. Surg Clin North Am 2005;85: 853–68.

82. Halverson JD. Micronutrient deficiencies after gastric bypass for morbid obesity. Am Surg 1986;52:594–8.

83. Halverson JD, Zuckerman GR, Koheler RE, et al. Gastric bypass for morbid obesity. A medical–surgical assessment. Ann Surg 1981;194:152–60.

84. Amaral JF, Thompson WR, Caldwell MD, et al. Prospective hematologic evaluation of gastric exclusion surgery for morbid obesity. Ann Surg 1985;201:186–93.

85. Brolin RE, Gorman JH, Gorman RC, et al. Are vitamin B12 and folate deficiency clinically important after Roux-en-Y gastric bypass? J Gastrointest Surg 1998;2: 436–42.

86. Berdainer CD. Advanced nutrition: micronutrients. Boca Raton: CRC; 1998.

87. Fairweather-Tait SJ. The concept of bioavailability as it relates to iron nutrition. Nutr Res 1987;7:319–25.

88. Avinoah E, Ovnat A, Charuzi I. Nutritional status seven years after Roux-en-Y gastric bypass surgery. Surgery 1992;111:137–42.

89. Mason EE. Starvation injury after gastric reduction for obesity. World J Surg 1998;22:1002–7.

90. MacLean LD, Rhode BM, Shizgal HM. Nutrition following gastric operations for morbid obesity. Ann Surg 1983;198:347–55.

91. Feit H, Glasberg M, Ireton C, et al. Peripheral neuropathy and starvation after gastric partitioning for morbid obesity. Ann Intern Med 1982;96:453–5.

92. Fawcett S, Young GB, Holliday RL. Wernicke's encephalopathy after gastric partitioning for morbid obesity. Can J Surg 1984;27:169–70.
93. Villar HV, Ranne RD. Neurologic deficit following gastric partitioning: possible role of thiamine. JPEN J Parenter Enteral Nutr 1984;8:575–8.
94. Brolin RE, Gorman JH, Gorman RC, et al. Prophylactic iron supplementation after Roux-en-Y gastric bypass: a prospective, double-blind, randomized study. Arch Surg 1998;122:740–4.
95. Decker GA, Swain JM, Crowell MD. Gastrointestinal and nutritional complications after bariatric surgery. Am J Gastroenterol 2007;102:1–10.
96. Parkes E. Nutritional management of patients after bariatric surgery. Am J Med Sci 2006;331(4):207–13.
97. Brolin RE, Leung M. Survey of vitamin and mineral supplementation alter gastric bypass and biliopancreatic diversion for morbid obesity. Obes Surg 1999;9:150–4.
98. Rhode BM, Arseneau P, Cooper BA, et al. Vitamin B-12 deficiency after gastric surgery for obesity. Am J Clin Nutr 1996;63:103–9.
99. Mallory GN, Macgregor AM. Folate status following gastric bypass surgery (the great folate mystery). Obes Surg 1991;1:69–72.
100. Updegraff TA, Neufeld NJ. Protein, iron, and folate status of patients prior to and following surgery for morbid obesity. J Am Diet Assoc 1981;78:135–40.
101. Dunlevy LP, Chitty LS, Burren KA. Abnormal folate metabolism in foetuses affected by neural tube defects. Brain 2007;130:1043–9.
102. Czeizel AE, Dudas I. Prevention of the first occurrence of neural tube defects by periconceptional vitamin supplementation. N Engl J Med 1992;327:1832–5.
103. Woodard CB. Pregnancy following bariatric surgery. J Perinat Neonatal Nurs 2004;18:329.
104. Goldner WS, O'Dorisio TM, Dillon JS, et al. Severe metabolic bone disease as a long-term complication of obesity surgery. Obes Surg 2002;12:685–92.
105. Amaral JF, Thompson WR, Caldwell MD, et al. Prospective metabolic evaluation of 150 consecutive patients who underwent gastric exclusion. Am J Surg 1984; 147:468–76.
106. Mahan LK, Escott-Stump S, editors. Krause's food, nutrition, diet therapy. 11th edition. Philadelphia: W.B. Saunders Company; 2004. p. 93–5.
107. Mejia LA. Role of vitamin A in iron deficiency anemia. In: Fomon SJ, Zlotkin S, editors. Nutritional anemias. New York: Raven Press; 1992. p. 93–104.
108. Shuster MH, Vázquez JA. Nutritional concerns related to Roux-en-Y gastric bypass: what every clinician needs to know. Crit Care Nurs Q 2005;28:227–60 [quiz: 261–2].
109. Somer H, Bergström L, Mustajoki P, et al. Morbid obesity, gastric plication and a severe neurologic deficit. Acta Med Scand 1985;217:575–6.
110. Paulson GW, Martin EW, Mojzisik C, et al. Neurologic complications of gastric partitioning. Arch Neurol 1985;42:675–7.
111. Oczkowski WJ, Kertesz A. Wernicke's encephalopathy after gastroplasty for morbid obesity. Neurology 1985;35:99–101.
112. Abarbanel JM, Berginer VM, Osimani A, et al. Neurologic complications after gastric restriction surgery for morbid obesity. Neurology 1987;37:196–200.
113. Singh S, Kumar A. Wernicke encephalopathy after obesity surgery: a systematic review. Neurology 2007;68:807–11.
114. Angstadt JD, Bodziner RA. Peripheral polyneuropathy from thiamine deficiency following laparoscopic Roux-en-Y gastric bypass. Obes Surg 2005;15:890–2.
115. Chaves LC, Faintuch J, Kahwage S, et al. A cluster of polyneuropathy and Wernicke-Korsakoff syndrome in a bariatric unit. Obes Surg 2002;12:328–34.

116. Primavera A, Brusa G, Novello P, et al. Wernicke-Korsakoff encephalopathy following biliopancreatic diversion. Obes Surg 1993;3:175–7.

117. Rindi G, Bordi C, Rappel S, et al. Gastric carcinoids and neuroendocrine carcinomas: pathogenesis, pathology, and behavior. World J Surg 1996;20:168–72.

118. Heye N, Terstegge K, Sirtl C, et al. Wernicke's encephalopathy: causes to consider. Intensive Care Med 1994;20:282–6.

119. Stocker DJ. Management of the bariatric surgery patient. Endocrinol Metab Clin North Am 2003;32:437–57.

120. Marceau S, Biron S, Lagacé M, et al. Biliopancreatic diversion, with distal gastrectomy, 250 cm and 50 cm limbs: long-term results. Obes Surg 1995;5:302–7.

121. Skroubis G, Sakellaropoulos G, Pouggouras K, et al. Comparison of nutritional deficiencies after Roux-en-Y gastric bypass and after biliopancreatic diversion with Roux-en-Y gastric bypass. Obes Surg 2002;12:551–8.

122. Lagacé M, Marceau P, Marceau S, et al. Biliopancreatic diversion with a new type of gastrectomy: some previous conclusions revisited. Obes Surg 1995;5:411–8.

123. Brolin RE, Gorman RC, Milgrim LM, et al. Multivitamin prophylaxis in prevention of postgastric bypass vitamin and mineral deficiencies. Int J Obes 1991;15:661–7.

124. Compston JE, Vedi S, Gianetta E, et al. Bone histomorphometry and vitamin D status after biliopancreatic bypass for obesity. Gastroenterology 1984;87:350–6.

125. Ernst B, Thurnheer M, Schmid SM, et al. Evidence for the necessity to systematically assess micronutrient status prior to bariatric surgery. Obes Surg 2009;19:66–73.

126. Shah M, Simha V, Garg A. Review: long-term impact of bariatric surgery on body weight, comorbidities, and nutritional status. J Clin Endocrinol Metab 2006;91:4223–31.

127. Carrodeguas L, Kaidar-Person O, Szomstein S, et al. Preoperative thiamine deficiency in obese population undergoing laparoscopic bariatric surgery. Surg Obes Relat Dis 2005;1:517–22.

128. Crowley LV, Seay J, Mullin G. Late effects of gastric bypass for obesity. Am J Gastroenterol 1984;79:850–60.

129. Saltzman E, Anderson W, Apovian CM, et al. Criteria for patient selection and multidisciplinary evaluation and treatment of the weight loss surgery patient. Obes Res 2005;13:234–43.

130. Shikora SA, Kim JJ, Tarnoff ME. Nutrition and gastrointestinal complications of bariatric surgery. Nutr Clin Pract 2007;22:29–40.

Complications of Laparoscopic Roux-en-Y Gastric Bypass

Ayman B. Al Harakeh, MD

KEYWORDS

• Bariatric surgery • Gastric bypass • Complications • Obesity

Morbid obesity is rapidly becoming a difficult to control epidemic and one of the most alarming public health problems in the United States.[1] In 2007, approximately 200,000 bariatric surgical procedures were performed in the United States, with gastric bypass being the most common.[2] With the advancement and use of minimally invasive techniques, laparoscopic Roux-en-Y gastric bypass (RYGB) has been performed in increasing volume. Since the first published case series in 1994, multiple studies have demonstrated the feasibility and safety of laparoscopic RYGB.[3]

Laparoscopy has revolutionized bariatric surgery worldwide. Prospective randomized studies have shown that laparoscopic RYGB results in less blood loss, pain, medication requirements, shorter return to daily activities, and fewer complications than the open approach.[4] Morbidly obese patients usually present with associated comorbidities at the time of evaluation and surgery. They are considered high-risk patients and should be evaluated thoroughly before their operation using a multidisciplinary team approach to select appropriate candidates. Laparoscopic RYGB remains one of the most advanced laparoscopic procedures currently performed worldwide.[3] In an effort to overcome the steep learning curve, formal fellowship training or prolonged monitoring is required by most centers to achieve good outcomes. In an effort to minimize postoperative morbidity and mortality and improve outcomes, "Center of Excellence" designations were developed by credentialing organizations. Nonetheless, laparoscopic RYGB is still associated with a unique set of postoperative complications and a risk of mortality. Therefore, patients must be educated about these possible complications and potential adverse outcomes. The same skills, knowledge, and experience needed to perform the surgery are also required to manage these complications.

The author has nothing to disclose.
Department of General and Vascular Surgery, Gundersen Lutheran Health System, 1900 South Avenue C05-001, La Crosse, WI 54601, USA
E-mail address: abalhara@gundluth.org

Surg Clin N Am 91 (2011) 1225–1237
doi:10.1016/j.suc.2011.08.011
0039-6109/11/$ – see front matter
surgical.theclinics.com

VENOUS THROMBOEMBOLISM

Deep venous thrombosis (DVT) and pulmonary embolism (PE) are infrequent but potentially fatal complications, and are two of the most feared causes of morbidity and mortality after any bariatric surgical procedure.[5,6] Venous thromboembolism (VTE) continues to be one of the top two causes of mortality in bariatric patients.[7] PE is the most common unexpected cause of death in the morbidly obese patient population and can occur anytime in the immediate or delayed postoperative period.[1]

No formal consensus or FDA-approved protocol exists for appropriate VTE prophylaxis in patients undergoing bariatric surgery.[6] Obesity is considered an important risk factor for perioperative DVT,[8] and most bariatric surgeons routinely use some form of thromboprophylaxis. The overall reported incidence of DVT/PE in this population ranges from 0.12% to 3.8%.[5] The prevalence of asymptomatic DVT in this group is undetermined. On postmortem evaluation, Melinek and colleagues[9] found microscopic evidence of PE in 80% of patients who underwent gastric bypass, whereas 20% were diagnosed clinically.

Morbidly obese patients often have multiple risk factors that can increase the incidence of VTE, including a sedentary lifestyle with significant history of degenerative disc and/or joint disease, and some are confined to a wheelchair. Obesity hypoventilation syndrome, with its associated hypoxemia and hypercarbia, can be another major predisposing factor. A history of peripheral venous insufficiency and moderate to severe venous stasis are also not uncommon. Smoking, older age, use of oral contraceptives, and obesity may increase the risk of VTE.[10] Any combination of these risk factors, along with general anesthesia, abdominal surgery, long operating time, increased intra-abdominal pressure from carbon dioxide insufflation, and decreased femoral venous flow,[11] can drastically increase the risk for VTE. Large multicenter trials are needed to formalize optimal preoperative and postoperative VTE prophylaxis recommendations. Currently, surgeons nationwide are depending on unpublished and experience-based data for management. Several approaches have been proposed to reduce the incidence of perioperative DVT in morbidly obese patients, including early ambulation, antiembolic stockings, intermittent pneumatic compression devices, and chemoprophylaxis, such as subcutaneous and intravenous unfractionated heparin (UFH) or low-molecular-weight heparin (LMWH). DVTs and PEs still occur despite widespread use of prophylaxis. Although almost all surgeons advocate the use of sequential compression devices, many also add chemoprophylaxis.

The choice and timing of chemoprophylaxis[12] are still debatable. Most advocates for postoperative chemoprophylaxis continue administration while patients are in the hospital, but fewer continue treatment after discharge. In contrast, others have reported good outcomes among patients not given chemoprophylaxis.[13] In the author's practice, all patients wear sequential compression devices during the procedure and while in the hospital when not ambulatory. They receive 5000 international units of subcutaneous UFH preoperatively, and three times per day postoperatively until discharge. Data from the author's institution has shown a lower risk of postoperative bleeding with UFH compared with LMWH.[12] Extended chemoprophylaxis is reserved for patients who are at higher risk (ie, history of VTE). Inferior vena cava filters are considered for patients with a history of recurrent DVTs while on anticoagulation, previously documented PE, and/or the presence of a hypercoagulable disorder.[14]

ANASTOMOTIC LEAKS

Anastomotic leaks (ALs) can be defined as inadequate tissue healing allowing for exit of gastrointestinal material through the staple or suture line. They are among the most feared and potentially devastating complications after laparoscopic RYGB, and are associated with a high morbidity and mortality. The incidence of this complication ranges from 0 to 5.6% in large series and does not differ significantly between laparoscopic and open RYGB.[15]

ALs remain the second leading cause of death after RYGB surgery,[16] and together with PEs account for more than 50% of the causes of death in patients undergoing bariatric surgery. Previous studies have reported mortality after AL to be as high as 37.5%.[15]

ALs can occur at five potential sites after laparoscopic RYGB; at the gastrojejunostomy, gastric pouch staple line, gastric remnant staple line, Roux limb staple line, and jejunojejunostomy. Clinical studies have identified several potentiating factors, both technical and patient-related.[15–17] Patients at higher risk are primarily those who are older super-obese, men, and those with multiple comorbidities and previous or revisional bariatric operations. Operative technique, including appropriate staple sizing, staple line reinforcement with biologic buttress material,[18] use of fibrin sealant,[19] intraoperative leak testing, anastomosis under tension, and ischemia can affect the incidence of ALs after laparoscopic RYGB.[20] Although most ALs occur 5 to 7 days after surgery and are thought to be related to ischemia, 95% of ALs that occur within 2 days of surgery probably result from technical error.[21] Choosing the appropriate staple height and inspecting the stapling devices and staple line for integrity and perfusion after firing are essential to minimize ALs. Another important factor in anastomotic integrity is creating a tension-free anastomosis. Anastomotic tension has been proposed as a risk factor for ALs after gastric bypass surgery because it may result in stress that exceeds the disruptive pressures of a stapled or sutured anastomosis. One technical factor that has been studied and reported is the role of Roux limb orientation in the development of ALs after laparoscopic RYGB. Theoretically, compared with the antecolic route, the retrocolic Roux limb has a more direct path to the gastric pouch and may be associated with lower gastrojejunal anastomotic tension. Although a prospective randomized study is still needed to prove this theory, a few studies have reported conflicting results. Edwards and colleagues[22] reported that ALs may occur more commonly after antecolic (3%) versus retrocolic (0.5%) laparoscopic RYGB. However, Bertucci and colleagues[23] reported no ALs after 141 retrocolic and 200 antecolic procedures, and Carrasquilla and colleagues[24] reported an AL rate of 0.1% after 1000 antecolic procedures versus 1.85% after 108 retrocolic procedures.

Diagnosis of an AL relies on a high index of clinical suspicion. Patients developing an AL will most likely require multiple diagnostic tests, prolonged hospitalization, intensive care settings, and operative interventions. A patient who does not progress favorably after the first postoperative day and experiences increasing abdominal pain, persistent tachycardia, fever, tachypnea, or any combination of these symptoms requires investigation. Radiographic findings such as fluid collections adjacent to the pouch, diffuse abdominal fluid, free intraperitoneal air, and trace amount of oral contrast in the drain tract can confirm the diagnosis.

Conservative management can be effective in nonseptic, hemodynamically stable patients with contained ALs that are accessible percutaneously, but others require reexploration, primary repair if possible, and adequate drainage. In many instances, the repair of ALs may not be feasible, especially if acute inflammatory changes are present around the gastrojejunostomy and adequate drainage is the only practical intervention. Surgical exploration is warranted in hemodynamically unstable patients. Many bariatric surgeons practice the routine use of drains after laparoscopic RYGB. Drains positioned near the gastrojejunostomy may be useful for detecting early and small-volume ALs or bleeding. Drain output may prompt surgeons to take preventive measures, such as discontinuing anticoagulation and initiating early fluid resuscitation.[25] Abdominal drains placed during the initial procedure may prevent collections and allow early diagnosis, resulting in effective control of leaks and fewer indications for early surgical treatment.

Some studies have reported very good outcomes with conservative management of gastrojejunostomy, excluded stomach, and pouch leaks.[16] A conservative approach requires adequate drainage, broad-spectrum antibiotics, and nutritional support. Enteral nutrition through a gastrostomy tube in the excluded stomach is preferred over total parenteral nutrition when possible. Endoscopic injection of fibrin sealant in controlled gastrojejunostomy ALs has also been anecdotally reported with variable success.[26]

GASTROINTESTINAL BLEEDING

The incidence of gastrointestinal bleeding (GIB) after laparoscopic RYGB has been reported to be between 1.1% and 4%.[27] Although its incidence is low, GIB can be life-threatening if not recognized and treated early. Podnos and colleagues[3] reported a higher rate of GIB after laparoscopic RYGB compared with open RYGB (1.9% vs 0.6%, respectively). The increased incidence of GIB post-RYGB in the minimally invasive surgery era can be explained partly by the decreased practice of oversewing the staple lines and the overuse of DVT chemoprophylaxis. GIB after laparoscopic RYGB can originate at one of five potential staple lines: the gastric pouch, excluded stomach, Roux limb staple line, gastrojejunostomy, and jejunojejunostomy. Bleeding from these sites can be intraperitoneal or intraluminal. Staple-line bleeding occurs at the transected tissue edges or at the sites of staple penetration of the tissue.[27] Additional sites of bleeding include the liver, spleen, and trocar sites.

Recognizing the clinical signs and symptoms of GIB is crucial in determining the most appropriate steps for managing this life-threatening complication. Primary treatment depends on the timing of onset and the clinical presentation.[26] The presence of pallor, dizziness, confusion, tachycardia, hypotension, hematemesis, bright red blood per rectum, and low urine output should alert the surgeon to ongoing postoperative bleeding that might necessitate urgent reexploration. Early postoperative bleeding, occurring within a few hours after the procedure, manifested by hematemesis or bright red blood per rectum in the presence of clinical signs of bleeding is a clear indication for urgent surgical intervention. Late presentation of GIB (>48 hours) after laparoscopic RYGB can be conservatively managed in most cases, especially when associated with no acute clinical symptoms, and melena, which might indicate the passage of old blood and inactive bleeding. Discontinuation of DVT chemoprophylaxis and watchful waiting with supportive therapy can be successful in most of these cases. Although hematemesis suggests a gastrojejunostomy origin, brisk, bright red blood per rectum might originate from the gastric remnant or jejunojejunostomy anastomosis.

A substantial amount of blood can be lost with an acute postoperative gastrointestinal hemorrhage before overt clinical abdominal signs develop. When intra-abdominal bleeding is suspected based on systemic clinical signs, such as hypotension, tachycardia, or a falling hematocrit, in the absence of any obvious GIB source, reexploration should not be delayed. Interventions are dictated by the timing and clinical scenario of the GIB. A proximal intraluminal GIB is best addressed by endoscopic intervention, which is invaluable in controlling bleeding from the gastric pouch or gastrojejunostomy. Thermal coagulation, injection of vasoconstrictors, and clipping are all effective ways of controlling bleeding from these sites. Endoscopy is a less-effective means of managing a jejunojejunostomy bleed because of difficult accessibility. Reexplorations can be performed either laparoscopically or via open surgery, depending on the patient's hemodynamic status. In unstable patients, laparoscopy is a relative contraindication, because the increased intra-abdominal pressure during pneumoperitoneum can result in worsening hemodynamics.[27] During reoperations, other potential bleeding sites, such as the excluded stomach, can be examined and the staple lines oversewn if needed. Finding a dilated excluded stomach, filled with thrombus, necessitates evacuation and gastric tube placement for continuous decompression. Not infrequently, no obvious source of bleeding can be determined during reexplorations, but the patient can still benefit from the evacuation of intraperitoneal hematoma, which might speed the recovery process through shortening the duration of postoperative ileus.

Use of appropriate staple heights and staple-line reinforcement with buttressing material are methods that have been advocated for decreasing the occurrence of GIB after laparoscopic RYGB.[18,20] Choice of chemoprophylaxis regimen may also influence GIB rates. Data from the author's institution has shown that UFH for DVT chemoprophylaxis was associated with a decreased risk for postoperative bleeding compared with enoxaparin.[12] Routine drain placement after laparoscopic RYGB can serve as an adjunct in diagnosing early intraperitoneal bleeding. Chousleb and colleagues[25] concluded that drain output may alert surgeons to take preventive measures for a suspected bleed, such as discontinuing anticoagulation and initiating early fluid resuscitation.

INTERNAL HERNIA AND INTESTINAL OBSTRUCTION
Internal Hernia

In the laparoscopic era, internal hernia is a feared and well-recognized complication after RYGB. An internal hernia can be defined as a protrusion of intestine through a defect within the abdominal cavity. Most internal hernias present later in the postoperative period rather than early. Compared with the open approach, the incidence of internal hernia is greater after laparoscopic RYGB, estimated between 3% and 4.5%.[28] Investigators have postulated that laparoscopic RYGB results in fewer postoperative adhesions, and therefore reduced fixation of small intestine to adjacent structures.[29] In addition, rapid weight loss after laparoscopic RYGB results in reduced intraperitoneal fat and larger mesenteric defects. An internal hernia can lead to clinically significant complications, such as a closed loop bowel obstruction with or without strangulation. It is considered the most common cause of small bowel obstruction (SBO) after laparoscopic RYGB.[29,30] Internal hernias typically occur at three potential locations: the jejunojejunostomy mesenteric defect, Petersen's space, and transverse mesocolic defect in the retrocolic approach (**Fig. 1**). In general, the Roux limb configuration plays a major role in determining the type of hernia. The most common location for internal hernias and its relation to Roux limb configuration has been a subject of debate, with no consensus thus far. Understandably, mesocolic defect hernias are unique to a retrocolic approach and are not seen with an antecolic approach. In some reports, mesocolic defects were the most common among all internal hernias. Garza and colleagues[28] reported that transverse mesocolic hernias were the most common, followed by jejunojejunostomy and Petersen's space hernias. In an antecolic approach, however, both Petersen's and jejunojejunostomy mesenteric defect hernias are reported, with hernias at the jejunojejunostomy defect being more common in some series.[31] Other investigators report a higher incidence of Petersen's and jejunojejunostomy hernias with a retrocolic approach.[30] Champion and Williams[29] reported a significant decrease in SBO after switching from a retrocolic to an antecolic technique.

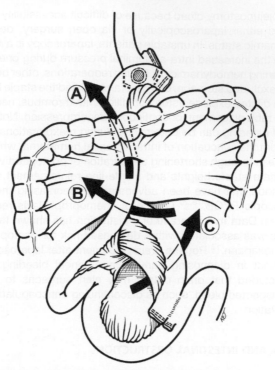

Fig. 1. Mesenteric defects: (A) transverse mesocolic, (B) Petersen's space, and (C) jejunojejunostomy mesentery. (*From* Kothari SN. Bariatric surgery and postoperative imaging. Surg Clin North Am 2011;91(1):155–72, with permission.)

Intestinal Obstruction

Abdominal pain with or without intestinal obstruction is the most common presentation of an internal hernia. Usually the presentation is delayed, occurring several months to years after the operation, but it can occur in the immediate postoperative period. Some patients report previous episodes of undefined gastrointestinal upset and frequent mild symptoms of self-limited intestinal obstruction before their main presentation. The small bowel may intermittently become trapped and then reduced at the site of the internal hernia, causing this subtle presentation and atypical bowel obstruction features. CT scanning is not always diagnostic, and therefore any patient with unexplained abdominal pain that does not correlate with physical findings should be considered to have an internal hernia. A high index of suspicion is crucial for early intervention and avoidance of an abdominal catastrophe, such as long segment of small bowel ischemia. Gandhi and colleagues[32] suggested that SBO from an internal hernia after laparoscopic RYGB is typically preceded by symptoms of intermittent obstruction. Patients who have these symptoms should be promptly offered elective laparoscopic exploration.

Other intraoperative factors besides the Roux limb configuration, such as closure of all potential defects with a nonabsorbable running suture, have been suggested to influence the incidence of internal hernia.[31] Some authors who have modified their technique from absorbable to nonabsorbable sutures and from an interrupted to a running technique have reported a reduction in the incidence of internal hernias.[33] Hope and colleagues[34] concluded that routine suture closure of mesenteric defects after laparoscopic RYGB may not be an effective permanent closure, likely because of the extensive loss of fat and weight loss within the mesentery. Some authors still report acceptable results when not closing mesenteric defects.[35]

In the author's practice, all laparoscopic RYGB procedures are performed with a retrocolic approach to create a tension-free gastrojejunostomy. All potential mesenteric defects are routinely closed with a running nonabsorbable suture. The rate of internal hernias at the author's institution is comparable to that reported in literature.[36]

The second most common cause of SBO after laparoscopic RYGB is obstruction at the jejunojejunostomy, occurring in approximately 1.8% of antecolic laparoscopic RYGB procedures.[37] It can also be a complication of the retrocolic approach. Early obstructions at the jejunojejunostomy can be caused by technical problems, such as bowel kinking, narrowing, or acute angulation of the anastomosis. Other causes include postsurgical anastomotic edema, stenosis, ischemia, and staple-line bleeding with intraluminal thrombus formation. Early SBOs at other locations usually result from edema or technical problems with the Roux limb position, such as an extrinsic compression of the Roux limb as it traverses the transverse mesocolic defect from thickened cicatrix formation in this area.[38]

Other less-common causes of SBO after laparoscopic RYGB include trocar site incisional hernias, adhesive bands, bezoars, anastomotic strictures, and jejunojejunostomy intussusception. Rarely, superior mesenteric artery syndrome might complicate the course of laparoscopic RYGB secondary to rapid weight loss and cause gastric outlet obstruction symptoms.[39]

MARGINAL ULCERATIONS

Marginal ulceration (MU) has been reported to be the most commonly found abnormality on endoscopy in symptomatic patients who underwent laparoscopic RYGB.[40] It is diagnosed in 1% to 16% of patients.[41] Most recent studies cite an incidence of around 2%.[42] Factors predisposing patients to MU have not been completely revealed, but the origin is likely multifactorial. Several factors, including pouch size and orientation, mucosal ischemia, staple-line disruption and gastrogastric fistula, foreign body reaction, exogenous substances, and *Helicobacter pylori* infection, have been all implicated as potential causes. Other intrinsic factors, such as hormonal and metabolic, versus extrinsic factors, such as tobacco and nonsteroidal anti-inflammatory drug (NSAID) use have also been suggested.

Larger pouch size (>50 mL) and orientation have been thought to predispose patients to MU,[43] and reducing its size has been shown to decrease its incidence.[44] Sapala and colleagues[45] found that creating a pouch limited to the cardia resulted in a 0.6% MU rate at 3-year follow-up among 173 patients. Thus, larger pouch size was postulated early on to be correlated with increased acid production, leading to increased incidence of marginal ulcers.

A pathway in which less acid reaches the antrum, leading to excessive stimulation of antral gastrin-secreting cells and higher gastrin levels, has been proposed.[46] Later investigators showed that little, if any, gastric acid is produced in the pouch.[47] However, the significant decrease in acid secretion after gastric bypass may not be universal, as concluded by Mason and colleagues,[48] who found that although gastric acid secretion is nearly absent in most patients after gastric bypass, 43% of their study patients had a low pH within the pouch. Thus, even with smaller pouch sizes, MU would be expected to occur despite the presumed absence of or decreased acid production.

A noteworthy finding was that serum gastrin levels were found to be universally low after gastric bypass.[48] It seems that gastric acid secretion is primarily stimulated by gastrin in most obese patients, but in patients who continue to have low gastric pH after surgery, vagal innervation may be the primary stimulus for acid secretion, putting them at higher risk for MU. This role of acid secretion in developing MU is supported by evidence that acid suppression alone is effective in healing most MUs.[41]

Another precipitating factor for MU after laparoscopic RYGB may be the prolonged irritation by foreign material, such as nonabsorbable sutures at the gastrojejunostomy. Sacks and colleagues[49] reported their data comparing the incidence of MU associated with the use of nonabsorbable sutures versus absorbable ones. They found a significant decrease in incidence from 2.6% to 1.3%, respectively, in a study cohort of 3285 patients. Local ischemia has also been suggested as a cause of MU, although it might more commonly lead to the development of stricture formation. H pylori is another contributing factor in the development of ulcer disease. Patients who present with upper gastrointestinal symptoms should undergo endoscopy before gastric bypass and should be treated if H pylori is diagnosed. However, Papasavas and colleagues[50] hypothesized and concluded that the prevalence of H pylori in patients undergoing RYGB is similar to that in the general population, and that preoperative H pylori testing and treatment does not decrease the incidence of anastomotic ulcer or pouch gastritis.

Tobacco use is also an important factor in the development of ulcer disease. Studies have shown significant compromise of the gastric mucosal barrier and impaired wound healing associated with smoking.[51] Decreased tissue oxygenation has been proposed as the factor responsible for the impaired wound healing. It is important to remember that the jejunum, unlike the native duodenum, does not possess an innate acid buffer, and this is probably the most important contributor to the development of MU at the gastrojejunostomy. In the era of minimally invasive bariatric surgery, staple-line disruption and gastrogastric fistula are encountered less frequently with the introduction of new stapling techniques and complete division/separation of the excluded stomach and gastric pouch staple lines.

Timing and presentation of MU after laparoscopic RYGB vary widely. One early study by Møller and colleagues[52] suggested that most ulcers developed in the first 3 months postoperatively, with a continued, lower risk up to 1 year. Another group reported a mean of 48 days (around 7 weeks) for the development of MU.[53] Nausea and vomiting may be common presenting complaints in patients with MU. Endoscopic evaluation, especially in the presence of epigastric pain and dysphagia, should be considered. In addition to MU, postoperative endoscopy for symptoms after laparoscopic RYGB may also reveal stenosis of the gastrojejunostomy or a gastrogastric fistula. Late presentation of GIB at the gastrojejunostomy is most commonly associated with MU.[54]

Treatment is primarily medical, consisting of antisecretory therapy with proton pump inhibitors (PPIs) and sucralfate, except in the presence of a gastrogastric fistula wherein surgery is warranted. When diagnosed, most cases of MU will respond to PPI, H2-blockade, or sucralfate therapy.[55] If not treated promptly, MU may lead to stricture formation and gastric pouch outlet obstruction, which will require endoscopic dilation. Unlike the more common peptic ulcers, these lesions tend to require prolonged therapy, usually for 3 to 4 months, and repeat endoscopy is recommended to confirm ulcer resolution. An attempt should be made to identify the causative factor if present, such as NSAID use, smoking, or a remnant suture, which should then be managed accordingly. Occasionally, revision of the gastrojejunostomy anastomosis will be required for patients with persistent symptoms and ulceration despite aggressive medical therapy.

ANASTOMOTIC STRICTURES

Gastrojejunal anastomotic stricture is one of the most commonly occurring complications after laparoscopic RYGB.[56] It is reported in 5% to 27% of cases, typically within 90 days after surgery.[57] Clinically, it manifests through persistent or worsening postprandial vomiting with or without pain. Although the origin of stricture formation is unclear, the possible mechanisms include ischemia causing scarring, nonischemic excessive scar formation, recurrent MU, tension or malposition of the anastomosis, and surgical technique. Causative technical factors that might contribute to increased stricture formation are type of stapler used (circular vs linear), stapler size, handsewing, and surgeon experience.

Circular staplers offer surgeons a reproducible anastomosis, which eliminates any technique-dependent variability that might make it difficult to scientifically assess the effect of anastomotic size on incidence of stenosis and on the eventual weight loss resulting from gastric bypass surgery. This fact was the basis of many studies designed to assess the effect of the diameter on long-term anastomotic patency. Fisher and colleagues[58] prospectively compared the incidence of gastrojejunostomy stenosis in laparoscopic RYGB using a 21- versus 25-mm circular stapler. They reported that the 29.6% increase in lumen with the 25-mm stapler compared with the 21-mm stapler significantly decreased stenosis rates by one-half, and significantly delayed the onset of symptoms. Nguyen and colleagues[59] reported a 26.8% incidence of strictures after laparoscopic RYGB using a 21-mm circular stapler (which gives an internal diameter of 11 mm) compared with 8.8% using the a 25-mm circular stapler (which gives an internal diameter of 15 mm).

In contrast, Frutos and colleagues[60] reported a 3.4% incidence of stenosis with the use of 21-mm circular staplers. They argued that restrictive procedures fail when the stoma is too wide. Therefore, they advocated the use of a 21-mm stapler instead of the 25-mm stapler, because the stapler is less difficult to insert through the abdominal wall and small intestine, but, more importantly, because the small diameter of the anastomosis delays gastric pouch emptying and consequently increases weight loss in the long-term.

Gonzalez and colleagues[61] previously published their results of a comparative study of the circular mechanical anastomosis versus a hand-sewn anastomosis, noting a significant increase in stenosis rates in the circular stapler group (31% vs 3%). Routine performance of early postoperative upper gastrointestinal series (UGIS) would not seem to help predict the occurrence or progression to strictures.[62] Daylami and colleagues[63] reported that a positive UGIS is 100% specific for the presence of stricture, whereas its sensitivity and negative predictive value is poor, making it unsatisfactory in definitively excluding the diagnosis. However, a possible role in predicting better postoperative weight loss in patients showing normal early gastric emptying has been reported.[64] Note that MU may also produce the same clinical symptoms of stenosis and can even be the cause.

Endoscopy, therefore, is considered the preferred diagnostic procedure and has the added benefit of being therapeutic. Several studies have shown that endoscopic balloon dilation is the first line of treatment. Findings have shown that 17% to 67% of cases responded to the first dilation, whereas 3% to 8% of cases required three or more dilations.[57] Early endoscopy and gentle dilatation are warranted once appropriate symptoms are suspected. Late scarring and fibrosis at the anastomotic stricture would be a prohibitive factor and put the patient at increased risk of perforation during balloon dilatation.

SUMMARY

Despite the well-documented safety of laparoscopic RYGB, several short-term and long-term complications, with varying degrees of morbidity and mortality risk, are known to occur. Bariatric surgeons, all too familiar with these complications, should be knowledgeable in risk-reduction strategies to minimize the incidence of complication occurrence and recurrence. Bariatric and nonbariatric surgeons who evaluate and treat abdominal pain should be familiar with these complications to facilitate early recognition and intervention, thereby minimizing the associated morbidity and mortality.

REFERENCES

1. Byrne TK. Complications of surgery for obesity. Surg Clin North Am 2001;81(5): 1181–93, vii–viii.
2. Mechanick JI, Kushner RF, Sugerman HJ, et al. American Association of Clinical Endocrinologists, The Obesity Society, and American Society for Metabolic & Bariatric Surgery Medical Guidelines for Clinical Practice for the perioperative nutritional, metabolic, and nonsurgical support of the bariatric surgery patient. Surg Obes Relat Dis 2008;4(Suppl 5):S109–84.
3. Podnos YD, Jimenez JC, Wilson SE, et al. Complications after laparoscopic gastric bypass: a review of 3464 cases. Arch Surg 2003;138(9):957–61.
4. Nguyen NT, Lee SL, Goldman C, et al. Laparoscopic versus open gastric bypass: a randomized study of outcomes, quality of life, and costs. Ann Surg 2001;234(3): 279–89 [discussion: 289–91].
5. Escalante-Tattersfield T, Tucker O, Fajnwaks P, et al. Incidence of deep vein thrombosis in morbidly obese patients undergoing laparoscopic Roux-en-Y gastric bypass. Surg Obes Relat Dis 2008;4(2):126–30.
6. Wu EC, Barba CA. Current practices in the prophylaxis of venous thromboembolism in bariatric surgery. Obes Surg 2000;10(1):7–13 [discussion: 14].
7. Sapala JA, Wood MH, Schuhknecht MP, et al. Fatal pulmonary embolism after bariatric operations for morbid obesity: a 24-year retrospective analysis. Obes Surg 2003;13(6):819–25.
8. De Pergola G, Pannacciulli N. Coagulation and fibrinolysis abnormalities in obesity. J Endocrinol Invest 2002;25(10):899–904.
9. Melinek J, Livingston E, Cortina G, et al. Autopsy findings following gastric bypass surgery for morbid obesity. Arch Pathol Lab Med 2002;126(9):1091–5.
10. Geerts WH, Bergqvist D, Pineo GF, et al. Prevention of venous thromboembolism: American College of Chest Physicians Evidence-Based Clinical Practice Guidelines (8th Edition). Chest 2008;133(Suppl 6):381S–453S.
11. Jorgensen JO, Lalak NJ, North L, et al. Venous stasis during laparoscopic cholecystectomy. Surg Laparosc Endosc 1994;4(2):128–33.
12. Kothari SN, Lambert PJ, Mathiason MA. Best Poster Award. A comparison of thromboembolic and bleeding events following laparoscopic gastric bypass in patients treated with prophylactic regimens of unfractionated heparin or enoxaparin. Am J Surg 2007;194(6):709–11.
13. Clements RH, Yellumahanthi K, Ballem N, et al. Pharmacologic prophylaxis against venous thromboembolic complications is not mandatory for all

laparoscopic Roux-en-Y gastric bypass procedures. J Am Coll Surg 2009;208(5): 917–21 [discussion: 921–3].

14. Keeling WB, Haines K, Stone PA, et al. Current indications for preoperative inferior vena cava filter insertion in patients undergoing surgery for morbid obesity. Obes Surg 2005;15(7):1009–12.

15. Fernandez AZ Jr, DeMaria EJ, Tichansky DS, et al. Experience with over 3,000 open and laparoscopic bariatric procedures: multivariate analysis of factors related to leak and resultant mortality. Surg Endosc 2004;18(2):193–7.

16. Ballesta C, Berindoague R, Cabrera M, et al. Management of anastomotic leaks after laparoscopic Roux-en-Y gastric bypass. Obes Surg 2008;18(6):623–30.

17. Livingston EH, Ko CY. Assessing the relative contribution of individual risk factors on surgical outcome for gastric bypass surgery: a baseline probability analysis. J Surg Res 2002;105(1):48–52.

18. Miller KA, Pump A. Use of bioabsorbable staple reinforcement material in gastric bypass: a prospective randomized clinical trial. Surg Obes Relat Dis 2007;3(4): 417–21 [discussion: 422].

19. Lee MG, Provost DA, Jones DB. Use of fibrin sealant in laparoscopic gastric bypass for the morbidly obese. Obes Surg 2004;14(10):1321–6.

20. Fullum TM, Aluka KJ, Turner PL. Decreasing anastomotic and staple line leaks after laparoscopic Roux-en-Y gastric bypass. Surg Endosc 2009;23(6):1403–8.

21. Baker RS, Foote J, Kemmeter P, et al. The science of stapling and leaks. Obes Surg 2004;14(10):1290–8.

22. Edwards MA, Jones DB, Ellsmere J, et al. Anastomotic leak following antecolic versus retrocolic laparoscopic Roux-en-Y gastric bypass for morbid obesity. Obes Surg 2007;17(3):292–7.

23. Bertucci W, Yadegar J, Takahashi A, et al. Antecolic laparoscopic Roux-en-Y gastric bypass is not associated with higher complication rates. Am Surg 2005; 71(9):735–7.

24. Carrasquilla C, English WJ, Esposito P, et al. Total stapled, total intra-abdominal (TSTI) laparoscopic Roux-en-Y gastric bypass: one leak in 1000 cases. Obes Surg 2004;14(5):613–7.

25. Chousleb E, Szomstein S, Podkameni D, et al. Routine abdominal drains after laparoscopic Roux-en-Y gastric bypass: a retrospective review of 593 patients. Obes Surg 2004;14(9):1203–7.

26. Kowalski C, Kastuar S, Mehta V, et al. Endoscopic injection of fibrin sealant in repair of gastrojejunostomy leak after laparoscopic Roux-en-Y gastric bypass. Surg Obes Relat Dis 2007;3(4):438–42.

27. Nguyen NT, Longoria M, Chalifoux S, et al. Gastrointestinal hemorrhage after laparoscopic gastric bypass. Obes Surg 2004;14(10):1308–12.

28. Garza E Jr, Kuhn J, Arnold D, et al. Internal hernias after laparoscopic Roux-en-Y gastric bypass. Am J Surg 2004;188(6):796–800.

29. Champion JK, Williams M. Small bowel obstruction and internal hernias after laparoscopic Roux-en-Y gastric bypass. Obes Surg 2003;13(4):596–600.

30. Capella RF, Iannace VA, Capella JF. Bowel obstruction after open and laparoscopic gastric bypass surgery for morbid obesity. J Am Coll Surg 2006;203(3): 328–35.

31. Ahmed AR, Rickards G, Husain S, et al. Trends in internal hernia incidence after laparoscopic Roux-en-Y gastric bypass. Obes Surg 2007;17(12):1563–6.

32. Gandhi AD, Patel RA, Brolin RE. Elective laparoscopy for herald symptoms of mesenteric/internal hernia after laparoscopic Roux-en-Y gastric bypass. Surg Obes Relat Dis 2009;5(2):144–9 [discussion: 149].

33. Higa KD, Ho T, Boone KB. Internal hernias after laparoscopic Roux-en-Y gastric bypass: incidence, treatment and prevention. Obes Surg 2003;13(3):350–4.

34. Hope WW, Sing RF, Chen AY, et al. Failure of mesenteric defect closure after Roux-en-Y gastric bypass. JSLS 2010;14(2):213–6.

35. Cho M, Pinto D, Carrodeguas L, et al. Frequency and management of internal hernias after laparoscopic antecolic antegastric Roux-en-Y gastric bypass without division of the small bowel mesentery or closure of mesenteric defects: review of 1400 consecutive cases. Surg Obes Relat Dis 2006;2(2):87–91.

36. Kothari SN, Kallies KJ, Mathiason MA, et al. Excellent laparoscopic gastric bypass outcomes can be achieved at a community-based training hospital with moderate case volume. Ann Surg 2010;252(1):43–9.

37. Lewis CE, Jensen C, Tejirian T, et al. Early jejunojejunostomy obstruction after laparoscopic gastric bypass: case series and treatment algorithm. Surg Obes Relat Dis 2009;5(2):203–7.

38. Ahmed AR, Rickards G, Messing S, et al. Roux limb obstruction secondary to constriction at transverse mesocolon rent after laparoscopic Roux-en-Y gastric bypass. Surg Obes Relat Dis 2009;5(2):194–8.

39. Baker MT, Lara MD, Kothari SN. Superior mesenteric artery syndrome after laparoscopic Roux-en-Y gastric bypass. Surg Obes Relat Dis 2006;2(6):667.

40. Huang CS, Forse RA, Jacobson BC, et al. Endoscopic findings and their clinical correlations in patients with symptoms after gastric bypass surgery. Gastrointest Endosc 2003;58(6):859–66.

41. Rasmussen JJ, Fuller W, Ali MR. Marginal ulceration after laparoscopic gastric bypass: an analysis of predisposing factors in 260 patients. Surg Endosc 2007;21(7):1090–4.

42. Schauer PR, Ikramuddin S, Gourash W, et al. Outcomes after laparoscopic Roux-en-Y gastric bypass for morbid obesity. Ann Surg 2000;232(4):515–29.

43. Mason EE, Munns JR, Kealey GP, et al. Effect of gastric bypass on gastric secretion. 1977. Surg Obes Relat Dis 2005;1(2):155–60 [discussion: 161–2].

44. Printen KJ, Scott D, Mason EE. Stomal ulcers after gastric bypass. Arch Surg 1980;115(4):525–7.

45. Sapala JA, Wood MH, Sapala MA, et al. Marginal ulcer after gastric bypass: a prospective 3-year study of 173 patients. Obes Surg 1998;8(5):505–16.

46. Mason EE. Ulcerogenesis in surgery for obesity. Obes Surg 1996;6(2):180–1.

47. Behrns KE, Smith CD, Sarr MG. Prospective evaluation of gastric acid secretion and cobalamin absorption following gastric bypass for clinically severe obesity. Dig Dis Sci 1994;39(2):315–20.

48. Mason EE, Munns JR, Kealey GP, et al. Effect of gastric bypass on gastric secretion. Am J Surg 1976;131(2):162–8.

49. Sacks BC, Mattar SG, Qureshi FG, et al. Incidence of marginal ulcers and the use of absorbable anastomotic sutures in laparoscopic Roux-en-Y gastric bypass. Surg Obes Relat Dis 2006;2(1):11–6.

50. Papasavas PK, Gagné DJ, Donnelly PE, et al. Prevalence of Helicobacter pylori infection and value of preoperative testing and treatment in patients undergoing laparoscopic Roux-en-Y gastric bypass. Surg Obes Relat Dis 2008;4(3):383–8.

51. Kurata JH, Nogawa AN. Meta-analysis of risk factors for peptic ulcer. Nonsteroidal antiinflammatory drugs, Helicobacter pylori, and smoking. J Clin Gastroenterol 1997;24(1):2–17.

52. Møller AM, Villebro N, Pedersen T, et al. Effect of preoperative smoking intervention on postoperative complications: a randomised clinical trial. Lancet 2002; 359(9301):114–7.

53. Sanyal AJ, Sugerman HJ, Kellum JM, et al. Stomal complications of gastric bypass: incidence and outcome of therapy. Am J Gastroenterol 1992;87(9): 1165–9.

54. Braley SC, Nguyen NT, Wolfe BM. Late gastrointestinal hemorrhage after gastric bypass. Obes Surg 2002;12(3):404–7.

55. Sugerman HJ. Gastric bypass surgery for severe obesity. Semin Laparosc Surg 2002;9(2):79–85.

56. Swartz DE, Gonzalez V, Felix EL. Anastomotic stenosis after Roux-en-Y gastric bypass: a rational approach to treatment. Surg Obes Relat Dis 2006;2(6):632–6 [discussion: 637].

57. Ryskina KL, Miller KM, Aisenberg J, et al. Routine management of stricture after gastric bypass and predictors of subsequent weight loss. Surg Endosc 2010; 24(3):554–60.

58. Fisher BL, Atkinson JD, Cottam D. Incidence of gastroenterostomy stenosis in laparoscopic Roux-en-Y gastric bypass using 21- or 25-mm circular stapler: a randomized prospective blinded study. Surg Obes Relat Dis 2007;3(2):176–9.

59. Nguyen NT, Stevens CM, Wolfe BM. Incidence and outcome of anastomotic stricture after laparoscopic gastric bypass. J Gastrointest Surg 2003;7(8):997–1003 [discussion: 1003].

60. Frutos MD, Luján J, García A, et al. Gastrojejunal anastomotic stenosis in laparoscopic gastric bypass with a circular stapler (21 mm): incidence, treatment and long-term follow-up. Obes Surg 2009;19(12):1631–5.

61. Gonzalez R, Lin E, Venkatesh KR, et al. Gastrojejunostomy during laparoscopic gastric bypass: analysis of 3 techniques. Arch Surg 2003;138(2):181–4.

62. Raman R, Raman B, Raman P, et al. Abnormal findings on routine upper GI series following laparoscopic Roux-en-Y gastric bypass. Obes Surg 2007;17(3):311–6.

63. Daylami R, Rogers AM, King TS, et al. Accuracy of upper gastrointestinal swallow study in identifying strictures after laparoscopic gastric bypass surgery. Surg Obes Relat Dis 2008;4(2):96–9.

64. Akkary E, Sidani S, Boonsiri J, et al. The paradox of the pouch: prompt emptying predicts improved weight loss after laparoscopic Roux-Y gastric bypass. Surg Endosc 2009;23(4):790–4.

Evolution of Laparoscopic Adjustable Gastric Banding

Corrigan L. McBride, MD[a],*, Vishal Kothari, MD[b]

KEYWORDS

• Gastric banding • Gastric bypass • Laparoscopy • Obesity

In the United States, obesity continues to be a major health issue.[1,2] The Centers for Disease Control and Prevention determined that more than 30% of Americans were obese in 2009.[3,4] Young Americans today are possibly heading toward the first decrease in life expectancy in the era of modern health care.[5] Obesity clearly is a chronic condition involving genetic, metabolic, and environmental factors.[6–8] Surgeons today are working harder than ever to offer patients bariatric procedures as a therapeutic tool in the fight against obesity.[9–11] Multiple studies have shown the efficacy of the laparoscopic Roux-en-Y gastric bypass (LRYGB) as the gold standard procedure in bariatric surgery.[12] Patients still, however, express concerns about the short-term and long-term consequences of changes to their anatomy and the possible disastrous complications of an anastomotic leak.[13] The creation of Bariatric Centers of Excellence was one way to combat these concerns by showing patients that higher-volume centers could perform these procedures with significantly less morbidity and mortality.[14] Even so, Americans still desired an alternative solution to surgical weight loss.[15] The introduction of laparoscopic adjustable banding in the last 2 decades became this new surgical tool, providing similar outcomes with limited morbidity and mortality.[16] As younger and younger patients are becoming obese and morbidly obese at earlier ages, there may be a role for banding as a preventive tool as well.[17,18] With the recent Food and Drug Administration (FDA) approval of the LAP-BAND in patients with a body mass index (BMI) greater than 30 (BMI is weight in kilograms divided by height in meters squared, ie, kg/m^2), this article looks at the evolution of laparoscopic adjustable gastric banding (LAGB).

[a] University of Nebraska Medical Center, 983280 Nebraska Medical Center, Omaha, NE 68198-3280, USA
[b] Department of General Surgery, Advanced Laparoscopic and Bariatric Surgery, University of Nebraska Medical Center, 983280 Nebraska Medical Center, Omaha, NE 68198-3280, USA
* Corresponding author.
E-mail address: clmcbride@unmc.edu

Surg Clin N Am 91 (2011) 1239–1247
doi:10.1016/j.suc.2011.08.006
0039-6109/11/$ – see front matter © 2011 Elsevier Inc. All rights reserved.

HISTORY OF GASTRIC BANDING

The FDA approved the first laparoscopic adjustable band in 2001.[19] The LAP-BAND, as it was named by Allergan (Irvine, CA), was a purely restrictive weight-loss tool that provided patients a safe outpatient procedure to help with weight loss. Its origins began in the 1980s when Szinicz and colleagues[20] discovered that creating restrictive pouches in dog and rabbit models created significant weight loss. This research eventually translated into the vertical banded gastroplasty (VBG) by Mason and colleagues in 1982.[21,22] The VBG was a restrictive procedure using staple lines to create safe sustained weight reduction. These staple lines, however, eventually became disrupted, causing significant weight regain over time, or the bands eroded, causing obstruction. Open gastric banding tried to eliminate the use of staples by placing polyester or polypropylene mesh around the proximal stomach to create restriction.[23] This attempt also failed, due to erosion and gastric outlet obstruction. Kuzmak and colleagues[24] translated this into humans with the first open adjustable band placement in 1986.[25] His contemporaries, Forsell and colleagues, began working on the Swedish Adjustable Gastric Band at this time as well.[26,27] As the laparoscopic era of surgery flourished in the early 1990s, Belachew and colleagues[28,29] solidified the LAGB with the first placement of a LAP-BAND in a human in September 1993. Subsequently, the LAP-BAND was approved internationally and became the most common surgery in European countries. The FDA initiated trials in the United States in 1995 and approved its use in 2001. Since that time, Ethicon EndoSurgery (Cincinnati, OH) has bought the Swedish Adjustable Band from the Swiss company Obtech Medical. Ethicon developed the REALIZE band, which became approved for use in the United States in 2008. As of February 2010, the FDA approved the LAP-BAND for use in patients with severe comorbidities and BMI of 30 to 35.[18] Both bands are currently available to patients in the United States, providing a safe procedure with minimal morbidity, quick recovery, and the possibility of reversibility.

SURGICAL TECHNIQUE OF LAGB PLACEMENT

Significant advances in the placement of the LAGB have occurred in the last 2 decades. Belachew's original technique for LAP-BAND placement was called the perigastric technique.[28,29] The band was placed 3 cm below the gastroesophageal junction. A tunnel was created from the lesser sac around the stomach to the greater curvature, creating a 25- to 30-cm pouch. The greater curvature was then plicated over the band. A gastrostenometer was used to inflate 1 to 2 mL of saline and determine proper pressure and position. Early international results of this technique found an extremely high prolapse rate of approximately 15% to 30% and erosion rate of 1% to 3%.[30] It seemed that partially inflating the band at the time of surgery and the creation of a large pouch led to worsening nausea and vomiting, predisposing patients to prolapse, deserosalization, and erosion.[31]

Due to the significant complication rate, Forsell's original technique for the Swedish Adjustable Gastric Band (SAGB), now the REALIZE Band, has become the standardized placement for LAGB.[32] This technique, known as the pars flaccida technique, creates a 1-cm virtual pouch below the esophagogastric junction. The gastrohepatic ligament is opened and a retrogastric tunnel is created above the omentalis bursa where the stomach is naturally fixed to its posterior attachments. The greater curve dissection is completed at the angle of His. A small retrogastric tunnel is created only large enough for the band to pass through. This action allows the stomach to stay fixated to the decussating fibers of the right and left diaphragmatic crura, keeping the band in a fixed position. Plication stitches are then placed anteriorly from the greater curvature to above the band to hold the band in place.[23,33] In addition, fluid is no longer recommended to fill the band during initial placement. Multiple studies comparing the two techniques have shown similar outcomes in weight loss and a dramatic decrease in prolapse and erosion rates with the pars flaccida technique, which is now standard practice for all LAGBs.[30,34]

PREOPERATIVE, INTRAOPERATIVE, AND POSTOPERATIVE CARE

Like all bariatric procedures, patients who wish to undergo LAGB require extensive preoperative preparation. The National Institutes of Health (NIH) requirements for bariatric surgery include a BMI greater than 40 without severe medical comorbidities, or BMI greater than 35 with severe medical comorbidities such as type 2 diabetes mellitus, hypertension, obstructive sleep apnea, and degenerative joint disease. Once these criteria are met, patients must undergo significant nutritional education, dietary counseling, and often psychological screening before surgery. Medical clearances may be obtained for patients who have significant cardiac and pulmonary risk factors.

Once the screening process is complete, the patient is taken to the operating room. Endotracheal intubation is required for LAGB. After this is completed, patients are positioned on a bariatric capacity operating table in supine position with a foot board to prevent patient sliding and lower extremity neuropathy. In general, 5 to 6 ports are placed in the upper abdomen to maintain adequate exposure during the procedure. One of the trocars is typically 15 mm in size, as this will accommodate introduction of the band. A Nathanson liver retractor or similar retracting device is placed in the epigastrium to lift the left lateral segment of the liver and expose the esophagus, hiatus, and stomach. Fatty attachments of the angle of His are dissected. Then the gastrohepatic ligament is opened and the base of the right crus is identified, and the peritoneum is incised. A grasper or band-passing device is passed through a retrogastric tunnel until it emerges behind the dissected angle of His. The band device is introduced through a 15-mm trocar into the abdomen. The end of the band is grasped, and the grasper or band-passing device is pulled back through the gastric tunnel until the entire band is around the stomach. Two graspers are used to fasten the buckle of the band. Two to 4 anterior plication stitches are placed from the greater curvature to the stomach above the band. The band is then rotated so there is no friction of the buckle against the plication. The tubing is pulled out of the 15-mm port. The tubing is connected to the subcutaneous reservoir.[35] Air is removed from the band and the subcutaneous reservoir is fastened to the abdominal wall fascia with sutures or a stapling device.

Postoperatively, patients are placed on a sugar-free liquid diet for approximately 2 weeks supplemented with protein drinks.[36] Patients are usually discharged the same day as surgery or kept overnight for an extended 23-hour observation.[37] Patients are then seen at a 2-week postoperative visit when their diets are advanced to soft puréed foods. Two to 4 weeks after this visit, the patients are scheduled for their first LAGB adjustment. Whether in the office or fluoroscopy suite, reservoirs are filled with 3 to 4 mL of fluid and patients are asked to test restriction by drinking fluids afterwards. Patients are instructed to remain on liquid diets for 24 to 48 hours to allow any edema to subside. Patients are asked to return every 4 to 6 weeks to assess restriction, and may require multiple visits in the first year until adequate restriction or "the sweet spot" is obtained.[32] At each visit, patients are asked about rapid loss of satiety, increased meal volume, and hunger between meals to assess the need for addition or subtraction of fluid.[38–40] Recent studies have shown that a more vigorous adjustment schedule results in better weight loss, better patient accountability, and decreases in complications including prolapse, obstruction, and/or erosion.[34] Ideal weight loss is gradual, at about 0.5 to 1 kg per week.

OUTCOMES OF LAGB, SHORT TERM AND LONG TERM

Safety is the major perioperative advantage of LAGB. LAGB is considerably safer than gastric bypass, with reported morbidity and mortality rates of 11.3% and 0.05%,[41,42] 10 times lower than the mortality rate of gastric bypass at approximately 0.5%.[41,43] Multiple studies have reported minimal complications with LAGB in properly trained hands.[44–46]

O'Brien and Dixon[30] reported a 1.5% perioperative complication rate that resulted in delayed discharge or readmission.[41] These complications included port site infections at 0.9%, acute gastric outlet obstruction at 0.4%, and deep venous thrombosis (DVT) at 0.09%.[30] Fielding and colleagues[45] reported a series of 335 LAGB patients with only 2 reoperations for malpositioning of the band, 1 subphrenic abscess, and 4 wound infections requiring antibiotics. Similar results have been published by Chevallier and colleagues[47] in a series of 1000 LAGB patients. Their results included a 0.4% gastric perforation rate, early prolapse rate of 0.3%, pulmonary embolism in 0.2%, and acute respiratory distress syndrome in 0.2%.[47]

Gastric perforation is the most detrimental complication, and rates are reported from 0.1% to 0.4% in multiple studies.[48] To decrease the likelihood of gastric perforation, both major companies, Allergan and Ethicon, require proctoring before surgeons can place bands in the operating room. A proctor is a skilled surgeon who is trained in the insertion of the LAGB. This individual must observe a surgeon place bands in 2 different patients. Once they feel these individuals can safely place the LAGB, the company allows the sale of the device to the hospital.

Successful LAGB placement does not eliminate the potential for reoperation in the patient's lifetime. Bueter and colleagues[49] showed a 23% reoperation rate in a series of 172 patients over a 56-month median follow-up. These reoperations included band replacements, repositions, and conversions to other bariatric procedures, due to failure of weight loss. The pars flaccida technique has significantly reduced some of these reoperation rates. Dargent[50] showed a significant decrease in prolapse rates, from 6.2% to 0.6%, using the pars flaccida technique. Erosion rates have also significantly decreased from 3% to 0.3%.[51,52] While improvements in technique have improved overall outcomes, there is still a significant reoperation rate that patients need to consider when choosing the LAGB as an option for bariatric surgery.[53,54]

WEIGHT LOSS OUTCOMES

Numerous studies have been performed to evaluate weight loss from LAGB. Using LRYGB as the gold standard, many of these studies showed that whereas early weight loss may be significantly less than for LRYGB in the first 6 months to a year, excess weight loss (EWL) does start to reach approximately 50% to 65% in 2 to 3 years,[41,55–57] then slowly approaches the 65% to 70% EWL seen in LRYGB.[12] This weight loss is gradual, and is dependent on adequate adjustments and more frequent follow-up.[58] A study by Shen and Ren[59] showed that patients with 6 or more visits at 1 year had an EWL of 50% compared with only 42% EWL for those patients with fewer than 6 visits. Belachew and Zimmermann[31] reported percent EWL to be 40% at 1 year and 50% at 2 years, with a range of 50% to 60% at 48 months in a large trial of 763 patients.

Early studies in the United States reported poor weight loss and high complication rates.[60,61] However, this was likely attributable to the perigastric technique of band placement and inadequate adjustment protocols. Ren and colleagues[52] formulated a multi-institutional study and reported a 44.3% EWL in 99 patients with mean preoperative BMI of 52. An American trial from Jan and colleagues[62] compared 154 LAGB patients with 219 LRYGB patients from October 2000 to November 2003. EWL was 36% for LAGB versus 64% for LRYGB after the first year, 45% for LAGB versus 70% for LRYGB after the second year, and then 60% for LAGB versus 57% for LRYGB at the third year. As seen in previous studies, whereas early weight loss was less when compared with LRYGB, 3-year EWL correlates well with that for LRYGB. Therefore, it seems from these results as well that Americans can succeed with LAGB surgery.

RESOLUTION OF COMORBIDITIES

The real benefit of weight loss surgery is the resolution of the significant comorbidities related to morbid obesity. LRYGB has clearly shown that significant weight loss can improve type 2 diabetes, hypertension, gastroesophageal reflux (GERD), hyperlipidemia, sleep apnea, asthma, polycystic ovarian syndromes, depression, arthritis, stress incontinence, and overall quality of life.[30,63] LAGB has been shown to improve these comorbidities as well.[64]

Dixon and O'Brien[20,65,66] have completed multiple studies showing improvements in diabetes after LAGB. These investigators reported significant normalization of glucose, hemoglobin A1c, and insulin resistance in 64% of type 2 diabetics and improvements in 26% after LAGB, and also noted resolution or improvements in hypertension with 92% of patients after LAGB. There were some reports of increasing rates of GERD after LAGB.[67] This phenomenon was thought to correlate with the presence of hiatal hernias that were not concomitantly repaired during the time of surgery, as well as adjustment difficulties such as overtightening of the band.[68] The pars flaccida technique and the adoption of the principle that all hiatal hernias should be repaired during LAGB changed these early outcomes.[46,69] Dixon and O'Brien found that 89% of patients had resolution of GERD after LAGB, 5% had improvement in symptoms, 2.5% had no change in symptoms, and 2.5% had worsening of symptoms.

SUMMARY

A systematic review from October 2007 put it best:

> LAGB has been shown to produce a significant loss of excess weight while maintaining low rates of short-term complications and reducing obesity-related comorbidities. LAGB may not result in the most weight loss but it may be an option for bariatric patients who prefer or who are better suited to undergo less invasive and reversible surgery with lower perioperative complication rates. One caution with LAGB is the uncertainty about whether the low complication rate extends past three years, given a possibility of increased band-related complications (eg, erosion, slippage) requiring re-operation.[70]

It is clear that there is a role for LAGB in bariatric surgery. LAGB has evolved through the decades to become an effective option for patients fighting the disease of obesity. Patients can receive a less invasive bariatric procedure and have similar weight loss to LRYGB patients as well as resolution of their comorbidities,[71–73] although it comes with the risk of possible reoperation rate for band slippage, erosion, port flips, and foreign-body infections.[74] Understanding these risks, patients can still make quality choices on bariatric procedures and still choose LAGB as an option. With recent FDA approval of the LAP-BAND for a BMI greater than 30, the next frontier will begin for LAGB. LABG may play a crucial role in primary prevention of obesity and morbid obesity for Americans in the near future.

REFERENCES

1. Athyros VG, Tziomalos K, Karagiannis A, et al. Cardiovascular benefits of bariatric surgery in morbidly obese patients. Obes Rev 2011;12(7):515–24.
2. Ayloo SM, Buchs NC, Bianco FM, et al. Cost and validity of early postoperative contrast swallow after laparoscopic adjustable gastric banding. Surg Obes Relat Dis 2011, Mar 21. DOI:10.1016/j.soard.2011.02.001.
3. Parikh MS, Shen R, Weiner M, et al. Laparoscopic bariatric surgery in super-obese patients (BMI>50) is safe and effective: a review of 332 patients. Obes Surg 2005;15(6):858–63.
4. Centers for Disease Control and Prevention (CDC). Vital signs: state-specific obesity prevalence among adults – United States, 2009. MMWR Morb Mortal Wkly Rep 2010;59:951–5.
5. Olshansky SJ, Passaro DJ, Hershow RC, et al. "A potential decline in life expectancy in the United States in the 21st century". N Engl J Med 2005;352(11):1138–45.
6. Benedix F, Westphal S, Patschke R, et al. Weight loss and changes in salivary ghrelin and adiponectin: comparison between sleeve gastrectomy and roux-en-Y gastric bypass and gastric banding. Obes Surg 2011;21(5):616–24.
7. Brunault P, Jacobi D, Leger J, et al. Observations regarding 'quality of life' and 'comfort with food' after bariatric surgery: comparison between laparoscopic adjustable gastric banding and sleeve gastrectomy. Obes Surg 2011;21(8):1225–31.
8. Calle EE, Thun MJ, Petrelli JM, et al. Body-mass index and mortality in a prospective cohort of U.S. adults. N Engl J Med 1999;341(15):1097–105.
9. Christou NV, Sampalis JS, Liberman M, et al. Surgery decreases long-term mortality, morbidity, and health care use in morbidly obese patients. Ann Surg 2004;240(3):416–23 [discussion: 423–4].
10. Ding D, Chen DL, Hu XG, et al. Outcomes after laparoscopic surgery for 219 patients with obesity. Zhonghua Wei Chang Wai Ke Za Zhi 2011;14(2):128–31 [in Chinese].
11. Padwal R, Klarenbach S, Wiebe N, et al. Bariatric surgery: a systematic review and network meta-analysis of randomized trials. Obes Rev 2011;12(8):602–21.
12. Wittgrove AC, Clark GW. Laparoscopic gastric bypass, Roux-en-Y—500 patients: technique and results, with 3-60 month follow-up. Obes Surg 2000;10(3):233–9.
13. Flum DR, Dellinger EP. Impact of gastric bypass operation on survival: a population-based analysis. J Am Coll Surg 2004;199(4):543–51.
14. Nguyen NT, Paya M, Stevens CM, et al. The relationship between hospital volume and outcome in bariatric surgery at academic medical centers. Ann Surg 2004;240(4):586–93 [discussion: 593–4].
15. Franco JV, Ruiz PA, Palermo M, et al. A review of studies comparing three laparoscopic procedures in bariatric surgery: sleeve gastrectomy, roux-en-Y gastric bypass and adjustable gastric banding. Obes Surg 2011;21(9):1458–68.
16. Buchwald H, Avidor Y, Braunwald E, et al. Bariatric surgery: a systematic review and meta-analysis. JAMA 2004;292(14):1724–37.
17. Hedley AA, Ogden CL, Johnson CL, et al. Prevalence of overweight and obesity among US children, adolescents, and adults, 1999-2002. JAMA 2004;291(23):2847–50.

18. Varela JE, Frey W. Perioperative outcomes of laparoscopic adjustable gastric banding in mildly obese (BMI <35 kg/m^2) compared to severely obese. Obes Surg 2011;21(4):421–5.

19. Cadiere GB, Himpens J, Vertruyen M, et al. Laparoscopic gastroplasty (adjustable silicone gastric banding). Semin Laparosc Surg 2000;7(1):55–65.

20. Szinicz G, Muller L, Erhart W, et al. "Reversible gastric banding" in surgical treatment of morbid obesity—results of animal experiments. Res Exp Med (Berl) 1989; 189(1):55–60.

21. Mason EE, Doherty C, Cullen JJ, et al. Vertical gastroplasty: evolution of vertical banded gastroplasty. World J Surg 1998;22(9):919–24.

22. Moschen AR, Molnar C, Enrich B, et al. Adipose and liver expression of IL-1 family members in morbid obesity and effects of weight loss. Mol Med 2011; 17(7–8):840–5.

23. Provost DA. Laparoscopic adjustable gastric banding: an attractive option. Surg Clin North Am 2005;85(4):789–805, vii.

24. Kuzmak LI, Yap IS, McGuire L, et al. Surgery for morbid obesity. using an inflatable gastric band. AORN J 1990;51(5):1307–24.

25. Martin MB, Earle KR. Laparoscopic adjustable gastric banding with truncal vagotomy: any increased weight loss? Surg Endosc 2011;25(8):2522–5.

26. Catona A, La Manna L, Forsell P. The Swedish adjustable gastric band: laparoscopic technique and preliminary results. Obes Surg 2000;10(1):15–21.

27. Forsell P, Hellers G. The Swedish adjustable gastric banding (SAGB) for morbid obesity: 9 year experience and a 4-year follow-up of patients operated with a new adjustable band. Obes Surg 1997;7(4):345–51.

28. Belachew M, Legrand M, Vincenti VV, et al. Laparoscopic placement of adjustable silicone gastric band in the treatment of morbid obesity: how to do it. Obes Surg 1995;5(1):66–70.

29. Belachew M, Legrand MJ, Defechereux TH, et al. Laparoscopic adjustable silicone gastric banding in the treatment of morbid obesity. A preliminary report. Surg Endosc 1994;8(11):1354–6.

30. O'Brien PE, Dixon JB. Laparoscopic adjustable gastric banding in the treatment of morbid obesity. Arch Surg 2003;138(4):376–82.

31. Belachew M, Zimmermann JM. Evolution of a paradigm for laparoscopic adjustable gastric banding. Am J Surg 2002;184(6B):21S–5S.

32. Favretti F, O'Brien PE, Dixon JB. Patient management after LAP-BAND placement. Am J Surg 2002;184(6B):38S–41S.

33. Ren CJ, Fielding GA. Laparoscopic adjustable gastric banding: surgical technique. J Laparoendosc Adv Surg Tech A 2003;13(4):257–63.

34. Shen R, Dugay G, Rajaram K, et al. Impact of patient follow-up on weight loss after bariatric surgery. Obes Surg 2004;14(4):514–9.

35. Favretti F, Cadiere GB, Segato G, et al. Laparoscopic adjustable silicone gastric banding: technique and results. Obes Surg 1995;5(4):364–71.

36. Dodsworth A, Warren-Forward H, Baines S. A systematic review of dietary intake after laparoscopic adjustable gastric banding. J Hum Nutr Diet 2011;24(4):327–41.

37. Thomas H, Agrawal S. Systematic review of same-day laparoscopic adjustable gastric band surgery. Obes Surg 2011;21(6):805–10.

38. Hudson SM, Dixon JB, O'Brien PE. Sweet eating is not a predictor of outcome after lap-band placement. Can we finally bury the myth? Obes Surg 2002;12(6):789–94.

39. King WC, Belle SH, Eid GM, et al. Physical activity levels of patients undergoing bariatric surgery in the longitudinal assessment of bariatric surgery study. Surg Obes Relat Dis 2008;4(6):721–8.

40. Kurrek MM, Cobourn C, Wojtasik Z, et al. Morbidity in patients with or at high risk for obstructive sleep apnea after ambulatory laparoscopic gastric banding. Obes Surg 2011. [Epub ahead of print]. DOI: 10.1007/s11695-011-0381-6.

41. O'Brien PE, Dixon JB. Lap-band: outcomes and results. J Laparoendosc Adv Surg Tech A 2003;13(4):265–70.

42. Shapiro K, Patel S, Abdo Z, et al. Laparoscopic adjustable gastric banding: is there a learning curve? Surg Endosc 2004;18(1):48–50.

43. Spivak H, Anwar F, Burton S, et al. The lap-band system in the United States: one surgeon's experience with 271 patients. Surg Endosc 2004;18(2):198–202.

44. Chapman AE, Kiroff G, Game P, et al. Laparoscopic adjustable gastric banding in the treatment of obesity: a systematic literature review. Surgery 2004;135(3):326–51.

45. Fielding GA, Rhodes M, Nathanson LK. Laparoscopic gastric banding for morbid obesity. Surgical outcome in 335 cases. Surg Endosc 1999;13(6):550–4.

46. Reynoso JF, Goede MR, Tiwari MM, et al. Primary and revisional laparoscopic adjustable gastric band placement in patients with hiatal hernia. Surg Obes Relat Dis 2011;7(3):290–4.

47. Chevallier JM, Zinzindohoue F, Douard R, et al. Complications after laparoscopic adjustable gastric banding for morbid obesity: experience with 1,000 patients over 7 years. Obes Surg 2004;14(3):407–14.

48. Eid I, Birch DW, Sharma AM, et al. Complications associated with adjustable gastric banding for morbid obesity: a surgeon's guides. Can J Surg 2011; 54(1):61–6.

49. Bueter M, Maroske J, Thalheimer A, et al. Short- and long-term results of laparoscopic gastric banding for morbid obesity. Langenbecks Arch Surg 2008;393(2): 199–205.

50. Dargent J. Pouch dilatation and slippage after adjustable gastric banding: is it still an issue? Obes Surg 2003;13(1):111–5.

51. Egberts K, Brown WA, O'Brien PE. Systematic review of erosion after laparoscopic adjustable gastric banding. Obes Surg 2011;21(8):1272–9.

52. Ren CJ, Weiner M, Allen JW. Favorable early results of gastric banding for morbid obesity: the American experience. Surg Endosc 2004;18(3):543–6.

53. Freeman L, Brown WA, Korin A, et al. An approach to the assessment and management of the laparoscopic adjustable gastric band patient in the emergency department. Emerg Med Australas 2011;23(2):186–94.

54. Robert M, Poncet G, Boulez J, et al. Laparoscopic gastric bypass for failure of adjustable gastric banding: a review of 85 cases. Obes Surg 2011. [Epub ahead of print]. DOI:10.1007/s11695-011-0391-4.

55. O'Brien PE, Dixon JB, Brown W, et al. The laparoscopic adjustable gastric band (lap-band): a prospective study of medium-term effects on weight, health and quality of life. Obes Surg 2002;12(5):652–60.

56. Weiner R, Blanco-Engert R, Weiner S, et al. Outcome after laparoscopic adjustable gastric banding—8 years experience. Obes Surg 2003;13(3):427–34.

57. Vertruyen M. Experience with lap-band system up to 7 years. Obes Surg 2002; 12(4):569–72.

58. Dixon JB, O'Brien PE. Selecting the optimal patient for LAP-BAND placement. Am J Surg 2002;184(6B):17S–20S.

59. Shen R, Ren CJ. Removal of peri-gastric fat prevents acute obstruction after lap-band surgery. Obes Surg 2004;14(2):224–9.

60. DeMaria EJ, Sugerman HJ. A critical look at laparoscopic adjustable silicone gastric banding for surgical treatment of morbid obesity: does it measure up? Surg Endosc 2000;14(8):697–9.

61. Puzziferri N, Nakonezny PA, Livingston EH, et al. Variations of weight loss following gastric bypass and gastric band. Ann Surg 2008;248(2):233–42.

62. Jan JC, Hong D, Pereira N, et al. Laparoscopic adjustable gastric banding versus laparoscopic gastric bypass for morbid obesity: a single-institution comparison study of early results. J Gastrointest Surg 2005;9(1):30–9 [discussion: 40–1].

63. Sesti G, Folli F, Perego L, et al. Effects of weight loss in metabolically healthy obese subjects after laparoscopic adjustable gastric banding and hypocaloric diet. PLoS One 2011;6(3):e17737.

64. Colucci RA. Bariatric surgery in patients with type 2 diabetes: a viable option. Postgrad Med 2011;123(1):24–33.

65. Dixon JB, O'Brien PE. Health outcomes of severely obese type 2 diabetic subjects 1 year after laparoscopic adjustable gastric banding. Diabetes Care 2002;25(2):358–63.

66. Dixon JB, O'Brien PE, Playfair J, et al. Adjustable gastric banding and conventional therapy for type 2 diabetes: a randomized controlled trial. JAMA 2008; 299(3):316–23.

67. DeMaria EJ, Sugerman HJ, Meador JG, et al. High failure rate after laparoscopic adjustable silicone gastric banding for treatment of morbid obesity. Ann Surg 2001;233(6):809–18.

68. Greenstein RJ, Nissan A, Jaffin B. Esophageal anatomy and function in laparoscopic gastric restrictive bariatric surgery: implications for patient selection. Obes Surg 1998;8(2):199–206.

69. Dolan K, Finch R, Fielding G. Laparoscopic gastric banding and crural repair in the obese patient with a hiatal hernia. Obes Surg 2003;13(5):772–5.

70. Boudreau R, Hodgson A. Laparoscopic adjustable gastric banding for weight loss in obese adults: clinical and economic review. Ottawa (Canada): Canadian Agency for Drugs and Technologies in Health; 2007 [Technology report number 90].

71. Garb J, Welch G, Zagarins S, et al. Bariatric surgery for the treatment of morbid obesity: a meta-analysis of weight loss outcomes for laparoscopic adjustable gastric banding and laparoscopic gastric bypass. Obes Surg 2009;19(10):1447–55.

72. Helmio M, Salminen P, Sintonen H, et al. A 5-year prospective quality of life analysis following laparoscopic adjustable gastric banding for morbid obesity. Obes Surg 2011. [Epub ahead of print]. DOI:10.1007/s11695-011-0425-y.

73. Himpens J, Cadiere GB, Bazi M, et al. Long-term outcomes of laparoscopic adjustable gastric banding. Arch Surg 2011;146(7):802–7.

74. Goitein D, Feigin A, Segal-Lieberman G, et al. Laparoscopic sleeve gastrectomy as a revisional option after gastric band failure. Surg Endosc 2011;25(8): 2626–30.

Complications of Adjustable Gastric Banding

Jay Michael Snow, MD, Paul A. Severson, MD*

KEYWORDS

- Adjustable gastric banding • Complications
- Revisional surgery

Although the initial success and proven safety of adjustable gastric banding (AGB) have led to near extinction of the vertical banded gastroplasty, more recent analyses of rising long-term complications of AGB show the need for ongoing careful study. The mortality is remarkably low,[1] the in-hospital mortality is only 0.02%, and the risk-adjusted mortality index 0.4%, compared with 0.08% and 0.7% for laparoscopic Roux-en-Y gastric bypass (LRNYGB) in a large randomized, prospective trial.[1,2] However, AGB is associated with a 13% hospital readmission rate[3] and up to a 52% revisional surgery rate.[4] Of patients, 73% would not agree to gastric banding again, after removal or deflation for a complication.[5]

Complications that range from band perforation to failure of weight loss are becoming increasingly apparent as the length of time bands are left indwelling increases. It has been suggested that each year the band is left in vivo increases the complication rate 3% to 4%,[6] with a major complication rate of 40% at 10 years. This situation is partially to blame for the tendency of surgeons worldwide to tame their initial enthusiasm for AGB and increasingly offer alternative procedures for surgical weight loss. Although the literature highlights many different complications, short-term studies clearly underreport the long-term incidence of complications, particularly gastric prolapse, pouch dilation, and esophageal failure. Failure of weight loss is considered by many as a complication, but is common to all surgical alternatives and is considered separately.

For the purposes of this discussion, complications are grouped as intraoperative, early postoperative, and late postoperative. The remarkably low mortality cannot overshadow the increasingly described life-altering complications that can occur years later. The increased morbidity and mortality associated with required revisional surgery need to be considered when offering the patient their initial options for surgical weight loss.

Minnesota Institute for Minimally Invasive Surgery, MIMIS Weight Loss Center, 320 East Main Street, Crosby, MN 56441, USA
* Corresponding author.
E-mail address: pseverson@cuyunamed.org

Surg Clin N Am 91 (2011) 1249–1264
doi:10.1016/j.suc.2011.08.008   **surgical.theclinics.com**
0039-6109/11/$ – see front matter © 2011 Elsevier Inc. All rights reserved.

INTRAOPERATIVE COMPLICATIONS

Intraoperative complications associated with AGB are likely underreported in the literature because there has been no requirement for tracking outcomes in bariatric centers until recently (Bariatric Outcomes Longitudinal Database for American Society of Metabolic and Bariatric Surgeons accredited Centers of Excellence, National Surgical Quality Improvement Program for Levels 1A and 2A American College of Surgeons Bariatric Surgery Center Network). Many surgeons who perform AGB are not affiliated with such centers and do not report complications. Nevertheless, in the studies that have been published, intraoperative complications are infrequent.

Technique in placement of the AGB has evolved since the time of its inception. What was first termed the perigastric technique was later modified to include the neurovascular tissue along the lesser curvature, termed the pars flaccida technique, as first described by Fielding in 2001.[7] This technique was particularly important in nearly eliminating posterior gastric prolapse. However, retrogastric dissection through the pars flaccida and along the left crus of the diaphragm toward the spleen is commonly performed blindly, risking damage to all surrounding structures. Splenic bleeding can be frustrating and necessitate use of hemostatic agents or even splenectomy in the most severe cases. Placement of the device through the gastric wall has been reported and has led to patient death.[8] Furthermore, it is theorized that subclinical gastric wall injury may result in later tendency toward erosion (intragastric band migration).

Later, in an effort to decrease the incidence of complications including obstruction and anterior prolapse, gastric fat pad removal was advocated and showed a decrease in the postoperative incidence of dysphagia and anterior gastric perforation. Multiple studies have been published regarding different techniques to optimize outcomes; perhaps the most notable was the recommendation to close the crura in cases of suspected hiatal hernia,[9–20] as popularized by Fielding and Ren. In Zagzag and colleagues'[21] recent study of 2334 AGB patients, the rate of prolapse dropped from 3.83% to 1.76% with routine cruroplasty at every band placement, although the study only had 22-month follow-up. More recently, a widely-practiced modification termed the antiprolapse stitch, a gastrogastric plication suture placed along the lesser curve distal to the band,[22] has been shown to provide no additional protection from prolapse complications.[21]

Inferior vena cava (IVC) inclusion in the band is rare but is described, as is inadvertent dissection into the mediastinum. Whereas the former can result in intra-abdominal catastrophe, the latter may simply present as pneumomediastinum or pneumothorax in the immediate postoperative period without clinical consequence. Tube thoracostomy may be advisable because many patients require positive pressure ventilation secondary to obesity-related obstructive sleep apnea. Damage to the device itself, particularly rupture of the balloon reservoir by suture needles during placement of plicating sutures, necessitates immediate explantation with replacement using a second device: a costly complication.

Early Postoperative Complications

Pulmonary

Pulmonary complications are a well-known source of morbidity in all bariatric procedures. Administration of general anesthesia is the most important risk factor and contributes to the development of pulmonary atelectasis, which most often responds to spirometry and early postoperative ambulation. Additional aggressive postoperative pulmonary toilet is needed because many patients carry the diagnosis of obstructive sleep apnea and use home positive pressure airway devices. As a result, continuous oximetry monitoring has become standard in the postoperative care of the bariatric patient.

In contrast to atelectasis, which does not significantly change the management of patients postoperatively, pulmonary embolism is said to be the most common cause of death, accounting for at least 23% of patient deaths after AGB.[23] Perioperative chemical and mechanical deep vein thrombosis prophylaxis should be instituted in all patients, and extension of treatment to include use after hospital discharge should be considered in those at increased risk, or with a previous history of thromboembolic disease. IVC filter placement may be indicated in selected patients at high risk, although complications associated with this procedure occur in up to 57% of patients.[24]

Cardiac

The risk of perioperative myocardial infarction is less than 1%, but the gravity of this complication requires preoperative preparation to lower the incidence of this dreaded complication. Placement of the AGB, like any major operative procedure requiring general anesthesia in a higher-risk population, requires that attention should be given to thorough preoperative evaluation and risk assessment, and specific cardiology consultation is advised when cardiac risk is increased. Coronary revascularization needs to be accomplished preoperatively to avert cardiac morbidity and mortality. For those higher-risk patients unable to undergo revascularization or with significant nonoperative valvular disease, medical optimization and careful continuous monitoring with transesophageal echocardiography should be considered during surgery. Perioperative and postoperative β-blockade should be continued in patients on that class of antihypertensives preoperatively.[25]

Early Obstruction

Although overfilling the band is a known cause of esophageal outlet obstruction, early obstruction (<24 hours) after band placement is reported in the literature.[26,27] A retrospective article published in 2007[28] reported the incidence to be 6% among a study group of 400 patients. Multiple causes for esophageal outlet obstruction exist, including postoperative edema, inappropriately small diameter band, and inclusion of perigastric fat pads.[10] For this reason, the design of the AGB has undergone evolutionary changes. The LAP-BAND (Allergan Inc, Irvine, CA, USA) has eliminated the smaller sizes, including the original 10-cm band, and replaced it with the LAP-BAND AP, which is 10.5 cm long and less likely to result in early obstruction. A larger size is also available at the surgeon's discretion. The addition of a low-pressure 360° balloon design with creased pillows was introduced to try to decrease the incidence of erosion. The other major product available in the United States is the improved Swedish Adjustable Gastric Band, now owned and marketed as the REALIZE Band-C (Ethicon Endo-Surgery Inc, Cincinnati, OH, USA). This product also has a low pressure and creased but triangular shape to the inflated balloon. There is only a smaller band length available, but the REALIZE has the widest (23 mm) platform, which is an antislip design. Despite the design improvements, most studies are not able to show a significant difference in the incidence of complications between the 2 band systems.

Patients with immediate postoperative obstruction experience intolerance to solids or liquids and in the most severe cases, their own secretions. Contrast esophagram reveals obstruction at the level of the band and the initial management includes intravenous (IV) fluids with nasoenteric decompression and antiinflammatory medications. For those who fail nonoperative management, operative exchange for a larger diameter band combined with perigastric fat pad excision is usually curative. Although conversion to another procedure has been suggested as an alternative, this should not be necessary unless the largest size band had already been used.

Late Postoperative Complications

Late postoperative complications of AGB are frequent and often lead to revisional procedures. The true incidence of long-term complications is not yet known, because the incidence is rising as long-term study results emerge. When patient frustrations mount or anatomic difficulties abound, explantation with replacement or conversion to other procedures is indicated. Patients should be informed that the choice of AGB likely results in future revisional procedures.

Infrequent complications such as gastric artery erosion with near fatal hemorrhage,[29–31] cecal volvulus around the tubing,[32] thrombosed band tubing,[33] paragastric Richter hernia,[34] chronic cough,[35] pouch necrosis,[36] and gastric bezoar formation[37–39] have all been reported in the literature, but are rare. Our discussion primarily focuses on common late complications such as port and tubing problems, gastroesophageal reflux disease (GERD), pouch dilation, prolapse, erosion, and esophageal failure.

Port and Tubing Complications

Port and tubing complications represent a significant source of morbidity. Although these complications are rarely life-threatening in nature, their incidence is reported between 4.3% and 24%,[40–42] and this seems to be related to length of follow-up.[40] Failure of the port and tubing may be related to mechanical forces associated with change in abdominal wall anatomy after weight loss, as well as physical changes in the silicone tubing. The initial compliant and flexible nature becomes increasingly firm and brittle over time, and is more likely to fracture. The rate of mechanical problems seems to correlate with weight loss and be directly related to the length of follow-up.[43] The banding device is composed of 2 separate pieces coupled together by a metal connector, most often situated inside the peritoneal cavity. Disconnection between these 2 parts of the device has been reported at a rate between 5%[44] and 9.4%.[45] This problem is easily appreciated at fluoroscopy, and is visualized by addition of the fluid to the band without evidence of increased restriction of contrast through the gastric pouch. This finding can be confirmed by contrast injection into the port with evidence of extravasation under fluoroscopy.

Although presenting in a similar fashion, the diagnosis of both reservoir leakage and tubing fracture is made more difficult with clinical adjustments alone, often necessitating multiple office visits and repeat band-fills until the diagnosis is confirmed with fluoroscopy. Termed a minor complication by most, operative intervention under a general anesthetic is usually required for replacement of the port, especially if entry into the abdominal cavity is needed to retrieve the disconnected tubing.

Further port complications include skin ulceration, persistent port-cutaneous sinus, and port infection/abscess. These complications are typically treated with port removal and subsequent replacement once the infection has cleared. The important consideration is that what seems to be a simple port infection may represent a devastating band erosion. This complication must be ruled out with endoscopy.

A frequent complaint, but not mentioned as a complication in most reports, is the patient who complains of port site pain. This complication can be bothersome to the patient and presents a challenge to the bariatric surgeon. Workup should include fluoroscopic radiologic evaluation to ensure normal port position and absence of a port site hernia by computed tomography scan. In an effort to eliminate port migration and inversion, application of mesh has been advocated to the underside of the port. The efficacy of this intervention is unknown and opinions are at best anecdotal.

Repositioning of the port further from the costal margin and out of natural flexion creases has resulted in resolution of chronic pain in some cases.

GERD

Exacerbation of preoperative GERD, as well as new development of reflux symptoms, has been described in as many as one-third of postoperative patients (who had been asymptomatic preoperatively).[46–48] This condition can be troubling and often leads to patient disappointment when fluid is removed from the band, which is the first-line treatment. The frequency of GERD symptoms can lead to delayed or poor weight loss. Similarly, development of Barrett's esophagus has been noted as a result of gastric banding,[49] as has adenocarcinoma of the esophagus.[50]

It is routine practice in our bariatric program to perform a preoperative endoscopy, because the incidence of asymptomatic morbidly obese patients with pathologic findings is 57% in 1 study, primarily erosive esophagitis and hiatal hernia.[51] The prevalence of GERD and esophageal motility disorder is higher in the morbidly obese, and is more often asymptomatic. As a result, it has been suggested that morbidly obese patients may have altered visceral sensation.[22] At preoperative endoscopy, if erosive GERD is present, it is our practice to recommend LRNYGB over AGB. If the endoscopic findings reveal hiatal hernia without erosive GERD, then esophageal manometry is performed. If esophageal function is normal without a motility disorder, then AGB with hiatal herniorrhaphy can be offered to the patient. Crural repair should always be performed in the presence of hiatal hernia, even if it is small in size. The presence of an anterior dimple has been described as a reliable guide to performing an anterior crurorhaphy at the time of AGB and has been shown in numerous studies to decrease the incidence of GERD postoperatively.

After placement of the band, should GERD symptoms develop, sequelae such as esophagitis, ulcerations, and Barrett's esophagus are easily appreciated on endoscopy. Treatment includes band deflation and proton pump inhibitor medical therapy. Most authorities agree that GERD recalcitrant to nonoperative management indicates the need for conversion to LRNYGB as the rescue procedure of choice.

Esophageal Failure

It is customary in many bariatric centers, including ours, to perform preoperative esophageal anatomy and function studies before placement of an AGB. It has been shown that preoperative manometry can predict development of esophageal dilation after AGB.[52] Furthermore, some form of esophageal dilation is seen in nearly half of patients and is believed to be only partially reversible.[53] When esophageal dilation is encountered in the symptomatic band patient, removal of the fluid allows reversal of the dilatation with recovery of esophageal function in most (87%) cases. However, in 13% of patients, no recovery from their achalasia-like dilatation was observed.[51] These patients regain their weight and fail, requiring conversion to a secondary bariatric procedure. Normal preoperative manometry does not preclude post-AGB esophageal complications. Normal manometry was found in 4 of 5 patients who developed megaesophagus 32 months postoperatively.[54]

Attenuation of the lower esophageal sphincter has been confirmed under manometric testing.[55] A 2010 study[56] revealed that an intact lower esophageal contractile segment was seen more often in successful band patients than in those with postoperative symptoms of poor weight loss, volume reflux, regurgitation, or fluid intolerance by mouth. Furthermore, esophageal dysmotility disorders are seen more commonly in symptomatic patients.[55] Despite the fact that more than two-thirds of AGB patients develop esophageal motility disorders at long-term follow-up and 25% develop significant dilatation of the esophagus, it remains difficult to predict these problems from preoperative manometry. Nevertheless, it is responsible to evaluate the prospective AGB patient fully and recommend an alternative bariatric procedure, such as LRNYGB, for the patient with a known esophageal motility disorder.

Slippage/Prolapse

Gastric band prolapse is reported in the literature to occur at a rate as little as 0.5%[57] or as frequently as 36%.[58] The broad range of frequency is explained by differences in definition of the term, differences in the technique and implant used, and duration and completeness of follow-up.[59] Early publications cited a decrease in the rate of prolapse after changing from the perigastric technique to the pars flaccida technique.[60–62] Further reduction was reported using gastrogastric sutures and gastropexy techniques.[63]

Band prolapse occurs when a portion of gastric wall herniates or prolapses under the band, causing clockwise or counterclockwise rotation of the band. Patients present with any combination of dysphagia, GERD exacerbation, food intolerance, or nausea and vomiting. Diagnosis is confirmed by contrast swallow, which reveals horizontal band positioning in the case of anterior prolapse or vertical positioning of the band in the case of posterior prolapse (**Fig. 1**). Contrast pools in the excess prolapsed stomach overhanging the band. Endoscopy can also be valuable and reveals enlargement of the pouch above the level of the band.

Theoretic causes of gastric prolapse are many and include failure of suture fixation of the stomach over the band. This situation can result from poor eating habits, or overstuffing the pouch, persistent vomiting, or any combination that causes mechanical stress on the sutures or the anchoring portions of the gastric wall. These causes may lead to disruption of the plication and subsequent allowance of stomach distal to the band to herniate in a cephalad direction under the band. The prolapsed stomach may then incarcerate above the level of the band, and even strangulate in some cases (**Fig. 2**).

Initial treatment of gastric prolapse requires band deflation. If initial nonoperative techniques are unsuccessful in relieving symptoms, surgery should ensue. The safety and feasibility of treatment using the laparoscopic approach has been shown.[64] Some surgeons prefer unbuckling, reduction of the prolapsed stomach, and then rebuckling the band. The rebuckling can also be performed at a second procedure to allow resolution of edema and ischemia. Most centers now understand that recurrence is common with this approach and recommend removal of the band, with replacement through a newly created retrogastric tunnel cephalad to the original tunnel. If repositioning or replacement is not feasible, simple removal is an acceptable alternative. Future plans for replacement or conversion to another weight loss procedure, such as LRNYGB or sleeve gastrectomy, can then be discussed with the patient. However, this approach can be problematic in that previous authorization for revisional surgery is not always granted by third-party payors until the patient has become morbidly obese again. As a result, this approach should be discussed with the patient in detail preoperatively.

Symptoms of prolapse overlap those of both band overtightening and gastroesophageal dilation. Acute prolapse is treated with hospital admission, pouch decompression with nasogastric tube, and IV fluid administration. Should the patient develop a concerning abdominal examination or pain out of proportion to the physical examination, the diagnosis of pouch ischemia or necrosis should be entertained and ruled out with emergent laparoscopic evaluation.

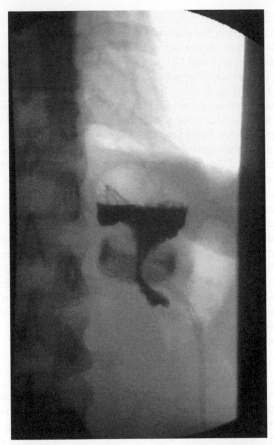

Fig. 1. Anterior prolapse as seen on contrast swallow. Note the horizontal position of the band.

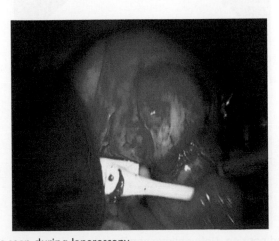

Fig. 2. Prolapse as seen during laparoscopy.

Pouch Dilation

Concentric pouch dilation is believed to be an entity separate from prolapse or slippage. A recently published review of the literature surrounding gastric band prolapse analyzed 40 studies from an initial 121 and revealed that 25% of these studies lumped concentric pouch dilation together with slippage data,[59] thus diluting the data. Normal positioning of the band (**Fig. 3**) along its axis is seen, which differentiates pouch dilation from a prolapse. Endoscopy reveals the symmetry of the concentric dilation and contrast swallow reveals poor flow across the band. Furthermore, treatment differs from that of prolapse in that band fluid removal is usually curative in the short-term.

Again reported are the symptoms of GERD, dysphagia, food intolerance, and vomiting, similar to prolapse. Dilation may be severe enough to weaken the lower esophageal sphincter and enable the patient to use the distal esophagus as a food reservoir. Concentric pouch dilation is most often caused by overtightening of the band, effectively causing a gastric outlet obstruction, in addition to the patient habitually overeating, or failing to stop eating at the first sensation of satiety.

As mentioned earlier, treatment is to give the patient a band holiday, consisting of complete fluid removal. Over a period of several weeks resolution of the dilation occurs in most patients. Should repeat contrast swallow reveal persistence of the dilation, additional time before a fill is recommended. If after slow and judicious reinstallation of fluid, pouch dilation becomes a chronic problem, then discussion about removal and possible alternative procedures should ensue. If the dilation resolves, attempts to reinstill fluid into the band can again be undertaken, although lower volumes and closer follow-up are indicated.

Erosion

Band erosion, or intragastric migration of the device, is a feared complication of AGB. The incidence ranges from 0% to 5.8%, with the average more often quoted between 0.6% and 3%. The risk of development of erosion remains as long as the device is indwelling. Foreign material surrounding a dynamic organ can lead to eventual erosion, a lesson learned from the historical experience of the Angelchik prosthesis in decades

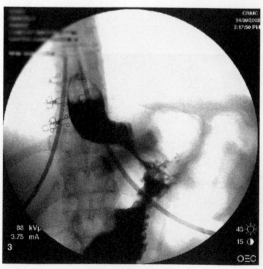

Fig. 3. Normal band position. Note oblique angulation.

past.[65–69] Unlike the Angelchik, which encircled the lower esophagus, the AGB is placed over the thicker and serosalized fundus of the stomach. In addition, chronic band erosions have not proved to be dangerous complications leading to mortality.

Theories regarding cause include subclinical gastric wall injury at the time of placement, plication over the buckle mechanism, overtightening, and abnormal reaction of gastric tissue in contact with the prosthesis. The diagnosis is surprisingly subtle and elusive. The patient may present initially with vague abdominal pain and weight regain, but rarely peritonitis. Some patients present with port site infections, which should always trigger endoscopy to assure that intragastric migration has not occurred. Diagnosis is made by endoscopic visualization of the prosthesis located within the lumen of the stomach on retroflexed endoscopic viewing (**Fig. 4**).

Treatment of the erosion includes removal of the band, repair of the gastric wall, and possible revision to another procedure at a later date. Band removal is normally accomplished by laparoscopy, but can also be successfully treated by endoscopic band removal.[70–72] Band replacement at the time of its removal is ill advised, because there is not enough evidence at this time to consider conversion to another procedure at the same time.

Failure of weight loss

AGB boasts many attractive benefits that led to an exponential increase in use over recent years. Hinojosa and colleagues[73] report a 329% increase in band usage over a 4-year period between 2004 and 2007. However, the most troublesome complication is likely underreported in the literature because patients who have failed with the device are often the ones lost to follow-up. Failure of weight loss is multifactorial and it is nearly impossible to predict which patients will fail before placement.

In a 2008 review of gastric banding versus gastric bypass, Tice and colleagues[58] highlight data from 14 studies published between 2000 and 2007 that reveal a range of 1-year excess weight loss (EWL) from 31% to 54% with the band. There was only 1 high-quality study (randomized, controlled) that compared banding to bypass. In this 5-year study by Angrisani and colleagues, preoperative body mass index (BMI), calculated as weight in kilograms divided by the square of height in meters, averaged 43.4 kg/m^2, and follow-up was 96% at 12 months. The AGB achieved a 35% EWL at 1 year, compared with 51% EWL with the LRNYGB. Weight loss failure (BMI >35 kg/m^2 at 5 years) was observed in 34.6% of AGB patients and in 4.2% of LRNYGB patients (P<.001).[74]

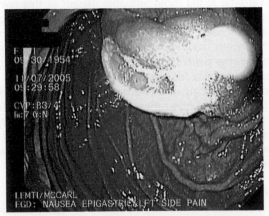

Fig. 4. Band erosion as identified on endoscopic retroflexion.

Although the slower weight loss associated with the band does not seem to be a problem in the short-term (because EWL continues to improve for several years), there is a large percentage of AGB patients who fail to lose weight over the long-term. Early reports indicated this percentage to be low but more recent reports reveal failure to lose more than 50% EWL in as many as 46% of patients at 5 years.[75]

Long-term data are surfacing that reveal 7-year success rate as defined by EWL of more than 50% to be present in 43% of patients.[6] Nguyen and colleagues[2] reported treatment failure (as defined by EWL <20%) in 16.7% of patients. Conversion to a different weight loss procedure occurs at an astonishing rate of 25% to 58% after as little as 7 years.[6,76]

The approach to the patient who fails to lose weight with an AGB is to initially ensure good function of the components of the device. This situation is investigated by aspiration of the fluid in the band. If no fluid returns, concern exists for the integrity of the system and the leak must be identified and addressed. If the system seems to be functioning well, an in-depth discussion is undertaken with the patient to evaluate eating habits, especially eating between meals and consumption of liquid calories. Review of a diet log in the presence of family members may elucidate the cause and direct therapy to include other members of the patient-care team such as the bariatric dietician and the bariatric psychologist. The psychologist must have specific knowledge of eating disorders in addition to experience in the diagnosis and treatment of bariatric patients.

Failure to lose weight after appropriate adjustments, device interrogation, and confirmation of patient compliance indicates failure of the device as a weight loss tool. Further debate surrounds management of the patient who has failed to lose weight with the AGB, and there is no consensus as to which procedure is most appropriate for the failed AGB.

Options after failed gastric banding include removal, replacement, or conversion to another procedure. Removal of the band leads to weight regain in most patients, with rapid recurrence of morbid obesity and return of comorbidities.

Replacement of the band after a failed band should be discouraged based on current literature. Muller and colleagues[77] describe a 45% reoperative rate in patients who undergo rebanding after having failed their first band.

Adjustment difficulty

The ability to titrate the volume of fluid within the band can be difficult and many algorithms have been published describing optimal technique. Finding the green zone or the sweet spot can be challenging in certain individuals who seem to have a narrow window between too much restriction and too little. However, detailed discussion with the patient over time is the most valuable aspect of this part of the patient's care. Patients with an indwelling band can become compulsive about the amount of fluid in the band, and the need to remove fluid for any reason can be met with resistance because of concern over weight gain. Frequent outpatient visits (monthly) with counseling to help the patient learn to stop eating when they begin to feel the sensation of fullness is essential for long-term success.

Overtightening of the band causes intolerance to food and sometimes even liquids in severe cases. Maladaptive eating then ensues, which can be frustrating for the patient, because this usually results in weight gain. Patients frequently present to clinic hours to days after instillation of fluid and require fluid removal for acute obstruction. Removal of all the fluid is not necessary. Many bariatric centers remove a quantity equivalent to the last 2 fills.[78]

Treatment of the failed adjustable gastric band

Treatment of late complications leading to failure of AGB has been discussed by numerous investigators, but to date there are no trials with sufficient numbers of patients to make firm conclusions regarding revisional surgery. The Weight Loss Center at the Minnesota Institute for Minimally Invasive Surgery has performed a retrospective review of late complications associated with AGB that required revisional surgery. Data were collected on all 296 AGB patients from June 2003 to March 2011 (7.75 years). The average follow-up measured 4.02 years. Of a total of 296 patients in our database, 16 were referred from outside practices for revisional procedures, and were excluded. A total of 62 of 280 (22.14%) of the patients who received their index procedure at our facility required 1 or more revisional procedures. A total of 77 procedures were performed in these 62 patients, for a revision rate of 27.5%. Follow-up data were obtained on 61 of 62 (98%) revisional surgery patients. In this subgroup of major late AGB complications requiring surgery, the average preoperative BMI was 42.3 and EWL was 39.3%.

Of the 62 patients who required band revision, 51 patients had the original 10-cm LAP-BAND, 6 had the LAP-BAND AP, and 5 had the 11-cm Vanguard.

Indications for revisions are summarized in **Fig. 5**. They consisted of 31 cases of prolapse (45%), 20 cases of port/tubing complications (29%), 6 cases of erosion (9%), 5 cases of weight loss failure (7%), and 1 case each (1%) of pouch dilation, GERD, and esophageal failure. Unusual indications consisted of 1 case of chronic pain, 1 case requiring dialysis, 1 case desiring to join the military (and unable to do so with the LAP-BAND in place), and a single case of port infection secondary to self-adjustments.

Revisional procedures consisted of 28 removal/replacements (36%), 20 port/tubing revisions (26%), 12 single-stage AGB to LRNYGB (16%), 3 2-stage AGB to LRNYGB (4%), and 14 band removals (18%) **(Fig. 6)**. All were successfully performed laparoscopically, without need for conversion to open.

Our conversion procedure of choice is the LRNYGB. Controversy exists regarding technical considerations, specifically as to where the gastrojejunostomy should be created (above, at, or below the band). We prefer transection of the stomach above the level of the band, which leaves a small gastric pouch but healthy tissue less prone to leak or stricture. Excision of the proximal stomach damaged by the previous surgery is performed. Of the 15 patients, initially 2 of 3 patients who had transection below the band suffered complications: 1 leak and 1 stricture (at the band site, despite release of the capsule). Since our dismal early experience below the band, all 12 patients had the

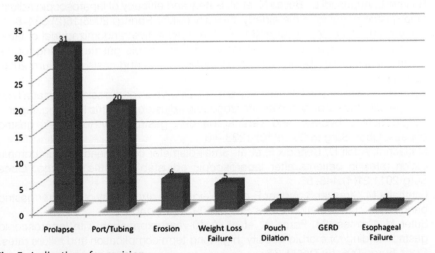

Fig. 5. Indications for revision.

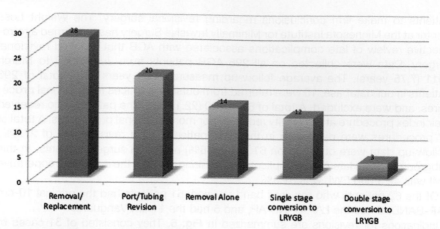

Fig. 6. Revisional procedures performed.

anastamosis above the band, and only 1 had a complication of stricture at the gastro-jejunostomy. This complication was successfully treated by endoscopic balloon dilation.

SUMMARY

The AGB is a popular, rapidly proliferating option for surgical weight loss. It has a remarkably low mortality rate and an excellent safety profile for intraoperative and early postoperative complications. However, late complications are frequent and lead to a high rate of revisional surgery. There is substantially increased risk for revisional surgery, and the incidence of late complications increases 3% to 4% per year. Prospective studies are needed to identify patients at risk for late complications. Certainly a subset of patients are successful with AGB, but the methodology for selection preoperatively remains elusive.

REFERENCES

1. Busetto L, Angrisani L, Basso N, et al. Safety and efficacy of laparoscopic adjustable gastric banding in the elderly. Obesity (Silver Spring) 2008;16(2):334–8.
2. Nguyen NT, Slone JA, Nguyen XM, et al. A prospective randomized trial of laparoscopic gastric bypass versus laparoscopic adjustable gastric banding for the treatment of morbid obesity: outcomes, quality of life, and costs. Ann Surg 2009; 250(4):631–41.
3. Saunders J, Ballantyne GH, Belsley S, et al. One-year readmission rates at a high volume bariatric surgery center: laparoscopic adjustable gastric banding, laparoscopic gastric bypass, and vertical banded gastroplasty-Roux-en-Y gastric bypass. Obes Surg 2008;18(10):1233–40.
4. Matlach J, Adolf D, Benedix F, et al. Small-diameter bands lead to high complication rates in patients after laparoscopic adjustable gastric banding. Obes Surg 2011;21(4):448–56.
5. Lanthaler M, Strasser S, Aigner F, et al. Weight loss and quality of life after gastric band removal or deflation. Obes Surg 2009;19(10):1401–8.
6. Suter M, Calmes JM, Paroz A, et al. A 10-year experience with laparoscopic gastric banding for morbid obesity: high long-term complication and failure rates. Obes Surg 2006;16(7):829–35.

7. Fielding GA. LAP-BAND persisting good result with slipped band by modified technique. Presented at the 6th World Congress of the International Federation for the Surgery of Obesity: Crete; 2001.
8. Loewe C, Diaz F, Jackson A. LAP-banding obesity: a case of stomach perforation, peritonitis, and death. Am J Forensic Med Pathol 2005;26(3):297–301.
9. Korenkov M, Kneist W, Heintz A, et al. Technical alternatives in laparoscopic placement of an adjustable gastric band: experience of two German university hospitals. Obes Surg 2004;14(6):806–10.
10. Shen R, Ren CJ. Removal of peri-gastric fat prevents acute obstruction after Lap-Band surgery. Obes Surg 2004;14(2):224–9.
11. Spivak H, Gold D, Guerrero C. Optimization of access-port placement for the lap-band system. Obes Surg 2003;13(6):909–12.
12. Ren CJ, Fielding GA. Laparoscopic adjustable gastric banding: surgical technique. J Laparoendosc Adv Surg Tech A 2003;13(4):257–63.
13. Furbetta F, Coli E. Codification of techniques for reoperation after Lap-Band. Obes Surg 2003;13(2):289–93.
14. Rubin M, Spivak H. Prospective study of 250 patients undergoing laparoscopic gastric banding using the two-step technique: a technique to prevent postoperative slippage. Surg Endosc 2003;17(6):857–60.
15. Fielding GA, Allen JW. A step-by-step guide to placement of the LAP-BAND adjustable gastric banding system. Am J Surg 2002;184(6B):26S–30S.
16. Belachew M, Zimmermann JM. Evolution of a paradigm for laparoscopic adjustable gastric banding. Am J Surg 2002;184(6B):21S–5S.
17. Favretti F, Segato G, De Marchi F, et al. An adjustable silicone gastric band for laparoscopic treatment of morbid obesity–technique and results. Surg Technol Int 2002;10:109–14.
18. Favretti F, Cadière GB, Segato G, et al. Laparoscopic banding: selection and technique in 830 patients. Obes Surg 2002;12(3):385–90.
19. Elias B, Staudt JP, Van Vyne E. The technical approach in banding to avoid pouch dilatation. Obes Surg 2001;11(3):311–4.
20. Weiner R, Wagner D, Blanco-Engert R, et al. [A new technique for laparoscopic placement of the adjustable gastric band (LAP-band) for preventing slippage]. Chirurg 2000;71(10):1243–50 [in German].
21. Zagzag J, SB, Youn H, Kurian M, et al. Should we do a cruroplasty in every laparoscopic gastric band placement? SAGES Poster Presentation. San Antonio (TX), April 1, 2011.
22. Koppman JS, Poggi L, Szomstein S, et al. Esophageal motility disorders in the morbidly obese population. Surg Endosc 2007;21(5):761–4.
23. Gagner M, Milone L, Yung E, et al. Causes of early mortality after laparoscopic adjustable gastric banding. J Am Coll Surg 2008;206(4):664–9.
24. Birkmeyer NJ, Share D, Baser O, et al. Preoperative placement of inferior vena cava filters and outcomes after gastric bypass surgery. Ann Surg 2010;252(2): 313–8.
25. Fleisher LA, Beckman JA, Brown KA, et al. ACC/AHA 2007 guidelines on perioperative cardiovascular evaluation and care for noncardiac surgery: executive summary: a report of the American College of Cardiology/American Heart Association Task Force on Practice Guidelines (Writing Committee to Revise the 2002 Guidelines on Perioperative Cardiovascular Evaluation for Noncardiac Surgery). Anesth Analg 2008;106(3):685–712.
26. Patel SM, Shapiro K, Abdo Z, et al. Obstructive symptoms associated with the Lap-Band in the first 24 hours. Surg Endosc 2004;18(1):51–5.

27. Bernante P, Francini Pesenti F, Toniato A, et al. Obstructive symptoms associated with the 9.75-cm Lap-Band in the first 24 hours using the pars flaccida approach. Obes Surg 2005;15(3):357–60.
28. Gravante G, Araco A, Araco F, et al. Laparoscopic adjustable gastric bandings: a prospective randomized study of 400 operations performed with 2 different devices. Arch Surg 2007;142(10):958–61.
29. Png KS, Rao J, Lim KH, et al. Lap-band causing left gastric artery erosion presenting with torrential hemorrhage. Obes Surg 2008;18(8):1050–2.
30. Iqbal M, Manjunath S, Seenath M, et al. Massive upper gastrointestinal hemorrhage: an unusual presentation after laparoscopic adjustable gastric banding due to erosion into the celiac axis. Obes Surg 2008;18(6):759–60.
31. Rao AD, Ramalingam G. Exsanguinating hemorrhage following gastric erosion after laparoscopic adjustable gastric banding. Obes Surg 2006;16(12):1675–8.
32. Agahi A, Harle R. A serious but rare complication of laparoscopic adjustable gastric banding: bowel obstruction due to caecal volvulus. Obes Surg 2009; 19(8):1197–200.
33. Sherwinter DA, Powers CJ, Geiss AC, et al. Thrombosis of the Lap-Band system. Surg Endosc 2008;22(12):2635–7.
34. Srikanth MS, Oh KH, Keskey T, et al. Critical extreme anterior slippage (paragastric Richter's hernia) of the stomach after laparoscopic adjustable gastric banding: early recognition and prevention of gastric strangulation. Obes Surg 2005;15(2):207–15 [discussion: 215].
35. Nemni J. Severe chronic cough after Lap-Band gastric surgery. Can Respir J 2007;14(3):171–2.
36. Foletto M, De Marchi F, Bernante P, et al. Late gastric pouch necrosis after Lap-Band, treated by an individualized conservative approach. Obes Surg 2005; 15(10):1487–90.
37. Parameswaran R, Ferrando J, Sigurdsson A. Gastric bezoar complicating laparoscopic adjustable gastric banding with band slippage. Obes Surg 2006;16(12): 1683–4.
38. Veronelli A, Ranieri R, Laneri M, et al. Gastric bezoars after adjustable gastric banding. Obes Surg 2004;14(6):796–7.
39. White NB, Gibbs KE, Goodwin A, et al. Gastric bezoar complicating laparoscopic adjustable gastric banding, and review of literature. Obes Surg 2003;13(6): 948–50.
40. Keidar A, Carmon E, Szold A, et al. Port complications following laparoscopic adjustable gastric banding for morbid obesity. Obes Surg 2005;15(3):361–5.
41. Busetto L, Segato G, De Marchi F, et al. Outcome predictors in morbidly obese recipients of an adjustable gastric band. Obes Surg 2002;12(1):83–92.
42. Szold A, Abu-Abeid S. Laparoscopic adjustable silicone gastric banding for morbid obesity: results and complications in 715 patients. Surg Endosc 2002; 16(2):230–3.
43. Lattuada E, Zappa MA, Mozzi E, et al. Injection port and connecting tube complications after laparoscopic adjustable gastric banding. Obes Surg 2010;20(4):410–4.
44. Holloway JA, Forney GA, Gould DE. The Lap-Band is an effective tool for weight loss even in the United States. Am J Surg 2004;188(6):659–62.
45. Fransis K, Deweer F, Vanrykel JP, et al. Experience with laparoscopic adjustable gastric banding (La-Band system) up to 8 years. Acta Chir Belg 2005;105(1): 69–73.
46. Suter M, Dorta G, Giusti V, et al. Gastric banding interferes with esophageal motility and gastroesophageal reflux. Arch Surg 2005;140(7):639–43.

47. de Jong JR, van Ramshorst B, Timmer R, et al. The influence of laparoscopic adjustable gastric banding on gastroesophageal reflux. Obes Surg 2004;14(3): 399–406.
48. Merrouche M, Sabate JM, Jouet P, et al. Gastro-esophageal reflux and esophageal motility disorders in morbidly obese patients before and after bariatric surgery. Obes Surg 2007;17(7):894–900.
49. Varela JE. Barrett's esophagus: a late complication of laparoscopic adjustable gastric banding. Obes Surg 2010;20(2):244–6.
50. Snook KL, Ritchie JD. Carcinoma of esophagus after adjustable gastric banding. Obes Surg 2003;13(5):800–2.
51. Naef M, Mouton WG, Naef U, et al. Esophageal dysmotility disorders after laparoscopic gastric banding–an underestimated complication. Ann Surg 2010; 253(2):285–90.
52. Klaus A, Gruber I, Wetscher G, et al. Prevalent esophageal body motility disorders underlie aggravation of GERD symptoms in morbidly obese patients following adjustable gastric banding. Arch Surg 2006;141(3):247–51.
53. de Jong JR, Tiethof C, van Ramshorst B, et al. Esophageal dilation after laparoscopic adjustable gastric banding: a more systematic approach is needed. Surg Endosc 2009;23(12):2802–8.
54. Arias IE, Radulescu M, Stiegeler R, et al. Diagnosis and treatment of megaesophagus after adjustable gastric banding for morbid obesity. Surg Obes Relat Dis 2009;5(2):156–9.
55. Burton PR, Brown W, Laurie C, et al. The effect of laparoscopic adjustable gastric bands on esophageal motility and the gastroesophageal junction: analysis using high-resolution video manometry. Obes Surg 2009;19(7):905–14.
56. Burton PR, Brown WA, Laurie C, et al. Pathophysiology of laparoscopic adjustable gastric bands: analysis and classification using high-resolution video manometry and a stress barium protocol. Obes Surg 2010;20(1):19–29.
57. Ponce J, Lindsey B, Pritchett S, et al. New adjustable gastric bands available in the United States: a comparative study. Surg Obes Relat Dis 2011;7(1):74–9.
58. Tice JA, Karliner L, Walsh J, et al. Gastric banding or bypass? A systematic review comparing the two most popular bariatric procedures. Am J Med 2008; 121(10):885–93.
59. Egan RJ, Monkhouse SJ, Meredith HE, et al. The reporting of gastric band slip and related complications; a review of the literature. Obes Surg 2010;21(8):1280–8.
60. Singhal R, Bryant C, Kitchen M, et al. Band slippage and erosion after laparoscopic gastric banding: a meta-analysis. Surg Endosc 2010;24(12):2980–6.
61. Ponce J, Paynter S, Fromm R. Laparoscopic adjustable gastric banding: 1,014 consecutive cases. J Am Coll Surg 2005;201(4):529–35.
62. O'Brien PE, Dixon JB, Laurie C, et al. A prospective randomized trial of placement of the laparoscopic adjustable gastric band: comparison of the perigastric and pars flaccida pathways. Obes Surg 2005;15(6):820–6.
63. Singhal R, Kitchen M, Ndirika S, et al. The "Birmingham stitch"–avoiding slippage in laparoscopic gastric banding. Obes Surg 2008;18(4):359–63.
64. Spivak H, Rubin M. Laparoscopic management of lap-band slippage. Obes Surg 2003;13(1):116–20.
65. Jalil O, Zia MK, Hassn A, et al. Laparoscopic Nissen fundoplication for the management of failed Angelchik prosthesis. J Laparoendosc Adv Surg Tech A 2011;21(1):77–80.
66. Carbonell AM, Maher JW. Laparoscopic transgastric removal of an eroded Angelchik prosthesis. Am Surg 2006;72(8):724–6 [discussion: 727].

67. Florez DA, Howington JA, Long JD. Esophageal obstruction secondary to erosion of an Angelchik prosthesis: the role of endoscopic management. Gastrointest Endosc 2003;58(4):624–6.
68. Varshney S, Kelly JJ, Branagan G, et al. Angelchik prosthesis revisited. World J Surg 2002;26(1):129–33.
69. Plaisier PW, Lange JF. Successful laparoscopic removal of a migrated Angelchik prosthesis. Surg Endosc 2000;14(6):592.
70. Cherian PT, Goussous G, Ashori F, et al. Band erosion after laparoscopic gastric banding: a retrospective analysis of 865 patients over 5 years. Surg Endosc 2010;24(8):2031–8.
71. Neto MP, Ramos AC, Campos JM, et al. Endoscopic removal of eroded adjustable gastric band: lessons learned after 5 years and 78 cases. Surg Obes Relat Dis 2010;6(4):423–7.
72. Blero D, Eisendrath P, Vandermeeren A, et al. Endoscopic removal of dysfunctioning bands or rings after restrictive bariatric procedures. Gastrointest Endosc 2010;71(3):468–74.
73. Hinojosa MW, Varela JE, Parikh D, et al. National trends in use and outcome of laparoscopic adjustable gastric banding. Surg Obes Relat Dis 2009;5(2):150–5.
74. Angrisani L, Lorenzo M, Borrelli V. Laparoscopic adjustable gastric banding versus Roux-en-Y gastric bypass: 5-year results of a prospective randomized trial. Surg Obes Relat Dis 2007;3(2):127–32 [discussion: 132–3].
75. Boza C, Gamboa C, Perez G, et al. Laparoscopic adjustable gastric banding (LAGB): surgical results and 5-year follow-up. Surg Endosc 2011;25(1):292–7.
76. Gustavsson S, Westling A. Laparoscopic adjustable gastric banding: complications and side effects responsible for the poor long-term outcome. Semin Laparosc Surg 2002;9(2):115–24.
77. Muller MK, Attigah N, Wildi S, et al. High secondary failure rate of rebanding after failed gastric banding. Surg Endosc 2008;22(2):448–53.
78. Allen JW. Laparoscopic gastric band complications. Med Clin North Am 2007; 91(3):485–97, xii.

Sleeve Gastrectomy

Stacy A. Brethauer, MD

KEYWORDS

• Bariatric • Sleeve gastrectomy • Vertical gastrectomy

HISTORY

Sleeve gastrectomy (SG) was originally performed as the restrictive component of the duodenal switch procedure. This partial vertical gastrectomy served to reduce gastric capacity and initiate short-term weight loss while the malabsorptive component of the operation (biliopancreatic diversion) provided the long-term weight loss. Some patients, however, could not undergo the intestinal bypass, and early investigations found that substantial weight loss occurred with the SG alone. The sleeve then developed into a risk management strategy for very large or high-risk patients who would not tolerate a longer or higher-risk procedure.[1]

In this staged approach, patients' medical conditions improved in the 1 or 2 years after SG, and many subsequently underwent a second-stage bypass procedure (gastric bypass or duodenal switch). In a study by Cottam and colleagues,[2] 126 high-risk super-obese patients with a mean preoperative body mass index (BMI) of 65.3 kg/m^2 underwent laparoscopic SG (LSG) as a first-stage procedure. The mean excess weight loss at 1 year was 43% and significant reductions were seen in the number of comorbidities and American Society of Anesthesiologists classification before the second-stage gastric bypass procedure. In the past 10 years, SG has increasingly been used as a stand-alone primary bariatric procedure and has gained popularity among patients and bariatric surgeons. Rapid growth has been seen in the number of SGs performed in the past 5 years, and it currently accounts for more than 5% of all bariatric operations performed worldwide.[3]

TECHNIQUE

LSG involves a vertical gastrectomy that results in a narrow, tubular stomach. The concept of SG is simple, but some components of the operation, if performed incorrectly, can result in serious complications. Five ports are placed across the upper abdomen identical to placement for a gastric bypass. If exposure is difficult because of a large amount of perigastric fat or a large liver, a sixth port can be placed in the left

Disclosures: Dr Brethauer is a speaker, advisory board member, and consultant for Ethicon Endo-Surgery, a speaker for Covidien, and a consultant for Apollo Endosurgery.
Cleveland Clinic Lerner College of Medicine, Bariatric and Metabolic Institute, Cleveland Clinic, 9500 Euclid Avenue, M61, Cleveland, OH 44195, USA
E-mail address: brethas@ccf.org

Surg Clin N Am 91 (2011) 1265–1279
doi:10.1016/j.suc.2011.08.012
0039-6109/11/$ – see front matter © 2011 Elsevier Inc. All rights reserved.

upper quadrant for the assistant (**Fig. 1**). The operating surgeon stands to the patient's right side and uses a footboard and tapes the patient to the operating table for placement in a steep reverse Trendelenburg position during the procedure. The first step of the procedure is to divide the vascular attachments of the gastroepiploic arcade and the short gastric vessels. This dissection is performed with ultrasonic shears, and is started along the greater curvature and extended proximally to the angle of His and distally to within 4 cm of the pylorus. The stomach and fundus must be fully immobilized during the dissection. The filmy posterior attachments should be divided so the entire posterior surface of the stomach can be seen. After the short gastric vessels are divided at the upper pole of the spleen, the attachments between the fundus and the left crus of the diaphragm must also be taken down. This technique is important to

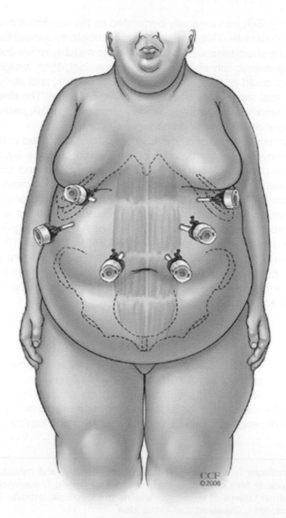

Fig. 1. Port placement for laparoscopic sleeve gastrectomy. The surgeon stands to the patient's right. The two middle ports are 12 mm and the lateral ports are 5 mm. (*Reprinted from* Cleveland Clinic Center for Medical Art & Photography © 2006–2011; with permission. All Rights Reserved.)

avoid leaving a large pouch of fundus at the top of the stomach and ensure that the gastroesophageal junction can be identified and avoided during the final staple firing.

Once this dissection is complete, the first stapler is placed tangentially across the antrum. The authors use green loads for the first two staple firings because of the increased thickness of the stomach in this area. The assistant should flatten the stomach with lateral retraction and the anesthesiologist should remove the temperature probe and orogastric tubes before the first staple firing. The angle of the first firing is determined by the patient's anatomy, but care should be taken to not use an angle that will narrow the lumen at the incisura. The authors fire the first staple load before placing the calibration tube and then close the stapler for the next firing, which helps guide the calibration tube distally into the antrum (**Fig. 2**). The authors use a diagnostic gastroscope (Olympus GIF-H180J, 9.9-mm outer diameter, Olympus, Center Valley, Pennsylvania) to calibrate the sleeve lumen and place the lighted tip of the scope into the antrum under laparoscopic guidance (no insufflation is used to place the endoscope initially).

If any concern exists that the lumen is too narrow at the incisura, the stapler is moved laterally before firing. This part of the procedure requires close attention, because a lumen that is too narrow at the incisura can result in severe dysphagia and food intolerance from stricture formation or, more commonly, kinking of the stomach in this area. Once the surgeon is satisfied with the lumen size, the stapler is fired. Blue loads of the stapler are then fired proximally along the calibration tube. Because the staple line is oversewn with an imbricating suture, several millimeters of lumen are left between the calibration tube (30 French gastroscope) and the staple line (ie, the calibration tube is not hugged tightly with the stapler). Care should be taken to create a straight staple line and avoid anterior or posterior "spiraling" of the staple line, which can also cause mechanical problems with the sleeve and can be avoided through good lateral retraction of the stomach by the assistant.

The position of the final staple firing is critical to avoid a leak. Leaving a significant portion of fundus will not be optimal in terms of weight loss or gastroesophageal reflux disease (GERD) in the long term, but care must be taken not to impinge on the gastroesophageal junction or esophagus during the final staple firing. Approximately 1 cm of gastric serosa should be seen to the left of the stapler cartridge before the stapler is fired. Mobilizing a large fat pad off of this area early in the case can help identify and avoid the gastroesophageal junction.

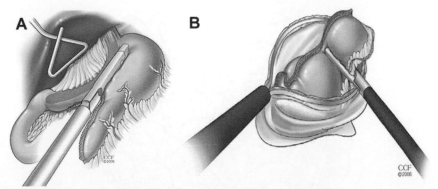

Fig. 2. The linear stapler is used to perform a vertical sleeve gastrectomy starting 4 cm from the pylorus. This technique is performed with a calibration tube in place (*A*). The resected gastric body and fundus are removed in a laparoscopic specimen bag (*B*). (*Reprinted from Cleveland Clinic Center for Medical Art & Photography © 2006–2011; with permission. All Rights Reserved.*)

The entire staple line is then oversewn with a continuous, imbricating suture. Caution must be taken not to imbricate too much tissue at the incisura, because this may also cause an obstruction in this area. If concern exists about the lumen size, a nonimbricating locking suture is placed in this area. After the suture line is completed, the endoscope is used to perform a leak test and evaluate the lumen for hemostasis and patency. Other methods of leak testing, such as the methylene blue dye test, can also be used, but the endoscopic view offers some reassurance that the lumen is uniform in size without obstruction. The omentum is then sewn to the entire suture line to provide another potential barrier if a leak occurs. Sewing the omentum or the gastrocolic fat back up to the distal sleeve may also anchor the sleeve and prevent kinking at the incisura. A closed-suction drain is placed under the omentum with its tip above the spleen. The 12-mm port sites are closed with a suture passer and the resected stomach is placed in a specimen bag and removed from the abdomen. **Fig. 3** shows the completed sleeve gastrectomy.

OUTCOMES
Weight Loss

The weight loss outcomes after SG have varied according to the population studied. Initial reports of SG used this operation to downstage high-risk medical patients

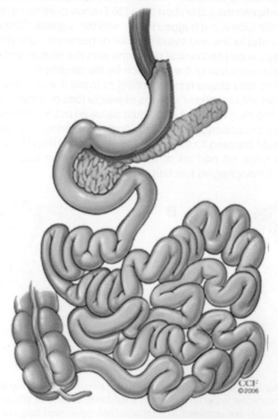

Fig. 3. Completed sleeve gastrectomy. (*Reprinted from* Cleveland Clinic Center for Medical Art & Photography © 2006–2011; with permission. All Rights Reserved.)

or super-obese patients before a staged bypass procedure.[1,2,4–14] Because many of these patients subsequently underwent a planned second-stage procedure, most of the early reports of SG did not provide follow-up beyond 1 or 2 years. As more experience was gained with this operation, many surgeons found it to be an effective primary bariatric procedure for patients with a lower BMI, and the more recent literature reflect this shift.[5,15–37] With this increasing experience over the past 5 years, longer-term outcome data are now emerging.

A systematic review of 36 studies recently evaluated overall weight loss after SG, and also assessed weight loss for the staged and primary patient groups.[38] The mean preoperative BMI for all patients included in the systematic review was 51.2 kg/m^2, and decreased to 37.1 kg/m^2 during the reported follow-up periods, which were predominantly 3 years or less. The mean excess weight loss (EWL) after SG was reported in 24 studies (n = 1662) and ranged from 33% to 85%, with an overall mean EWL of 55.4%. The mean preoperative BMI was 60.0 kg/m^2 (range, 49.1–69.0 kg/m^2) for the staged/high-risk patient group, and 46.6 kg/m^2 (range, 37.2–54.5 kg/m^2) for the patients undergoing SG as a primary procedure. The reduction in BMI and the EWL reported after SG in these two groups is shown in **Table 1**.

Several studies compare SG with other bariatric procedures. In a randomized, controlled trial comparing LSG and laparoscopic adjustable gastric banding, Himpens and colleagues[22] reported greater EWL (66% vs 48%; P = .025), greater loss of hunger (46.7% of patients vs 2.9%), and greater loss of craving for sweets

Table 1
Outcomes of sleeve gastrectomy in high-risk/staged patients versus primary procedure

	High-Risk Patients/Staged Approach[1,2,4–14]	Primary Procedure[5,15–37]
Number of studies[a] (number of patients)	13 (821)	24 (1749)
Preoperative BMI range (mean) kg/m^2	49.1–69.0 (60.0)	37.2–54.5 (46.6)
Postoperative BMI range (mean) kg/m^2	36.4–53.0 (44.9)	26.0–39.8 (32.2)
Follow-up	4 mo to 5 y	3 mo to 3 y
Percent excess weight loss range (mean)	33.0%–61.4% (46.9) IVW mean = 46.6% (43.8%–49.5%)	36.0%–85.0% (60.4) IVW mean = 60.7% (55.1%–66.3%)
Complication rate all studies (mean)	0–23.8% (9.4%)	0–21.7% (6.2%)
Studies with n>100	3.3%–15.3%	0–14.1%
Leaks[b]	8/686 (1.2%)	45/1681 (2.7%)[c]
Bleeding[b]	11/686 (1.6%)	17/1681 (1.0%)[d]
Strictures[b]	6/686 (0.9%)	9/1681 (0.5%)
Mortality	2/821 (0.24%)	3/1749 (0.17%)

Abbreviation: IVW, inverse variance weighted.
[a] One study included clearly defined patients in both groups.
[b] Includes studies with detailed complication data only.
[c] P = .02 compared with high-risk group.
[d] P not significant compared with high-risk groups.
From Brethauer SA. Systematic review of sleeve gastrectomy as staging and primary bariatric procedure. Surg Obes Relat Dis 2009;5:473; with permission.

(23.3% of patients vs 2.9%) in patients treated with LSG at 3 years. Two patients in that trial (5%) experienced insufficient weight loss 3 years after LSG and underwent a duodenal switch.

Another small randomized trial also showed superior weight loss and decreased ghrelin levels 6 months after LSG compared with laparoscopic adjustable gastric banding.[39]

Several studies have compared LSG and Roux-en-Y gastric bypass (RYGB). In a prospective, double-blind study with 16 patients in each group, Karamanakos and colleagues[23] reported better weight loss with LSG at 1 year compared with RYGB (EWL, 69.7% vs 60.5%, respectively; $P = .05$). The authors attributed this difference to more pronounced changes in specific gut hormones after the sleeve, resulting in decreased hunger. In a nonrandomized study, Vidal and colleagues[37] matched patients who were treated with LSG (n = 39) and RYGB (n = 52) for duration and severity of diabetes and, 1 year after surgery, found that weight loss was similar for the groups (31% of initial weight).

Despite being widely adopted in the past 5 years, the long-term durability of SG has remained a concern. Weiner and colleagues[14] published the first 5-year weight loss data in 2007, reporting their weight loss outcomes related to the calibration of the sleeve as their practice evolved. In their early experience, no calibration tube was used and they subsequently used a 40 French and then a 32 French Bougie to create a tighter sleeve. They also measured the volume of the resected stomach and the sleeve volume intraoperatively. After 2 years, patients who had tube calibration of their sleeve had better weight loss than those who underwent the uncalibrated procedures. They also reported that a volume of the resected stomach less than 500 mL predicted weight loss failure or weight regain. Overall, BMI decreased from 60.7 to 45.0 kg/m^2. A trend has been seen in the literature toward using smaller calibration tubes as more primary procedures are performed, and Weiner's study presents compelling data that long-term weight loss success is related to the calibration of the sleeve. Similar findings related to calibration were reported with the Magenstrasse and Mill procedure (a nonresectional form of the vertical sleeve procedure), in which weight regain was noted with larger calibration tubes early in the investigators' experience, prompting the use of smaller calibration tubes over time to achieve durable weight loss.[40]

Since the publication of the systematic review in 2009,[38] several important studies have been published that report longer-term follow-up (**Table 2**). Himpens and colleagues[41] reported long-term weight loss data on 41 patients who underwent SG intended as a primary procedure. These patients were not part of the randomized trial comparing LSG and adjustable banding. The median preoperative BMI in this study

Table 2
Long-term results after sleeve gastrectomy

Author	Patients (n)	Preoperative BMI	Follow-Up	Weight Loss
Johnston et al[40] (M+M procedure)	16	46	5 y	61% EWL
Weiner et al[14]	8	62	5 y	−17 BMI
Himpens et al[41]	41	39	6 y	53% EWL
Bohdjalian et al[42]	26	48	5 y	55% EWL
Eid et al[56]	69	66	6 y	52% EWL

Abbreviations: BMI, body mass index; EBMI, excess body mass index; EWL, excess weight loss; M+M, Magenstrasse and Mill.

was 39 kg/m^2. At 3 years after surgery, the mean EWL overall was 72.8%, and after the sixth year of follow-up the mean EWL overall was 57.3%. Eleven patients underwent a second-stage duodenal switch procedure and improved their EWL to 70.8% at 6 years (mean BMI 27 kg/m^2). The stand-alone LSG patient group (n = 30) had a 53% EWL and a mean BMI of 31 kg/m^2 at 6 years. This report shows that some patients regain weight long-term after LSG when it is used as a primary procedure, and that weight loss can be improved with a second-stage procedure in selected patients. Despite these issues, patient acceptance of the LSG procedure remained good at 6+ years in this study.

Another report of long-term outcomes after LSG was recently published by Bohdjalian and colleagues.[42] The authors provide 5-year weight loss data for 26 patients who underwent LSG. Mean BMI before surgery was 48.2 kg/m^2 and one-third of the patients were super-obese (BMI>50 kg/m^2). Mean EWL at 5 years was 55%. Four patients (15%) underwent a second-stage gastric bypass for weight regain (n = 3) and GERD (n = 1).

Comorbidity Improvement

Diabetes remission has been reported to different degrees after all of the currently performed bariatric procedures. A recent systematic review by Gill and colleagues[43] evaluated the rates of diabetes improvement after SG and found 28 studies that met their inclusion criteria. The patient population included 673 patients with a mean preoperative BMI of 47.4 kg/m^2. In this analysis, LSG resulted in diabetes remission in 66.2% of patients. Of those studies that reported improvement and remission of diabetes, 97% of patients had either improvement or remission. The mean hemoglobin A1c (HbA1c) decreased from 7.9 to 6.2 in the 11 studies that included this measure of glucose control.

A randomized, controlled trial by Lee and colleagues[44] from Taiwan compared gastric bypass (n = 30) and SG (n = 30) for the treatment of type 2 diabetes (remission defined as fasting glucose <126 mg/dL and HbA1c <6.5% off glycemic therapy). LSG resulted in remission of diabetes in 47% of patients at 1 year and was associated with an average 3% reduction in HbA1c levels. Gastric bypass, however, had more powerful effects on weight loss, waist circumference, the remission rate of type 2 diabetes (93%), and improvements in the metabolic syndrome in this study. In an analysis of patients undergoing LSG and RYGB who were matched for severity and duration of diabetes, Vidal and colleagues[37] found that both groups had 84% remission of diabetes and comparable rates of resolution of the metabolic syndrome at 1 year (62% for SG; 67% for RYGB).

Improvement in other major obesity-related comorbidities after LSG are shown in **Fig. 4.** In addition to improvements in the components of the metabolic syndrome, significant improvement or resolution of sleep apnea, joint pain, depression, and leg edema have been reported.[2,10,12,14,24,27]

MECHANISMS OF ACTION

The mechanisms of action through which SG produces early satiety, hunger control, and improvement in metabolic parameters are still controversial. Initially thought to be a purely restrictive operation, some studies reporting changes in gut hormones and the metabolic effects of this procedure have challenged that concept. Ghrelin, an orexigenic hormone produced primarily in the gastric fundus, is significantly decreased after SG[39] and this decrease has been shown to persist 5 years after the procedure.[42] Although ghrelin may affect changes in hunger, satiety, and even

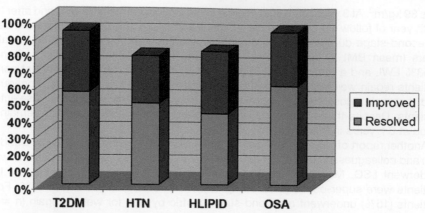

Fig. 4. Improvement and remission rates of major comorbidities after sleeve gastrectomy. HLIPID, hyperlipidemia; HTN, hypertension; OSA, obstructive sleep apnea; T2DM, type 2 diabetes mellitus. (*Data from* Brethauer SA, Hammel JP, Schauer PR. Systematic review of sleeve gastrectomy as staging and primary bariatric procedure. Surg Obes Relat Dis 2009;5:469–75.)

glucose metabolism after SG, it is unlikely the only mechanism that contributes to the long-term effects of this procedure.

Rapid nutrient transit to the distal bowel is one of the mechanisms responsible for early satiety and improvements in glucose metabolism after gastric bypass. These effects are mediated by gut hormones (PYY$_{3-36}$ and GLP-1) produced in the L cells located in the distal bowel. Evidence shows that nutrient transit is also increased after SG. Melissas and colleagues[26,45] showed increased gastric emptying after SG, and this rapid transit of solid food to the distal bowel may have similar effects on the L cell mass as the gastric bypass. In a small randomized trial comparing RYGB and LSG, Karamanakos and colleagues[23] showed similar increases in fasting and post-prandial PYY$_{3-36}$ after these two procedures. Weight loss was greater at 12 months after LSG in this study (69.7% vs 60.5%; $P = .05$), however, and the investigators attributed this to the lower ghrelin levels and decreased appetite seen after LSG compared with RYGB. Although further studies are needed to define the mechanisms of weight loss and diabetes remission after LSG, early evidence suggests that this operation has metabolic effects beyond weight loss.

COMPLICATIONS

Leaks are the most concerning complication after SG. The most common site of a leak is near the angle of His or at the gastroesophageal junction. This complication may be from placement of the final staple line across the gastroesophageal junction or distal esophagus with resultant staple line disruption. Another potential factor that can contribute to a proximal leak is mid-sleeve stenosis. This complication can be from a truly stenotic lumen or, more commonly, twisting or kinking of the sleeve at the incisura that causes a functional obstruction. This relative downstream obstruction in the setting of a proximal leak can lead to a persistent fistula that does not resolve with conservative management (**Fig. 5**). Leaks occur less than 2% of the time in most published series, and the leak rates associated with primary and staged SG are shown in **Table 1**. The higher leak rate reported among primary procedures performed in

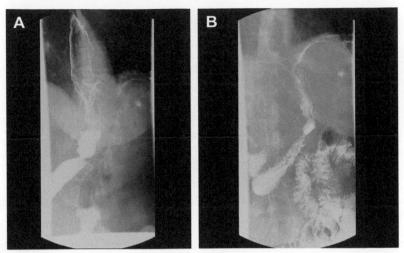

Fig. 5. Upper gastrointestinal contrast study showing extravasation of contrast from the upper stomach into the left subphrenic space (*A*). Stenosis of the mid portion of the sleeve is present where the barium tablet is lodged (*B*).

patients with lower BMIs may be related to some of the authors reporting their early experience with this procedure (several multicenter studies in this group included lower case volumes with higher complication rates).

A high index of suspicion and early identification of leaks after LSG are critical to achieving an acceptable outcome after this complication. Unexplained tachycardia, fevers, abdominal pain, or persistent hiccups after the procedure should alert surgeons to investigate for a leak. The authors perform routine upper gastrointestinal contrast studies the morning after the procedure to evaluate for leaks before starting the patient on clear liquids. This approach, however, should be at the discretion of the surgeon, and no compelling evidence shows that routine imaging is warranted. If the surgeon becomes concerned about a leak and a drain was left in place at the time of surgery, the drain fluid can be sent for an amylase level. If the fluid amylase level is much higher than normal serum levels (in the 1000s), this suggests that saliva is entering the drain. Regardless of the drain amylase level, early imaging is warranted if clinical suspicion of a leak exists. Upper gastrointestinal contrast studies are often ordered first, but CT scans can provide more information about fluid collections in the left upper quadrant (**Fig. 6**).

The management of the leak depends on the patient's clinical condition. The surgeon managing this complication must have a clear treatment strategy or algorithm based on the patient's status, the duration of the leak, and the resources available.[46,47] If the leak presents as a well-defined abscess several days or weeks after surgery and the patient is clinically stable, percutaneous image-guided drainage, antibiotics, and nutritional support with parenteral nutrition or a nasojejunal tube is appropriate.[48] If drainage is adequate, endoluminal therapies can be used to facilitate closure of the leak. This process often includes placement of endoscopic clips, fibrin glue, or bioabsorbable fistula plugs, and endoluminal stenting across the leak. Stenting has been shown to be effective in small series of selected cases,[48–51] but results can be variable depending on the size and duration of the leak. Although placement of self-expanding, covered, or partially covered stents (Polyflex or Wallflex stents,

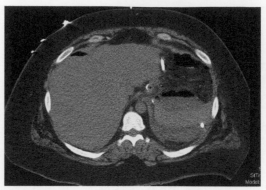

Fig. 6. CT scan of a postoperative leak after sleeve gastrectomy resulting in a left upper quadrant abscess.

Boston Scientific, Natick, Massachusetts) may be beneficial,[50] the current stent technology is not ideal for this anatomy that involves two different lumen diameters with curvature of the gastric lumen (**Fig. 7**). Before attempts at stenting, the extraluminal collection must be adequately addressed in all cases and surgical placement of drains

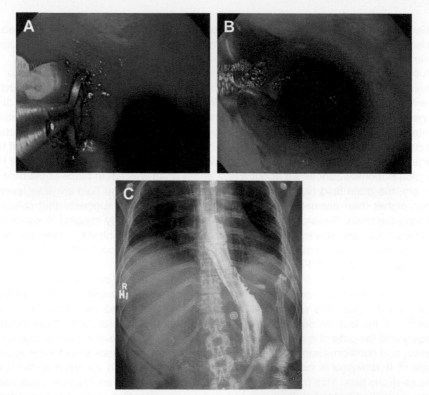

Fig. 7. Endoscopic placement of fibrin glue and clips across a small leak at the gastroesophageal junction after sleeve gastrectomy (*A*) followed by placement of a stent across the leak (*B*). Follow-up contrast study after stenting shows a small persistent leak of contrast refluxing up around the stent (*C*).

with washout of the infected field is often warranted to promote closure of the leak. Because successful outcomes after stenting often occur in carefully selected patients, evidence is currently insufficient to make any broad claims that stenting accelerates or promotes closure of leaks for all patients. Nevertheless, stenting may be a useful therapeutic adjunct in some patients and is associated with little risk. One advantage of stent placement in these patients is that it may allow patients to resume oral intake while the leak heals.

Patients who are manifesting signs of sepsis or are unstable should be managed operatively with laparoscopy or laparotomy. Drainage and washout of the infected collection and wide drainage of the area is the primary goal of the operation. Primary closure of the defect can be performed if discovered early, but the surrounding inflammatory reaction typically prohibits effective closure of the hole. Closed suction or sump drains should be placed and the omentum can be sewn over the defect to help contain the contamination. If the patient is stable during the case, a feeding jejunostomy should be placed for long-term enteral access.

A chronic fistula after LSG is a challenging problem. If a leak or gastrocutaneous fistula persists for months despite adequate surgical drainage, endoluminal therapy, and nutritional support, reoperation may be the only solution. The patient's gastrointestinal anatomy should be evaluated for a distal obstruction or stricture that would also jeopardize any revisional procedure. Several surgical options have been reported for these chronic fistulas, including resection of the proximal stomach with the fistula and creation of a Roux-en-Y esophagojejunostomy, bringing a Roux limb up and creating a gastrojejunal anastomosis directly on the leak site, placing a jejunal patch over the leak site, or placing a T tube into the leak site.[47,52] Evidence is insufficient to support one approach over another, and the type of salvage procedure should be determined by the patient's anatomy and the surgeon's judgment and experience.

Bleeding complications requiring transfusion or reoperation occur less than 2% of the time after LSG. Common sites of bleeding include the sleeve staple line, short gastric vessels, the spleen, and omental vessels that have been divided during the dissection of the greater curvature. Some evidence suggests that the use of staple-line buttressing can decrease intraoperative and postoperative blood loss after LSG, but these studies include small numbers of patients and do not provide definitive evidence that staple-line reinforcement is superior to oversewing or no reinforcement in terms of preventing postoperative complications.[53,54]

Strictures requiring endoscopic dilation or surgical revision occur less than 1% of the time after SG. The most common site of luminal narrowing is at the incisura. Although true strictures can occur, this problem after LSG is typically not a true mucosal or luminal stricture as much as it is an angulation or kinking of the stomach in this area (**Fig. 8**). This functional obstruction presents as persistent dysphagia to solids and liquids, with nausea and vomiting. When creating the SG initially, this complication can be prevented through avoiding sharp angulation of the staple line and allowing for adequate lumen size as the stapler approaches the incisura. Treatment includes symptom control with antiemetics and repeated endoscopic balloon dilations of the area. Laparoscopic seromyotomy has been reported to treat long strictures that are refractory to dilation[55] and conversion to gastric bypass is occasionally necessary to alleviate the obstruction.

GERD remains a concern after SG, and the onset of severe refractory GERD after LSG may be an indication to revise the procedure to gastric bypass. Often early improvement of GERD symptoms occurs after LSG,[22] but late onset of GERD symptoms has been reported after LSG. In the report by Himpens and colleagues[41] with 6-year follow-up, the overall incidence of new-onset GERD (defined as symptoms

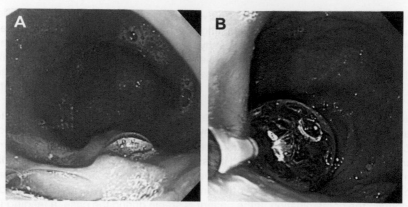

Fig. 8. Endoscopic view of a narrowing at the incisura after sleeve gastrectomy in a patient with persistent postoperative nausea and dysphagia (A). The scope passed easily through this area, but the angulation of the lumen resulted in a functional obstruction. Repeated endoscopic dilations were performed to alleviate her symptoms (B).

requiring proton pump inhibitor use) was 26%. The investigators attribute some of the new-onset GERD symptoms to the appearance of a neofundus (dilated pouch of fundus at the proximal sleeve) that occasionally requires reoperation. In patients in whom this dilated fundus was resected, GERD symptoms improved. Additionally, after 5 years of follow-up in the study by Bohdjalian and colleagues,[42] 31% of patients were taking chronic acid suppression medication for GERD. This long-term complication must be evaluated further with objective testing, but the possibility of new or recurrent GERD symptoms should be considered when discussing this procedure with patients.

The overall 30-day mortality rate in the published literature (n = 2570 patients) includes five deaths, for an overall mortality rate of 0.19%.[38] The mortality rates for the staged/high-risk and primary groups are shown in **Table 1**.

SUMMARY

LSG is an accepted bariatric procedure that can be used for many different patient populations. It has been effectively used as part of a staged risk-management strategy for high-risk patients and has gained popularity as a primary bariatric procedure. The evidence supporting the safety and efficacy of SG continues to increase and long-term data are emerging that report excess weight loss greater than 50%. A second-stage gastric bypass or duodenal switch promotes further weight loss in selected patients with weight regain or inadequate weight loss after LSG. Attractive features of LSG are rapid weight loss, comorbidity reduction, and avoidance of long-term complications of bypass procedures or implantable devices. Concerns remain regarding the risks of leak after LSG, the long-term incidence of GERD symptoms, and weight loss durability beyond 5 years. Management of leaks after LSG is a formidable challenge for the bariatric surgeon, and early diagnosis followed by a multidisciplinary treatment strategy is key. The precise mechanism of sustained weight loss and diabetes remission after SG is unclear, but early evidence suggests that this is a metabolic procedure that affects nutrient transit, gut hormones, and the enteroinsular axis in a favorable way.

REFERENCES

1. Regan JP, Inabnet WB, Gagner M, et al. Early experience with two-stage laparoscopic Roux-en-Y gastric bypass as an alternative in the super-super obese patient. Obes Surg 2003;13:861–4.
2. Cottam D, Qureshi FG, Mattar SG, et al. Laparoscopic sleeve gastrectomy as an initial weight-loss procedure for high-risk patients with morbid obesity. Surg Endosc 2006;20:859–63.
3. Buchwald H, Oien DM. Metabolic/bariatric surgery worldwide 2008. Obes Surg 2009;19:1605–11.
4. Almogy G, Crookes PF, Anthone GJ. Longitudinal gastrectomy as a treatment for the high-risk super-obese patient. Obes Surg 2004;14:492–7.
5. Baltasar A, Serra C, Perez N, et al. Laparoscopic sleeve gastrectomy: a multipurpose bariatric operation. Obes Surg 2005;15:1124–8.
6. Gagner M, Gumbs AA, Milone L, et al. Laparoscopic sleeve gastrectomy for the super-super-obese (body mass index >60 kg/m(2)). Surg Today 2008;38:399–408.
7. Hamoui N, Anthone GJ, Kaufman HS, et al. Sleeve gastrectomy in the high-risk patient. Obes Surg 2006;16:1445–9.
8. Milone L, Strong V, Gagner M. Laparoscopic sleeve gastrectomy is superior to endoscopic intragastric balloon as a first stage procedure for super-obese patients (BMI > or = 50). Obes Surg 2005;15:612–7.
9. Mognol P, Chosidow D, Marmuse JP. Laparoscopic sleeve gastrectomy as an initial bariatric operation for high-risk patients: initial results in 10 patients. Obes Surg 2005;15:1030–3.
10. Ou Yang O, Loi K, Liew V, et al. Staged laparoscopic sleeve gastrectomy followed by Roux-en-Y gastric bypass for morbidly obese patients: a risk reduction strategy. Obes Surg 2008;18:1575–80.
11. Parikh M, Gagner M, Heacock L, et al. Laparoscopic sleeve gastrectomy: does bougie size affect mean %EWL? Short-term outcomes. Surg Obes Relat Dis 2008;4:528–33.
12. Silecchia G, Boru C, Pecchia A, et al. Effectiveness of laparoscopic sleeve gastrectomy (first stage of biliopancreatic diversion with duodenal switch) on co-morbidities in super-obese high-risk patients. Obes Surg 2006;16:1138–44.
13. Takata MC, Campos GM, Ciovica R, et al. Laparoscopic bariatric surgery improves candidacy in morbidly obese patients awaiting transplantation. Surg Obes Relat Dis 2008;4:159–64.
14. Weiner RA, Weiner S, Pomhoff I, et al. Laparoscopic sleeve gastrectomy—influence of sleeve size and resected gastric volume. Obes Surg 2007;17:1297–305.
15. Braghetto I, Korn O, Valladares H, et al. Laparoscopic sleeve gastrectomy: surgical technique, indications and clinical results. Obes Surg 2007;17:1442–50.
16. Dapri G, Vaz C, Cadiere GB, et al. A prospective randomized study comparing two different techniques for laparoscopic sleeve gastrectomy. Obes Surg 2007; 17:1435–41.
17. Felberbauer FX, Langer F, Shakeri-Manesch S, et al. Laparoscopic sleeve gastrectomy as an isolated bariatric procedure: intermediate-term results from a large series in three Austrian centers. Obes Surg 2008;18:814–8.
18. Frezza EE, Reddy S, Gee LL, et al. Complications after sleeve gastrectomy for morbid obesity. Obes Surg 2009;19(6):684–7.
19. Fuks D, Verhaeghe P, Brehant O, et al. Results of laparoscopic sleeve gastrectomy: a prospective study in 135 patients with morbid obesity. Surgery 2009; 145:106–13.

20. Gan SS, Talbot ML, Jorgensen JO. Efficacy of surgery in the management of obesity-related type 2 diabetes mellitus. ANZ J Surg 2007;77:958–62.

21. Hakeam HA, O'Regan PJ, Salem AM, et al. Inhibition of C-reactive protein in morbidly obese patients after laparoscopic sleeve gastrectomy. Obes Surg 2009;19(4):456–60.

22. Himpens J, Dapri G, Cadiere GB. A prospective randomized study between laparoscopic gastric banding and laparoscopic isolated sleeve gastrectomy: results after 1 and 3 years. Obes Surg 2006;16:1450–6.

23. Karamanakos SN, Vagenas K, Kalfarentzos F, et al. Weight loss, appetite suppression, and changes in fasting and postprandial ghrelin and peptide-YY levels after Roux-en-Y gastric bypass and sleeve gastrectomy: a prospective, double blind study. Ann Surg 2008;247:401–7.

24. Kasalicky M, Michalsky D, Housova J, et al. Laparoscopic sleeve gastrectomy without an over-sewing of the staple line. Obes Surg 2008;18(10):1257–62.

25. Lee CM, Cirangle PT, Jossart GH. Vertical gastrectomy for morbid obesity in 216 patients: report of two-year results. Surg Endosc 2007;21(10):1810–6.

26. Melissas J, Koukouraki S, Askoxylakis J, et al. Sleeve gastrectomy: a restrictive procedure? Obes Surg 2007;17:57–62.

27. Moon Han S, Kim WW, Oh JH. Results of laparoscopic sleeve gastrectomy (LSG) at 1 year in morbidly obese Korean patients. Obes Surg 2005;15:1469–75.

28. Mui WL, Ng EK, Tsung BY, et al. Laparoscopic sleeve gastrectomy in ethnic obese Chinese. Obes Surg 2008;18(12):1571–4.

29. Nocca D, Krawczykowsky D, Bomans B, et al. A prospective multicenter study of 163 sleeve gastrectomies: results at 1 and 2 years. Obes Surg 2008;18:560–5.

30. Quesada BM, Roff HE, Kohan G, et al. Laparoscopic sleeve gastrectomy as an alternative to gastric bypass in patients with multiple intraabdominal adhesions. Obes Surg 2008;18:566–8.

31. Rubin M, Yehoshua RT, Stein M, et al. Laparoscopic sleeve gastrectomy with minimal morbidity early results in 120 morbidly obese patients. Obes Surg 2008;18(12):1567–70.

32. Skrekas G, Lapatsanis D, Stafyla V, et al. One year after laparoscopic "tight" sleeve gastrectomy: technique and outcome. Obes Surg 2008;18:810–3.

33. Stroh C, Birk D, Flade-Kuthe R, et al. Results of sleeve gastrectomy-data from a nationwide survey on bariatric surgery in Germany. Obes Surg 2009;19(5):632–40.

34. Tagaya N, Kasama K, Kikkawa R, et al. Experience with laparoscopic sleeve gastrectomy for morbid versus super morbid obesity. Obes Surg 2009;19(10):1371–6.

35. Tucker ON, Szomstein S, Rosenthal RJ. Indications for sleeve gastrectomy as a primary procedure for weight loss in the morbidly obese. J Gastrointest Surg 2008;12:662–7.

36. Uglioni B, Wolnerhanssen B, Peters T, et al. Midterm results of primary vs. secondary laparoscopic sleeve gastrectomy (LSG) as an isolated operation. Obes Surg 2009;19(4):401–46.

37. Vidal J, Ibarzabal A, Romero F, et al. Type 2 diabetes mellitus and the metabolic syndrome following sleeve gastrectomy in severely obese subjects. Obes Surg 2008;18:1077–82.

38. Brethauer SA, Hammel JP, Schauer PR. Systematic review of sleeve gastrectomy as staging and primary bariatric procedure. Surg Obes Relat Dis 2009;5:469–75.

39. Langer FB, Reza Hoda MA, Bohdjalian A, et al. Sleeve gastrectomy and gastric banding: effects on plasma ghrelin levels. Obes Surg 2005;15:1024–9.

40. Johnston D, Dachtler J, Sue-Ling HM, et al. The Magenstrasse and Mill operation for morbid obesity. Obes Surg 2003;13:10–6.
41. Himpens J, Dobbeleir J, Peeters G. Long-term results of laparoscopic sleeve gastrectomy for obesity. Ann Surg 2010;252:319–24.
42. Bohdjalian A, Langer FB, Shakeri-Leidenmuhler S, et al. Sleeve gastrectomy as sole and definitive bariatric procedure: 5-year results for weight loss and ghrelin. Obes Surg 2010;20:535–40.
43. Gill RS, Birch DW, Shi X, et al. Sleeve gastrectomy and type 2 diabetes mellitus: a systematic review. Surg Obes Relat Dis 2010;6:707–13.
44. Lee WJ, Chong K, Ser KH, et al. Gastric bypass vs sleeve gastrectomy for type 2 diabetes mellitus: a randomized controlled trial. Arch Surg 2011;146:143–8.
45. Melissas J, Daskalakis M, Koukouraki S, et al. Sleeve gastrectomy-a "food limiting" operation. Obes Surg 2008;18:1251–6.
46. Lalor PF, Tucker ON, Szomstein S, et al. Complications after laparoscopic sleeve gastrectomy. Surg Obes Relat Dis 2008;4:33–8.
47. Tan JT, Kariyawasam S, Wijeratne T, et al. Diagnosis and management of gastric leaks after laparoscopic sleeve gastrectomy for morbid obesity. Obes Surg 2010; 20:403–9.
48. Casella G, Soricelli E, Rizzello M, et al. Nonsurgical treatment of staple line leaks after laparoscopic sleeve gastrectomy. Obes Surg 2009;19:821–6.
49. de Aretxabala X, Leon J, Wiedmaier G, et al. Gastric leak after sleeve gastrectomy: analysis of its management. Obes Surg 2011;21(8):1232–7.
50. Eubanks S, Edwards CA, Fearing NM, et al. Use of endoscopic stents to treat anastomotic complications after bariatric surgery. J Am Coll Surg 2008;206: 935–8.
51. Nguyen NT, Nguyen XM, Dholakia C. The use of endoscopic stent in management of leaks after sleeve gastrectomy. Obes Surg 2010;20:1289–92.
52. Court I, Wilson A, Benotti P, et al. T-tube gastrostomy as a novel approach for distal staple line disruption after sleeve gastrectomy for morbid obesity: case report and review of the literature. Obes Surg 2010;20:519–22.
53. Consten EC, Gagner M, Pomp A, et al. Decreased bleeding after laparoscopic sleeve gastrectomy with or without duodenal switch for morbid obesity using a stapled buttressed absorbable polymer membrane. Obes Surg 2004;14: 1360–6.
54. Dapri G, Cadiere GB, Himpens J. Reinforcing the staple line during laparoscopic sleeve gastrectomy: prospective randomized clinical study comparing three different techniques. Obes Surg 2010;20:462–7.
55. Dapri G, Cadiere GB, Himpens J. Laparoscopic seromyotomy for long stenosis after sleeve gastrectomy with or without duodenal switch. Obes Surg 2009;19: 495–9.
56. Eid G, Brethaner SA, Mattar SG, et al. Laparoscopic sleeve gastrectomy: outcomes after 6–8 years with 93% follow-up. Abstract 23rd Annual International Consensal Summit for Sleeve Gastrectomy. New York, NY, 2010.

Biliopancreatic Diversion with Duodenal Switch

Ranjan Sudan, MD[a],*, Danny O. Jacobs, MD, MPH[b]

KEYWORDS

- Bariatric • Biliopancreatic diversion
- Duodenal switch • Obesity

HISTORY

The biliopancreatic diversion with duodenal switch (BPD-DS) is often referred to as the duodenal switch operation and is a modification of the original biliopancreatic diversion described by Scopinaro in 1979.[1] The essential difference between these two operations is that in the BPD-DS version, a sleeve gastrectomy is performed and the pylorus is preserved, whereas in the original Scopinaro operation, a distal gastrectomy sacrifices the pylorus. In both operations, the stomach pouch has a capacity of 250 mL and malabsorption results from a distal Roux-en-Y reconstruction of the bowel, with a common channel of 50 to 100 cm and an alimentary limb of 250 cm.[2,3] The Scopinaro BPD has excellent long-term weight loss[4] but, unlike the BPD-DS, has a greater risk of postgastrectomy symptoms that are related to the distal gastrectomy, including diarrhea, dumping, and marginal ulceration.

Postgastrectomy syndrome, which includes anastomotic ulceration, early and late dumping, bowel disturbance, and nutritional deficiencies, has been a problem with other general surgical operations, such as the Billroth hemigastrectomy or the radical pancreatoduodenectomy (Whipple procedure). To avoid these symptoms, several surgeons considered preserving the pylorus. Longmire and Traverso described the pylorus-preserving Whipple procedure in 1978.[5] Critchlow, in 1985, bypassed the duodenum beyond the pylorus to reduce mortality associated with a duodenal diverticulectomy.[6] In 1987, DeMeester, when conducting experiments for reflux disease in dogs, demonstrated that preserving the pylorus prevented marginal ulceration.[7] In bariatric surgery, Marceau and colleagues[8] were the first to describe a reduction in postgastrectomy symptoms associated with the BPD by preserving the pylorus in

The authors have nothing to disclose.
a Department of Surgery, Duke University Medical Center, Box 2834, Durham, NC 27710, USA
b Department of Surgery, Duke University Medical Center, Duke University School of Medicine, Box 3704, Suite 7690 HAFS 7th floor, Durham, NC 27710, USA
* Corresponding author.
E-mail address: ranjan.sudan@duke.edu

Surg Clin N Am 91 (2011) 1281–1293
doi:10.1016/j.suc.2011.08.015
0039-6109/11/$ – see front matter © 2011 Elsevier Inc. All rights reserved.

surgical.theclinics.com

1993. They modified the Scopinaro BPD by making a tube along the lesser curvature of the stomach, preserving the pylorus, and stapling the duodenum shut proximal to the ampulla of Vater. The first part of the duodenum was then anastomosed to the alimentary limb enabling gastric contents to bypass the pancreatic and biliary secretions. This operation was successful in reducing postgastrectomy symptoms; but the duodenal staple line broke down, and the continuity with the rest of the duodenum was reestablished in several patients.[8] Hess and Hess, in 1988, preserved the pylorus and completely divided the first part of the duodenum by cutting across it in a patient with a failed horizontal stapled gastroplasty and, later that year, performed the same operation as a primary bariatric procedure but they did not publish their results until 10 years later, in 1998.[9] That year, Marceau and colleagues[3] also published their results of the BPD-DS with a divided duodenum and demonstrated that weight loss was equivalent but the postgastrectomy symptoms were significantly reduced compared with the BPD. These findings contributed to the BPD-DS becoming the preferred version of the operation in North America.

The BPD-DS has traditionally been performed by midline laparotomy, and although the first laparoscopic Roux-en-Y gastric bypass was described by Wittgrove and colleagues[10] in 1994, it was not until 2000 that the results of the first human laparoscopic BPD-DS series were reported by Ren and colleagues.[11] The first robotically assisted BPD-DS was also performed in 2000 by a totally intracorporeal approach.[12] Currently, several methods of performing the laparoscopic BPD-DS have been described and differ primarily in the manner that the duodenoileostomy is created. These methods include the hand-assist technique using a linear stapler[13] and totally intracorporeal techniques using the circular stapler,[11] linear stapler,[14] robotically hand sewn,[15] and a conventional laparoscopic hand-sewn approach.[16]

Despite several good descriptions of the technique and its excellent weight-loss results, the BPD-DS is an infrequently performed procedure. A recent review of the patient registry of the American Society for Bariatric and Metabolic Surgery showed that over a 23-month period immediately before May of 2009, only 517 (.87%) of the 57,918 registered patients underwent either a BPD or a BPD-DS and most of them were performed by laparotomy.[17]

The possible reasons for the slow adoption of the BPD-DS in the United States include an apprehension about its malabsorptive side effects and its technical complexity. Apprehension about severe malabsorption is a carryover from the jejunoileal bypass (JIB) era. However, there are major differences between the JIB and the BPD-DS. In the JIB, the stomach was not resected and weight loss resulted from severe malabsorption by connecting the proximal 35 cm of jejunum to the distal 10 cm of the terminal ileum. The rest of the small bowel was a blind intestinal limb. The side effects associated with the JIB included severe diarrhea, nephropathy, and cirrhosis. Therefore, the procedure was largely abandoned by the 1980s. In contrast, the BPD-DS has no blind limb, stomach resection provides a restrictive component, and the 250-cm alimentary limb has not been associated with nephropathy or liver disease since the BPD-DS was first performed in 1988.

PHYSIOLOGIC BASIS

The clinical benefits and side effects of the BPD-DS have become known through observational studies. However, the underlying mechanisms of actions are not very well understood. It is thought that restriction from the sleeve gastrectomy provides early weight loss but fat malabsorption provides long-term weight loss. This explanation may be simplistic because significant gut hormonal changes have also been demonstrated in patients after a BPD-DS. These changes include reduced ghrelin and increased peptide YY levels.[18,19] Ghrelin is produced by the D cells of the stomach and by epsilon cells in the pancreas. Low levels of this hormone are associated with satiety. Peptide YY is released from the ileum and colon in response to feeding and also increases the sense of satiety. The sleeve component of the BPD-DS is most likely responsible for the changes in ghrelin because levels of this gut hormone have been shown to decline after isolated sleeve gastrectomy.[20] The rapid entry of nutrients in the distal gut is likely responsible for the increase in peptide YY levels seen after a distal bypass. Hence, not only mechanical but potent gut hormonal factors may be responsible for the weight loss associated with the BPD-DS.

The mechanism of action for reducing marginal ulceration is thought to be the result of a reduced parietal cell mass from the sleeve gastrectomy, which leads to lower acid production. The Brunner's glands in the duodenum may also play a role by producing mucus that serves to protect the ileal mucosa from marginal ulceration. Experimental animal models with the first part of the duodenum and the pylorus preserved have confirmed these findings,[7] and observational studies with the BPD-DS have shown a reduced incidence of marginal ulceration. In a follow-up study of more than 1000 patients over 15 years, Marceau and colleagues[21] had only 1 confirmed case of marginal ulceration, and Hess and colleagues[22] reported a 0.3% marginal ulceration rate after more than 10 years of follow-up.

Besides reducing the incidence of marginal ulceration and other postgastrectomy symptoms, such as dumping, the ability to tolerate larger quantities and wider varieties of food have led many patients and surgeons to think that the quality of life is better after a BPD-DS than the Roux-en-Y gastric bypass or other restrictive bariatric operations. Although the evidence does favor fewer dumping symptoms, the evidence for improved quality of life is equivocal in patients undergoing the BPD-DS versus other bariatric operations. A technetium-labeled omelet study in 20 patients after a BPD-DS demonstrated that half-time for emptying the remaining stomach was 28 ± 16 minutes, which was faster than the intact stomach (91 ± 20 minutes), but self-reported dumping symptoms in these patients were rare and minor.[18] Nevertheless, a survey of patients comparing food tolerance or quality of eating after 4 different bariatric operations failed to show a benefit for the BPD-DS patients.[23] Further, a health-related quality-of-life survey failed to show significant differences between patients undergoing the BPD-DS, laparoscopic adjustable gastric band, and Roux-en-Y gastric bypass. Another interpretation of these studies could be that the quality of life of patients undergoing a BPD-DS is not impaired by malabsorption. However, the proportion of BPD-DS patients in both these studies was relatively small and larger studies are needed.[24]

A bias also exists regarding the bowel habits of patients undergoing a BPD-DS. Patients are thought to have frequent malodorous stool and flatus. However, a study comparing the bowel habits of patients after a BPD-DS (n = 28) or a Roux-en-Y gastric bypass (n = 18) using a self-reported questionnaire showed no statistical difference in urgency, incontinence, episodes of waking from sleep, or stool consistency even though the BPD-DS patients reported more bowel movements (23.5 vs 16.5 over a 14-day period).[25] A greater amount of flatus is attributed to carbohydrate malabsorption and some of the bowel disturbance in BPD-DS patients is related to an increased incidence of lactose intolerance. Lactase is a brush border enzyme in the mammalian small bowel that digests dietary lactose and its levels decrease with age. The reduced length of the alimentary limb after a BPD-DS further decreases the ability of the bowel to tolerate a lactose load. Supplemental intake of the oral enzyme can mitigate some of these effects. Steatorrhea would also be expected in

BPD-DS patients because of fat malabsorption. Marceau and colleagues[26] showed that patients with the BPD-DS had an average of 2.7 soft bowel movements a day, but this frequency was less than that reported by patients who had undergone a BPD with a distal gastrectomy. These studies suggest that bowel habits alone should not be a reason to withhold the BPD-DS operation from patients as long as they are well informed about the effects of their dietary choices.

The effects of steatorrhea are not entirely negative. Absorption of dietary fat depends on emulsification by bile salts and can only take place in the common channel. The malabsorption of fat and the excretion of bile acids with a BPD-DS or a BPD cause a significant reduction in cholesterol and have been proposed for familial hypercholesterolemia even in the nonobese.[27] However, fat malabsorption also predisposes patients to deficiencies of vitamins, such as A, D, E, and K. A study comparing the vitamin status of patients after a BPD-DS or a Roux-en-Y gastric bypass found that patients undergoing a BPD-DS were at greater risk for vitamin A, D, and thiamine deficiency in the first year.[28] Another study found that patients undergoing either a BPD or a BPD-DS were at a higher risk for vitamin A, D, K, and calcium deficiency with concomitant elevation of parathormone levels, but did not differentiate between the BPD-DS and the BPD patients, and preoperative vitamin levels were not measured.[29] Based on the results of published studies, it is fair to say that the patients undergoing BPD-DS are at an increased risk for deficiency of fat-soluble vitamins. Therefore, supplementation with the water-soluble analogues of vitamins A, D, E, and K is recommended in addition to supplementation of other vitamins and minerals, including B12, iron, and calcium.

On the other hand, BPD-DS patients do not seem to suffer from as much protein-calorie malnutrition as is commonly thought. The remaining stomach after a BPD-DS produces acid and pepsinogen and should enhance protein digestion. The absorption of peptides and carbohydrates is also preserved along the length of the alimentary limb because of the presence of brush border enzymes. The BPD-DS has in fact been shown to be associated with less protein malnutrition compared with the BPD while facilitating excellent weight loss. By preserving the pylorus and making the common channel 100 cm in length in the BPD-DS in contrast to the 50 cm for the BPD with distal gastrectomy, Marceau and colleagues[30] have been able to reduce the incidence of revisions from 18% in BPD with distal gastrectomy patients to 2% in the BPD-DS group over an observation period of 10 years. The percentage of patients needing reversals for excessive diarrhea and malnutrition also decreased from 2.7% for the BPD to 0.5% for the BPD-DS over this period. Anthone and colleagues[31] have reported a higher reversal rate of 5.8% caused by protein malnutrition or diarrhea but they created a smaller stomach tube with a capacity of 100 mL, which may have predisposed their patients to more malnutrition. Protein malabsorption has not been a major issue in the authors' personal series of more than 400 BPD-DS patients, and they have not had to reverse any operation for malnutrition over the last 10 years.

INDICATIONS FOR PROCEDURE

In the American Society for Metabolic and Bariatric Surgery's 2005 consensus conference, the BPD-DS was recognized as an established bariatric operation.[32] The Centers for Medicare and Medicaid Services also reimburses for BPD-DS if a patient meets medical necessity for any bariatric operation (body mass index [BMI] ≥ 35 kg/m^2, has one major comorbidity, and has failed previous medical weight-loss attempts).[33] Other third-party payers variably cover the procedure and may have stipulations, such as BMI criteria (>50 kg/m^2), that must be met for preauthorization of a BPD-DS operation. Although it has been shown that patients with a BMI greater than 50 kg/m^2 will lose more weight[34] and have faster resolution of diabetes and hypertension[35] with a BPD-DS than after a Roux-en-Y gastric bypass, a recent review of 810 BPD-DS patients with a BMI less than 50 kg/m^2 also demonstrated excellent weight loss and resolution of other comorbid conditions. Patient satisfaction was also excellent, with acceptable complication rates.[36] Therefore, the authors think it is reasonable to offer the BPD-DS to patients who desire the operation as a primary bariatric operation even if their BMI is less than 50 kg/m^2 and are well informed of their choices as long as they meet criteria for a bariatric operation. Although rare, patients who have malrotation of the gut may also be good candidates for either an open or a laparoscopic BPD-DS because the small bowel lays on the patients' right side and a duodenoileostomy created in the right upper quadrant places less stretch on the mesentery of the alimentary limb.[37]

The BPD-DS may also be performed as a revision operation for other failed bariatric operations. Previously, these operations were performed by laparotomy.[38] More recently, laparoscopic revision of the laparoscopic adjustable gastric band[39–42] and the Roux-en-Y gastric bypass[43,44] to the BPD-DS have been described. Laparoscopic revision surgery to BPD-DS carries a higher morbidity.[40–42] Therefore, it is suggested that surgeons should only undertake revisions after they have surpassed the learning curve for primary laparoscopic BPD-DS procedure.

CURRENT PROCEDURE

The BPD-DS can be performed by either an open or laparoscopic approach. The operation has 3 main components: the creation of the stomach tube with pylorus preservation, the distal ileoileal anastomosis, and the proximal duodenal-ileal anastomosis.

The sleeve gastrectomy is performed by mobilizing the greater curvature of the stomach distally to about 4 cm past the pylorus and proximally to the angle of His, using a thermal sealing and cutting device (**Fig. 1**). This dissection preserves the lesser curvature blood supply and vagal innervations. Traction on the stomach should be gentle to avoid avulsing the short gastric vessels. The stomach reservoir should also be protected from thermal injury to prevent a delayed leak. To create the stomach tube, resection is typically begun along the greater curvature about 5 cm proximal to

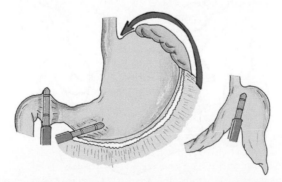

Fig. 1. Mobilization of the proximal 4 cm of duodenum and the greater curvature of stomach is followed by transection of the duodenum and resection of the greater curvature of the stomach to result in a gastric remnant with a capacity of 150 mL. (*From* Sudan R, Puri V, Sudan D. Robotically assisted biliary pancreatic diversion with a duodenal switch: a new technique. Surg Endosc 2007;21(5):729–33; with permission.)

the pylorus. In this location, the stomach wall is thick and, therefore, longer leg-length staples (4.5 mm) are used. A gentle curve is then created using additional stapler loads to complete the resection at the angle of His. The staple line may be further secured by either oversewing or the use of buttress material at the surgeon's discretion. Care is taken to ensure that the stomach is not narrowed, such as in an hourglass deformity, because this may cause functional obstruction and predispose to leaks and reflux.[45] The goal is to create a stomach tube with a capacity of 150 to 250 mL. A variety of bougie sizes have been used to determine the volume of the stomach tube. However, no difference in weight loss was found at 6 months when the stomach was sized using a 40F or a 60F bougie.[46] Another study measured gastric volume after surgery using computerized tomography and also found no correlation between the stomach tube volume and weight loss.[45] Because the BPD-DS is conceptualized as a combined restrictive and malabsorptive operation, there is probably a range of stomach volumes within which the operation is effective.

To perform the bypass, the bowel is divided 250 cm proximal to the ileocecal valve and the biliary limb is anastomosed to the common channel 100 cm proximal to the ileocecal valve (**Fig. 2**). The resulting enterotomy created by the stapler can be closed by staplers or by suturing, ensuring that the lumen of the bowel is not narrowed. Many investigators use these standard limb lengths for bypass; however, others have proposed making the common channel 10% and the alimentary limb 40% of the total length of the small bowel.[22]

The duodenal-ileal anastomosis can be performed using several techniques, including either the circular stapler,[11] the linear cutter,[13,14] the hand-sewn laparoscopic technique,[16] or the robot.[15] The position of the alimentary limb can be antecolic or retrocolic. A study comparing the circular stapler, linear stapler, and hand-sewn technique found that the leak rates and local wound complications rate were higher with the circular stapler compared with the other two methods.[47]

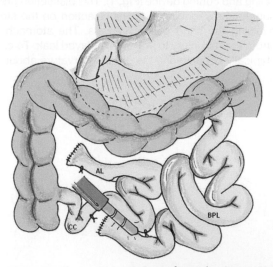

Fig. 2. The distal entero-enteric anastomosis is performed using a 60-mm vascular load endoscopic stapler. The 100-cm long common channel (CC) is shown. (AL, eventual alimentary limb; BPL, eventual biliopancreatic limb). (*From* Sudan R, Puri V, Sudan D. Robotically assisted biliary pancreatic diversion with a duodenal switch: a new technique. Surg Endosc 2007;21(5):729–33; with permission.)

Typically, the mesenteric defects between the biliary limb, the common channel, and the mesentery of the alimentary limb are closed using a running permanent suture, and the completed procedure is demonstrated in **Fig. 3.**

Many surgeons also perform an appendectomy, cholecystectomy, and a liver biopsy.[9,13,15] To evaluate the need for incidental cholecystectomy, a recent publication described performing a cholecystectomy selectively in patients with gallstones. The remaining patients did not undergo a cholecystectomy and were placed on ursodeoxycholic acid for 6 months. Only 8.7% of these patients required a cholecystectomy subsequently and, therefore, the investigators concluded that routine cholecystectomy was not necessary.[48] When making the decision to perform a cholecystectomy selectively, it is important to remember that the chances of gallstone formation after a BPD-DS may be higher than the Roux-en-Y gastric bypass or other purely restrictive operations because of the greater loss of bile salts from interruption of their enterohepatic recirculation. Also, if patients develop choledocholithiasis, access to the bile duct by endoscopic retrograde cholangiopancreatography is more challenging after a BPD-DS because of the absence of a remnant stomach pouch and a very long biliopancreatic limb. A subsequent cholecystectomy may also be more difficult in the presence of an inflamed gallbladder and adhesions in the area of the duodenal-ileal anastomosis.

In the postoperative period, many surgeons tend to be conservative with diet advancement after a BPD-DS and usually wait for ileus to resolve before initiating oral feeding. This practice usually results in a longer average length of hospital stay

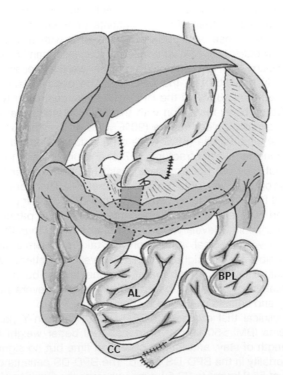

Fig. 3. The final configuration results in a 100-cm long common channel (CC). The alimentary limb (AL) and the biliopancreatic limb (BPL) are demonstrated. The length of the AL is 150 cm. (*From* Sudan R, Puri V, Sudan D. Robotically assisted biliary pancreatic diversion with a duodenal switch: a new technique. Surg Endosc 2007;21(5):729–33; with permission.)

of about 4 days for the BPD-DS patients compared with 2 days after a Roux-en-Y gastric bypass.[49] A well-balanced meal with 200% of the daily value of vitamin and mineral supplementation is required, and patients are advised to take 10,000 units of vitamin A, 2000 units of vitamin D, and 300 micrograms of vitamin K in the form of water-soluble analogues of these vitamins. Daily supplementation should include 1800 to 2400 mg/d of calcium citrate in 3 to 4 divided dosages. Guidelines for nutritional evaluation and vitamin supplementation for bariatric patients have been published.[50] Laboratory testing to detect nutritional deficiencies, including serum fat-soluble vitamin levels, should be performed at least annually.

RESULTS

The operative mortality for large BPD-DS series by laparotomy is approximately 1% with a range of 0.57% to 1.9%.[3,9,21,51] These series have also reported a leak rate of 2.7% to 3.75%. The operative mortality rate in the first reported laparoscopic BPD-DS series was 2.5%,[11] and for patients with a BMI more than 60 kg/m^2, a rate as high as 6.5% has been reported.[52] This finding has been the basis for offering a staged approach for performing a BPD-DS in high-risk patients (**Table 1**). However, other investigators have safely performed the operation in patients with a BMI greater than 50 kg/m^2 as a single-stage procedure with no significant increase in mortality.[53] Others have shown that patients' BMI becomes less predictive of complications after the learning curve for laparoscopic BPD-DS is overcome.[42]

In long-term studies with a follow-up greater than 10 years, Marceau and colleagues[21,30] have shown that BPD-DS patients continue to have 25% greater mean weight loss than those who underwent the BPD with a distal gastrectomy. Also, there were few patients (1.3%) who failed to lose less than 25% of their excess weight. Serum calcium, iron, and hemoglobin levels were higher and parathormone levels were lower in patients with the BPD-DS. The need for revisions was also dramatically lowered from 18.5% in the BPD with distal gastrectomy to 2.7% in the BPD-DS group. Comorbidity resolution with the BPD-DS was excellent for diabetes (92% were off medication), sleep apnea (90% were off continuous positive airway pressure machines), and asthma (88% were on a reduced dosage of medications). The incidence of long-term bone fractures (17%) and urolithiasis (14%) were similar in both groups, but they did not compare these results to either the nonbariatric surgery population or those with other bariatric operations. Therefore, the significance of this incidence of fractures is not known. Although 20% of their patients had lower serum calcium and 50% had a mild to moderate increase of parathormone levels, overall their serum vitamin D levels were higher after surgery than their preoperative levels. Compliance with medical instructions to take supplemental vitamins may have been responsible for the higher vitamin D levels. In patients with low serum vitamin D or calcium levels or high parathormone levels, bone density can be measured with dual-emission x-ray absorptiometry scans. Severe bone damage or vitamin deficiency and anemia were rare in their series.

A randomized clinical trial comparing BPD-DS to Roux-en-Y gastric bypass in superobese patients (BMI >50 kg/m^2) demonstrated better weight loss at 1 year, longer hospital length of stay, and longer operating time but no significant increase in morbidity or mortality in the BPD-DS group. The BPD-DS patients decreased their BMI from a mean of 55.2 kg/m^2 to 32.5 kg/m^2, whereas the Roux en Y gastric bypass patients decreased their BMI from 54.8 kg/m^2 to 38.5 kg/m^2.[49]

Another study compared the results of the BPD-DS with the Roux-en-Y gastric bypass for patients with a BMI greater than 50 kg/m^2 and found that the weight loss

Table 1
Comparison of results of open versus laparoscopic BPD-DS

Author, Year	Access	Cases (N)	Female (%)	Age (Years)	BMI (kg/m²)	Surgery Duration (minutes)	Convert to Open (%)	EBL (mL) Mean	Leaks (%)	Mortality <30 Days (%)	EWL %
Hess[51] 2005	O	1150	77	33.9a	50.9a	158–199b	NA	300	0.7	0.57c	75d
Marceau et al,[3] 1998	O	465	80	37a	47a	NR	NA	NR	2.7	1.7	73e
Ren et al,[11] 2000	L	40	70	43a	42–85b	360–110b	2.5	NR	2.5	2.5	58f
Kim et al,[52] 2003	L	26	58	42g	66.9g	210g	NR	100	3.8	7.6	76.7
Sudan et al,[15] 2007	R	47	87	38	45a	514g	6	118a	8	0	NR

Abbreviations: EBL, estimated blood loss; EWL, excess weight loss; L, laparoscopy; NR, not reported; O, laparotomy; R, robot assisted.
a Mean.
b Range.
c N = 1300 patients.
d N = 182 patients with more than 10 years postsurgery, with 92% follow-up.
e N = 1356 patients.[21]
f Median follow-up of 9 months.
g Median.

following a BPD-DS was superior.[34] In the same weight category, patients who underwent the BPD-DS were more likely to resolve type II diabetes (100% vs 60%), hypertension (68.0% vs 38.6%), and dyslipidemia (72.0% vs 26.3%) but the Roux en Y gastric bypass was superior for the resolution of gastroesophageal reflux disease (76.9% vs 48.57%).[35] In the future, based on patients' BMI and medical comorbidities, factors such as these may be used to inform the choice of procedure for patients.

SUMMARY

From mostly retrospective literature and one randomized study, some conclusions regarding the BPD-DS can be made. Compared with the BPD, patients who undergo BPD-DS are less likely to suffer adverse postgastrectomy symptoms, especially marginal ulcer and dumping. Furthermore, some patients may lose more weight than they would after a Roux-en-Y gastric bypass and have better resolution of diabetes, hypercholesterolemia, and hypertension. The Roux-en-Y gastric bypass may be more effective for the treatment of reflux disease. In any event, outcomes after the BPD-DS for patients with a BMI either greater than or less than 50 kg/m^2 are excellent. The reported operative mortality of the BPD-DS is currently higher than the Roux-en-Y bypass but this may decrease as surgeons gain more experience with the technical aspects of the procedure. Vitamin supplementation and monitoring are crucial for preventing postoperative nutritional deficiencies.

REFERENCES

1. Scopinaro N, Gianetta E, Civalleri D, et al. Bilio-pancreatic bypass for obesity: II. Initial experience in man. Br J Surg 1979;66(9):618–20.
2. Scopinaro N, Gianetta E, Civalleri D, et al. Bilio-pancreatic bypass for obesity: 1. An experimental study in dogs. Br J Surg 1979;66(9):613–7.
3. Marceau P, Hould FS, Simard S, et al. Biliopancreatic diversion with duodenal switch. World J Surg 1998;22(9):947–54.
4. Scopinaro N, Adami GF, Marinari GM, et al. Biliopancreatic diversion. World J Surg 1998;22(9):936–46.
5. Longmire WP Jr, Traverso LW. The Whipple procedure and other standard operative approaches to pancreatic cancer. Cancer 1981;47(Suppl 6):1706–11.
6. Critchlow JF, Shapiro ME, Silen W. Duodenojejunostomy for the pancreaticobiliary complications of duodenal diverticulum. Ann Surg 1985;202(1):56–8.
7. DeMeester TR, Fuchs KH, Ball CS, et al. Experimental and clinical results with proximal end-to-end duodenojejunostomy for pathologic duodenogastric reflux. Ann Surg 1987;206(4):414–26.
8. Marceau P, Biron S, Bourque RA, et al. Biliopancreatic diversion with a new type of gastrectomy. Obes Surg 1993;3(1):29–35.
9. Hess DS, Hess DW. Biliopancreatic diversion with a duodenal switch. Obes Surg 1998;8(3):267–82.
10. Wittgrove AC, Clark GW, Tremblay LJ. Laparoscopic gastric bypass, Roux-en-Y: preliminary report of five cases. Obes Surg 1994;4(4):353–7.
11. Ren CJ, Patterson E, Gagner M. Early results of laparoscopic biliopancreatic diversion with duodenal switch: a case series of 40 consecutive patients. Obes Surg 2000;10(6):514–23 [discussion: 524].
12. Sudan R, Sudan D. Development of a totally intracorporeal robotic assisted biliary pancreatic diversion with duodenal switch. Obes Surg 2002;12:205.
13. Rabkin RA, Rabkin JM, Metcalf B, et al. Laparoscopic technique for performing duodenal switch with gastric reduction. Obes Surg 2003;13(2):263–8.

14. Ramos AC, Galvao Neto M, Santana Galvao M, et al. Simplified laparoscopic duodenal switch. Surg Obes Relat Dis 2007;3(5):565–8.
15. Sudan R, Puri V, Sudan D. Robotically assisted biliary pancreatic diversion with a duodenal switch: a new technique. Surg Endosc 2007;21(5):729–33.
16. Baltasar A. Hand-sewn laparoscopic duodenal switch. Surg Obes Relat Dis 2007;3(1):94–6.
17. DeMaria EJ, Pate V, Warthen M, et al. Baseline data from American Society for Metabolic and Bariatric Surgery-designated bariatric surgery centers of excellence using the bariatric outcomes longitudinal database. Surg Obes Relat Dis 2010;6(4):347–55.
18. Hedberg J, Hedenstrom H, Karlsson FA, et al. Gastric emptying and postprandial PY response after biliopancreatic diversion with duodenal switch. Obes Surg 2011;21(5):609–15.
19. Kotidis EV, Koliakos G, Papavramidis TS, et al. The effect of biliopancreatic diversion with pylorus-preserving sleeve gastrectomy and duodenal switch on fasting serum ghrelin, leptin and adiponectin levels: is there a hormonal contribution to the weight-reducing effect of this procedure? Obes Surg 2006;16(5):554–9.
20. Bohdjalian A, Langer FB, Shakeri-Leidenmuhler S, et al. Sleeve gastrectomy as sole and definitive bariatric procedure: 5-year results for weight loss and ghrelin. Obes Surg 2010;20(5):535–40.
21. Marceau P, Biron S, Hould FS, et al. Duodenal switch: long-term results. Obes Surg 2007;17(11):1421–30.
22. Hess DS, Hess DW, Oakley RS. The biliopancreatic diversion with the duodenal switch: results beyond 10 years. Obes Surg 2005;15(3):408–16.
23. Schweiger C, Weiss R, Keidar A. Effect of different bariatric operations on food tolerance and quality of eating. Obes Surg 2010;20(10):1393–9.
24. Strain GW, Faulconbridge L, Crosby RD, et al. Health-related quality of life does not vary among patients seeking different surgical procedures to assist with weight loss. Surg Obes Relat Dis 2010;6(5):521–5.
25. Wasserberg N, Hamoui N, Petrone P, et al. Bowel habits after gastric bypass versus the duodenal switch operation. Obes Surg 2008;18(12):1563–6.
26. Marceau P, Hould FS, Lebel S, et al. Malabsorptive obesity surgery. Surg Clin North Am 2001;81(5):1113–27.
27. Mingrone G, Henriksen FL, Greco AV, et al. Triglyceride-induced diabetes associated with familial lipoprotein lipase deficiency. Diabetes 1999;48(6):1258–63.
28. Aasheim ET, Bjorkman S, Sovik TT, et al. Vitamin status after bariatric surgery: a randomized study of gastric bypass and duodenal switch. Am J Clin Nutr 2009;90(1):15–22.
29. Slater GH, Ren CJ, Siegel N, et al. Serum fat-soluble vitamin deficiency and abnormal calcium metabolism after malabsorptive bariatric surgery. J Gastrointest Surg 2004;8(1):48–55 [discussion: 54–5].
30. Marceau P, Biron S, Hould FS, et al. Duodenal switch improved standard biliopancreatic diversion: a retrospective study. Surg Obes Relat Dis 2009;5(1):43–7.
31. Anthone GJ, Lord RV, DeMeester TR, et al. The duodenal switch operation for the treatment of morbid obesity. Ann Surg 2003;238(4):618–27 [discussion: 627–8].
32. Buchwald H. Consensus conference statement bariatric surgery for morbid obesity: health implications for patients, health professionals, and third-party payers. Surg Obes Relat Dis 2005;1(3):371–81.
33. Medicare national coverage determinations manual Chapter 1, Part 1, Sections 40.5 and 100.1. 2006. Available at: www.cms.gov/manuals/downloads/ncd103c1_Part1.pdf. Accessed August 18, 2011.

34. Prachand VN, Davee RT, Alverdy JC. Duodenal switch provides superior weight loss in the super-obese (BMI > or = 50 kg/m2) compared with gastric bypass. Ann Surg 2006;244(4):611–9.

35. Prachand VN, Ward M, Alverdy JC. Duodenal switch provides superior resolution of metabolic comorbidities independent of weight loss in the super-obese (BMI > or = 50 kg/m2) compared with gastric bypass. J Gastrointest Surg 2010;14(2): 211–20.

36. Biertho L, Biron S, Hould FS, et al. Is biliopancreatic diversion with duodenal switch indicated for patients with body mass index <50 kg/m2? Surg Obes Relat Dis 2010;6(5):508–14.

37. Puri V, Ramachandran J, Sudan R. Experience with the duodenal switch operation in the presence of intestinal malrotation. Obes Surg 2008;18(5): 615–7.

38. Keshishian A, Zahriya K, Hartoonian T, et al. Duodenal switch is a safe operation for patients who have failed other bariatric operations. Obes Surg 2004;14(9): 1187–92.

39. de Csepel J, Quinn T, Pomp A, et al. Conversion to a laparoscopic biliopancreatic diversion with a duodenal switch for failed laparoscopic adjustable silicone gastric banding. J Laparoendosc Adv Surg Tech A 2002;12(4):237–40.

40. Dapri G, Cadiere GB, Himpens J. Laparoscopic conversion of adjustable gastric banding and vertical banded gastroplasty to duodenal switch. Surg Obes Relat Dis 2009;5(6):678–83.

41. Dolan K, Fielding G. Bilio pancreatic diversion following failure of laparoscopic adjustable gastric banding. Surg Endosc 2004;18(1):60–3.

42. Topart P, Becouarn G, Ritz P. Biliopancreatic diversion with duodenal switch or gastric bypass for failed gastric banding: retrospective study from two institutions with preliminary results. Surg Obes Relat Dis 2007;3(5):521–5.

43. Parikh M, Pomp A, Gagner M. Laparoscopic conversion of failed gastric bypass to duodenal switch: technical considerations and preliminary outcomes. Surg Obes Relat Dis 2007;3(6):611–8.

44. Baltasar A. Laparoscopic conversion from Roux-en-Y gastric bypass to biliopancreatic diversion/duodenal switch. Surg Obes Relat Dis 2008;4(2):210 [author reply: 210–1].

45. Sanchez-Pernaute A, Rodriguez R, Rubio MA, et al. Gastric tube volume after duodenal switch and its correlation to short-term weight loss. Obes Surg 2007; 17(9):1178–82.

46. Parikh M, Gagner M, Heacock L, et al. Laparoscopic sleeve gastrectomy: does bougie size affect mean %EWL? Short-term outcomes. Surg Obes Relat Dis 2008;4(4):528–33.

47. Weiner RA, Blanco-Engert R, Weiner S, et al. Laparoscopic biliopancreatic diversion with duodenal switch: three different duodeno-ileal anastomotic techniques and initial experience. Obes Surg 2004;14(3):334–40.

48. Bardaro SJ, Gagner M, Consten E, et al. Routine cholecystectomy during laparoscopic biliopancreatic diversion with duodenal switch is not necessary. Surg Obes Relat Dis 2007;3(5):549–53.

49. Sovik TT, Taha O, Aasheim ET, et al. Randomized clinical trial of laparoscopic gastric bypass versus laparoscopic duodenal switch for superobesity. Br J Surg 2010;97(2):160–6.

50. Aills L, Blankenship J, Buffington C, et al. ASMBS Allied Health nutritional guidelines for the surgical weight loss patient. Surg Obes Relat Dis 2008;4(Suppl 5): S73–108.

51. Hess DS. Biliopancreatic diversion with duodenal switch. Surg Obes Relat Dis 2005;1(3):329–33.
52. Kim WW, Gagner M, Kini S, et al. Laparoscopic vs. open biliopancreatic diversion with duodenal switch: a comparative study. J Gastrointest Surg 2003;7(4):552–7.
53. Buchwald H, Kellogg TA, Leslie DB, et al. Duodenal switch operative mortality and morbidity are not impacted by body mass index. Ann Surg 2008;248(4): 541–8.

Impact of Bariatric Surgery on Comorbidities

Ashutosh Kaul, MD, MS, FRCS(Edin)[a,b,]*, Jyoti Sharma, MD, MPH[a]

KEYWORDS

- Bariatric surgery • Comorbidity • Diabetes mellitus
- Hypertension • Sleep apnea

The challenges of the obesity epidemic are not limited to concerns about bulk and weight but also to the associated physiologic, psychosocial, and economic disabilities.[1] A small amount of weight loss, approximately 10 kg, carries significant benefits. including resolution of comorbid conditions,[2] and 10% of initial weight loss has been shown to improve long-term comorbidity control.[3] The likelihood of comorbidity resolution depends on many factors, including the length and severity of disease, the amount of weight loss attained, and the contribution of obesity to the severity of the disease. Bariatric surgery (BS) can significantly reduce body weight, resolve obesity-related comorbidities, and improve long-term survival.[4,5] Overall mortality of BS in a meta-analysis was 0.28%,[6] placing these procedures in the lowest category of mortality for elective operations performed in the United States.[7,8]

An observational cohort study based on submitted claims for reimbursement of services or medication showed that, after a mean of 5.3 years, BS was associated with a mean excess weight loss (EWL) of 67.1%; produced significant relative risk reductions in cardiovascular, endocrine, respiratory, infectious, and psychiatric diseases, as well as cancers; and was associated with an 89% reduction in the relative risk of mortality.[9] These benefits improved patients' quality of life and significantly decreased (71.6%) obesity-related claims to insurance companies as early as 4 months following BS.[10] The impact on comorbidities depends on the type of procedure, amount of weight loss achieved, alterations in hormones and incretins, degree of malabsorption, change in motility, and effect on eating habits.

This article reviews published literature on the impact of BS on some major obesity-associated comorbidities.

The authors gratefully acknowledge the help of Mr Donald A. Risucci PhD in editing this manuscript.

[a] Department of Surgery, Westchester Medical Center, 100 Woods Road PMB 583, Valhalla, NY 10595, USA
[b] New York Medical College, Valhalla, NY, USA
* Corresponding author. 19 Bradhurst Avenue, Suite 1700, Hawthorne, NY 10532.
E-mail address: kaulmd@hotmail.com

TYPE 2 DIABETES MELLITUS

The prevalence of type 2 diabetes mellitus (DM) is increasing worldwide and, from an epidemiologic point of view, almost 90% of diabetes cases could be prevented by avoiding obesity.[11,12] The estimated attributable risk of excess body weight leading to development of type 2 DM is extremely high and no other modifiable factor has such an impact on the health of the general population.[12] Total costs of diabetes care were estimated to be $132 billion in 2002.[13] Most (67%) people with type 2 DM have a body mass index (BMI) greater than or equal to 30, and thus diabetes is a key source of morbidity in the obese.[14] Roux-en-Y gastric bypass (RYGB) greatly ameliorates obesity-related type 2 DM.[15]

In the Swedish Obese Subjects (SOS) study, surgery, compared with nonsurgical interventions, decreased the risk of developing diabetes by more than 3 times, whereas resolution of diabetes was 3 times more frequent at 10 years.[16] Other studies have shown similar significant, sustained advantages of BS compared with medical management.[17,18] In a landmark article, Pories and colleagues[19] found substantial and maintained long-term control of DM after RYGB in 121 of 146 patients (82.9%) with DM, and 150 of 152 patients (98.7%) with glucose impairment maintained normal levels of plasma glucose, glycosylated hemoglobin, and insulin.[19]

A meta-analysis of all BS studies from 1990 to 2006[7] assessing type 2 DM resolution after BS found that 78.1% of diabetic patients had complete resolution, and diabetes improved or resolved in 86.6% of patients. Diabetes resolution was greatest for patients undergoing biliopancreatic diversion (BPD)/duodenal switch (95.1% resolved), followed by RYGB (80.3%), gastroplasty (79.7%), and adjustable gastric banding (AGB; 56.7%). The proportion of patients with diabetes resolution or improvement was constant at time points less than, equal to, and greater than 2 years. Insulin levels declined significantly after surgery, as did hemoglobin A1c and fasting glucose.

Resolution of DM is related to weight loss after surgery[7] but it is not a direct cause-and-effect relationship because resolution can occur within days after surgery, even before any significant weight loss.[19,20] Mechanisms underlying these results are interesting, although only partially understood. These mechanisms include caloric reduction,[21] appetite suppression,[22] weight loss after surgery,[7] decreased hepatic glucose production,[23] increase in glucose uptake,[24] changed gastric emptying,[25] decreased leptin levels,[26] increased leptin sensitivity,[27] decreased insulin resistance,[28,29] increased insulin levels, enhanced insulin sensitivity and β-cell responsiveness to glucose,[30] reduction in ghrelin levels,[31] change in gastric inhibitory peptide (GIP) levels,[32] and increased levels of derivatives of L-cells (GLP-1, PYY).[22,33,34] GLP-1 and its agonists promote β-cell replication and differentiation, increase β-cell mass, stimulate insulin secretion, and have an antiapoptotic effect on β-cells in the pancreas.[35,36] In addition, peptide YY (PYY) might ameliorate insulin resistance.[37] RYGB has been shown to decrease the activity of an incretin-inactivating enzyme called dipeptidyl peptidase-4 (DPP-4).[38] This may result in higher incretin levels, and improved incretin levels may result in better blood sugar control.[38] Both rat models[39,40] and human studies[41,42] have shown the role of nutrients being excluded from the foregut or rapidly delivered to the hindgut in controlling DM.

The cost of diabetic medications after BS is significantly lower compared with controls, likely because of decreased use.[43,44] A retrospective review of reimbursement claims of 5502 obese patients comparing presurgery and postsurgery data reported a statistically significant decrease in DM at 3 years (19.9% vs 7.7%, respectively).[10] In another cohort study at 12 months follow-up, diabetic medication use decreased 76% in patients undergoing surgery compared with an increase of 4% in the control.[45]

Metabolic surgery is equally effective in patients with low BMI (<35 kg/m^2) type 2 DM, producing postoperative euglycemia in a high proportion (85.3%) of these patients without undesirable weight loss. A desirable level of change was obtained with some patients moving from the overweight category into the normal weight category.[46]

Patients with DM typically have more preoperative comorbidities, despite having no difference in preoperative weight, than those without DM.[47] Patients with preoperative DM had lower EWL after RYGB at 1 year (67.6% for those without DM, 63.5% for those with diet-controlled DM, 60.5% for those with DM controlled by oral hypoglycemic agents, and 57.5% for those requiring insulin). Nevertheless, DM resolved in 89.8% of those with diet-controlled DM, 82.7% of those taking oral hypoglycemic medication, and 53.3% of those requiring insulin.[47] Duration of DM and preoperative C peptide levels also affect resolution rates. Subpopulations within the obese also have remission of DM after BS. For example, older populations have adequate resolution of type 2 DM after BS.[48] Compared with RYGB, duodenal switch showed better DM resolution at 3 years in superobese patients, with BMI greater than 50 kg/m^2 (60% vs 100% respectively, $P = .04$).[49] Studies have also shown that type 2 diabetics who underwent an RYGB have fewer disease complications.[50] Moreover, morbidly obese individuals after BS–induced DM resolution tend to have a longer lifespan.[9,51] Case-control studies have reported late-onset severe hyperinsulinemic hypoglycemia after BS, implying that these procedures may have a β-cell stimulatory effect.[52,53]

BS is an effective and sustained treatment of obesity-induced type 2 DM. The best results are achieved with, in decreasing order, BPD, RYGB, gastroplasty, and AGB. BS reduces DM-induced complications and costs. Comorbidity remission rates are best if surgery is performed early in the disease process.

HYPERTENSION

Hypertension is one of the most common comorbidities associated with obesity. About 40% to 70% of patients undergoing BS are hypertensive.[7,54] Mechanisms proposed to explain the contribution of obesity to the development of hypertension include an altered renin-angiotensin-aldosterone system, increased intra-abdominal pressure,[55] increased sympathetic nervous system activity, development of insulin resistance, hyperleptinemia, leptin resistance, altered coagulation factors, as well as inflammation and endothelial dysfunction.[54,56]

The SOS study, in which most of the BS procedures were vertical-banded gastroplasty (VBG) and banding, showed a reduction of systolic blood pressure at 2 years in the surgical group. The pulse-pressure increase was less pronounced in the surgery group than in the control group even after 10 years.[16] BS substantially improved and/or resolved hypertension in most patients (37%–53%) or reduced the need for antihypertensive agents (18%–36%).[54,57–59] This trend persisted in people more than 60 years of age.[58] Patients with vitamin D deficiency have significantly lower rates of resolution of hypertension compared with those with adequate vitamin D levels (42% vs 61%; $P = .008$).[59] Correction of deficiency with vitamin D supplementation (50,000 IU weekly) resulted in resolution of hypertension (75% vs 32%; $P = .029$).[60]

Obesity and hypertension places patients at a higher cardiovascular risk, which can be markedly reduced (risks of coronary arterial disease [CAD] decreased by 39% in men and 25% in women) after weight loss–induced resolution of hypertension.[61] BS decreases CAD risk to rates lower than the age-adjusted and gender-adjusted estimates for the general population.[61]

Cremieux and colleagues[10] found that the incidence of hypertension decreased from 38.8% in the preoperative period to 21.1% in the postoperative period (up to 4 months) and was only 12.3% at 3 years after surgery (P<.05). Sjostrom and colleagues[62] reported that the postoperative prevalence of hypertension after 8 years of follow-up was no different between VBG cases and controls, whereas a statistically significant decrease in hypertension occurred in the group that underwent RYGB compared with the control group. Magee and colleagues[63] found a 25% reduction or improvement of hypertension at 1 year in patients who had sleeve gastrectomy (SG). Reported rates of hypertension resolution differed across studies depending on the procedure. In the literature, after AGB resolution, rates of hypertension ranged between 48% and 62.95% in different studies[64,65]; after SG, between 78% and 93.8%[57,64,66,67]; after RYGB, between 65%[54] and 90.7%[68]; and, after duodenal switch in super morbid obese patients, resolution rates were more than 68%.[49]

Significant reduction in blood pressure can be seen within 1 month after surgery, with up to 25% showing resolution and 36% having improvement of hypertension.[54] In superobese patients (BMI>50 kg/m^2), similarly to DM patients, duodenal switch shows better resolution of hypertension at 3 years compared with RYGB (68% vs 38.6%).[49] An insurance data review showed a 51% decrease in hypertensive medication use at 12 months for patients undergoing surgery, compared with an increase of 8% in the patients who did not have surgery.[45]

Normotensive patients who were not on any blood pressure medications showed no reduction in systolic BP after surgery and only a small, gradual decline in diastolic pressure.[69] The best results were seen in hypertensive patients not on active treatment.[69] Resolution rates of hypertension are dependent on length of preexisting hypertension, with better results in those having hypertension for less than 4 years.[54,70]

In conclusion, hypertension is one of the most common morbid obesity–associated comorbidities and BS is an effective and sustained treatment. Resolution results are the best in BPD, followed by RYGB, gastroplasty, and AGB. These procedures reduce hypertension-induced complications and costs. Remission rates are best if surgery is performed early.

HYPERLIPIDEMIA

Hyperlipidemia is present in up to 50% of morbidly obese patients and is a major modifiable risk factor in development of atherosclerosis and CAD.[71] Hyerlipidemia refers to high levels of low-density lipoprotein (LDL), triglycerides (TG), and/or total cholesterol, as well as low high-density lipoprotein (HDL). BS greatly improves secondary hypercholesterolemia and mixed forms of hyperlipidemia. There is a relationship among measures of central obesity, insulin resistance, and impaired glucose metabolism with dyslipidemia in severely obese subjects.[72] Nonsurgical weight loss may lead to a decrease in serum TG and only a modest increase in HDL; however, serum total cholesterol (TC) and LDL remain unchanged.[73–75]

Ten-year follow-up in the SOS study revealed that TG reduction was 18% after AGB, 15% after VBG, and 28% after RYGB. TC reduction was 5% after AGB, 5% after VBG, and 12.6% after RYGB. The increase in HDL cholesterol was 20.4% after AGB, 23.5% after VBG, and 47.5% after RYGB. These findings were more significant in the surgically treated group than the control group.[16] In another study,[72] 1 year after AGB, mean TG concentration decreased by 23% and mean TC by 3.3%. Percentage EWL was not an important predictor of lipid profile improvement in this study. Those with insulin resistance and its associated metabolic problems had less weight loss, but greater improvement in dyslipidemia.[72]

SG results in marked improvement in hyperlipidemia, with improvement or resolution rates of more than 70% in most studies.[57,67,68,76] By causing malabsorption of fats to reduce enterocolic circulation and reabsorption of cholesterol, both RYGB and BPD lead to marked improvement in lipid profile.[48,77,78] A retrospective study[73] of 94 patients who had RYGB and who were diagnosed with hyperlipidemia showed optimization of serum TC, TG, and LDL profiles in all patients within 6 months after surgery. The HDL cholesterol levels improved more slowly, reaching desirable levels within 12 months after surgery, and reached the greatest level at 4 years. None of the patients taking lipid-lowering agents required the medication at the end of the study period. The overall improvement in serum lipid levels included a 27% improvement in serum TC, 47% improvement in serum TG, 40% improvement in serum LDL cholesterol, and a 12% increase in serum HDL cholesterol at the end of the 6-year follow-up period.[73] A Veterans Affairs study[48] of 298 patients with hyperlipidemia found a 40% medication discontinuation rate at 1 year after BS. The veterans with hyperlipidemia were more likely to discontinue medication if they had only been taking fibrates (odds ratio [OR] 6.15, P<.01) as opposed to statins and fibrates. Another insurance data review showed a 59% reduction of hyperlipidemia medication use in patients undergoing BS compared with a 20% increase in those without surgery at 12 months.[45] When comparing SG with RYGB, some studies showed comparable results (75% and 78%, respectively),[67] whereas others found that the improvement/resolution rate was significantly higher in the RYGB group (100%) than in the SG group (75%). BPD with duodenal switch shows marked improvement, if not complete resolution, of hyperlipidemia after surgery in most cases.[77,79] In superobese patients (BMI>50 kg/m^2), duodenal switch shows better resolution of dyslipidemia at 3 years compared with RYGB (72% vs 26.3%, P = .01).[49] Even in mildly obese or nonobese patients, duodenal switch without gastric resection has shown better results.[80]

In conclusion, hyperlipidemia is a major modifiable factor in development of atherosclerosis, and BS greatly improves secondary hypercholesterolemia and mixed forms of hyperlipidemia and leads to improved HDL cholesterol levels. This is associated with significant reduction in need of medications for hyperlipidemia.

CARDIOVASCULAR DISORDER
Congestive Heart Failure

The combination of increased adipose cells and increased lean muscle mass in obese patients results in high cardiac output and an increased circulating volume. Weight loss caused by caloric restriction or surgery promotes favorable hemodynamic changes referred to as reverse remodeling. Regression of left ventricle (LV) mass and chamber size has been shown universally.[81]

BS in morbidly obese patients decreases the thickness of the LV wall and the overall ventricular mass,[82,83] promotes both structural and functional myocardial changes that improve cardiac performance,[84] improves the right ventricle (RV) end-diastolic area, and might prevent progression to RV dysfunction.[85] The benefits of BS on LV mass continue even when weight loss has stopped, and these effects may be caused by neurohumoral factors. These factors may contribute to improved long-term survival.[86]

In patients undergoing BS with left ventricular ejection fraction (LVEF) less than or equal to 35%, mean LVEF at 6 months had significantly improved from 23% (±2%) to 32% (±4%) (P = .04) with subjective and objective improvement in cardiac function.[87] Surgical weight loss could therefore provide a bridge to heart transplantation in patients with morbid obesity.[87] Some evidence suggests that the greatest regression of LV mass and hypertrophy may occur when weight loss is combined with β-adrenergic blocker therapy.[81]

Coronary Artery Disease

Morbid obesity is an independent risk factor for CAD and, after BS, these risks have been shown to decrease. Both coronary microvascular function and peripheral vascular dilator function were found to significantly improve after BS.[88] Coronary microvascular function was assessed by measuring coronary blood flow velocity response to intravenous adenosine and to cold pressor test in the left anterior descending coronary artery by transthoracic Doppler echocardiography. Peripheral vascular dilator function was assessed by brachial artery diameter changes in response to postischemic forearm hyperemia (ie, flow-mediated dilation).[88] The favorable vascular effects of BS were independent of the presence and changes of other known cardiovascular risk factors and of basal values and changes of serum C-reactive protein levels.[88]

Ventricular repolarization abnormalities are significantly increased in subjects with morbid obesity. These QT abnormalities (QT interval and QT interval dispersion) improve substantially after BPD.[89] This change is independent of weight loss and may be related to surgical interruption of the enteroinsular axis. These changes may also be the cause of the survival advantage seen after BS. For patients less than 65 years of age, this survival advantage started at 6 months after surgery and, for patients more than 65 years of age, at 11 months.[90] Donadelli and colleagues[78] reported a significant overall reduction of 10-year cardiovascular disease (CVD) risk starting 1 year after RYGB surgery, with a 1.1% reduction of absolute risk and a 2.3% reduction of percent risk as a result of surgery in patients being observed for 2 years after the operation.[78] The SOS study, comparing a control with a surgical group, found that BS seemed to be a safe and feasible treatment in improving cardiovascular risk factors and may be used as a strategy for secondary prevention in CVD.[91] Recent data suggest that vitamin D might also reduce CVD risk through BP-independent mechanisms.[92]

Atherosclerosis

BS results in significant improvements in inflammatory, structural, and functional markers of coronary atherosclerosis.[93] By reversing some of the risk factors for development of atherosclerosis, including insulin resistance, lipid levels, diabetes, and hypertension, BS can reverse or decrease plaque progression.[94] Eighteen months after BS, carotid intima media thickness diminished from 0.56 to 0.53 mm (n = 37; $P = .004$), whereas brachial flow-mediated dilation improved from 5.81 to 9.01 (n = 25; $P<.001$).[95]

A growing body of evidence suggests that the broadly acting neurotrophic adipokine pigment epithelium–derived factor (PEDF) is associated with visceral adiposity, metabolic syndrome, diabetes, and atherosclerosis. BS reduces levels of PEDF.[96] Similarly, the increase in serum nitric oxide levels and decrease in elevated L-arginine concentration,[97] as well as decreasing C-reactive proteins,[93] may contribute to the diverse beneficial effects of weight loss after BS, especially in the context of atherosclerosis risk.

BS causes significant improvements in LVEF, leads to regression of left ventricular mass and chamber size, decreases risk factors for CAD, and improves ventricular repolarization abnormalities. BS also results in significant improvements in inflammatory, structural, and functional markers of coronary atherosclerosis. All these improvements may contribute to improved long-term survival.

OBSTRUCTIVE SLEEP APNEA AND ASTHMA

Obstructive sleep apnea (OSA) is a common problem among obese patients,[7] with a prevalence rate as high as 77%.[98] Neck circumference more than 17 inches in men and 16 inches in women is a good predictor of OSA.[99] Some studies suggest that, despite availability of prediction models, the diagnosis of OSA cannot be made easily[98,100] without routine polysomnography testing for all patients considering BS.[98] Chronic obstructive pulmonary disease (COPD) and other pulmonary disorders (including OSA) decrease significantly after BS (from 57.7% to 16.2% after surgery at 3 years).[10]

A study investigating the effects of surgical weight loss on inflammatory biomarkers associated with OSA reported that BS resulted in significant decrease in apnea-hypopnea index, cytokines (eg, interleukin-6, soluble tumor necrosis factor [sTNF] αR1, and sTNFαR2), and leptin levels. Of all the biomarkers, BS-related amelioration of sleep apnea independently determined the decrease in sTNFαR2. These results suggest that sTNFαR2 may be a specific OSA biomarker.[101]

High rates of OSA resolution after BS have been shown in many studies.[66,76] Continuous positive airway pressure (CPAP) use ceased in 52.9% of patients with OSA who had undergone SG at 1 year.[102] Two retrospective studies found complete resolution of OSA after BS in an Indian morbidly obese population at 1 or 3 years after surgery.[67,103]

Obesity and increased neck circumference lead to difficult intubation and management of the airway. After BS, patients had an increased interincisor gap, thyromental distance, and reduction in neck circumference.[104] A meta-analysis to identify the effects of surgical weight loss on the apnea-hypopnea index showed a reduction from a random-effects pooled baseline value of 54.7 events/h to 38.2 events/h and subsequent final value of 15.8 events/h. BS thus significantly reduces the apnea-hypopnea index, but postoperative apnea-hypopnea index was consistent with moderately severe OSA. Thus, these patients likely need continued treatment to minimize their future OSA-associated morbidity and complication rate.[105]

Excess BMI increases both the risk and severity of asthma. In a follow-up questionnaire, BS was found to decrease the number of medications required to control patients' asthma symptoms, although AGB seems to produce less significant effects.[106] BS thus shows significant improvement in OSA and other pulmonary diseases.

RENAL DISORDERS

The pathophysiology underlying obesity-associated renal disorders includes insulin resistance, adiponectin deficiency, hyperaldosteronism, and many other pathogenetic factors.[107] The abnormalities of renal structure in obese and morbidly obese individuals include increased kidney weight, glomerulomegaly, disorder of podocytes, mesangial expansion, and abnormalities of the renal interstitium. These abnormalities are accompanied by functional abnormalities like renal hyperperfusion, increased renal plasma flow, increased filtration fraction, and albuminuria.[108-110] Both obesity and metabolic syndrome have been identified as powerful predictors of chronic kidney disease and end-stage renal disease.[107]

Obesity is an independent risk factor for developing chronic or end-stage renal disease with 23% increased odds in patients with high BMI (>30 kg/m^2).[111] The mechanism and mediators of obesity's effects on renal function are not yet well known. A possible mechanism may be that obesity leads to a proinflammatory milieu, renal lipotoxicity, and altered renal hemodynamics, causing glomerulosclerosis and hyperfiltration.[108] Obesity seems to magnify the effect of hypertension on albuminuria.[112] This overall kidney dysfunction improves after BS, which may prevent the development of overt obesity-related glomerulopathy.[108–110] Moreover, these improvements, mainly observed in the first year after surgery with most of the weight loss, seem to occur in patients both with and without established chronic renal impairment.

Twenty-four hour albuminuria continues to improve during the second year of follow-up after BS. Agrawal and colleagues[113] found significant reduction in the median urine albumin/creatinine ratio and microalbuminuria in obese diabetic patients 1 year after RYGB. Saliba and colleagues[114] found that creatinine clearance decreased 15% in diabetics ($P = .02$) and 21% in nondiabetics ($P = .03$) 12 months after RYGB. A significant change in glomerular filtration rate was seen earlier in the nondiabetics (-29% after 6 months, $P = .003$). Tubular function remained unchanged in the nondiabetic subjects, but worsening occurred in the diabetic subjects. These results underscore the importance of reversal of excessive obesity before the onset of frank diabetes.[108,114]

In patients with established renal disease, 20% resolution, improvement, or stabilization of renal disease was seen at 1 year after RYGB, with complete resolution in 1 patient followed for 9 years.[115] Several case reports describing patients with established renal dysfunction have also shown either improvement or stabilization in proteinuria and creatinine at several months follow-up after RYGB.[116–120]

BS can lead to postoperative acute kidney injury (AKI) in up to 8.5% of all cases undergoing BS. Risk factors predisposing to AKI include higher BMI, hyperlipidemia, and preoperative use of angiotensin-converting enzyme inhibitors (ACE-I) or angiotensin receptor blockers.[121] However, BS in morbidly obese patients on dialysis can improve their comorbidities and prepare them for transplantation.[122]

Thus, BS has recently emerged as a successful intervention for obesity-associated renal disease for both prevention of further damage and improvement/resolution of renal dysfunction.

DIGESTIVE DISORDERS

Obese patients have up to 2.4 times more gastroesophageal symptoms compared with nonobese patients.[123] They also have higher distal esophageal acid exposure[124] and a higher number of gastroesophageal reflux episodes.[125] Cremieux and colleagues[10] found a significant decrease (39.4% before surgery vs 13.5% after BS) in medication use for gastroenterologic disorders after BS.

As expected, different BS procedures have varying effects on gastroesophageal reflux disease (GERD). A recent meta-analysis[126] found decrease in reflux symptoms (from 32.9% to 7.7%), decrease in antireflux medications (from 27.5% to 9.5%), and decreased prevalence of erosive esophagitis (from 33.3% to 27%) after AGB. However, they reported new reflux symptoms in 15% and new esophagitis in 22.9%.

SG seems to increase reflux compared with both banding[127] and silastic ring–banded RYGB.[128] The shape of the remaining stomach has an impact because preservation of the antrum may decrease reflux in contrast with a tubular pattern or a superior pouch.[129] RYGB significantly improves heartburn, acid regurgitation, eructation, flatus, and abdominal pain.[130] RYGB has shown excellent results in recalcitrant GERD in morbidly obese patients[131] and has been used to salvage reflux symptoms after restrictive surgery. A prospective study in which SG and RYGB were used as staged procedures found 78% of patients after stage I and 80% patients after stage II had resolution or improvement of GERD symptoms.[76] In superobese patients

(BMI>50 kg/m^2), RYGB showed better resolution of GERD at 3 years compared with duodenal switch (76.9% vs 48.6%, P = .04).[49]

To summarize, SG may increase GERD symptoms, whereas AGB shows conflicting results, but RYGB seems to have significant positive effects on GERD.

Obesity is a significant risk factor for the development of hepatic steatosis, nonalcoholic steatohepatitis (NASH), and nonalcoholic fatty liver disease (NAFLD). Steatosis of the liver is exacerbated with hyperlipidemia. Obesity surgery improves steatosis, necroinflammatory activity, and hepatic fibrosis in patients with morbid obesity and NASH.[132,133] NAFLD-related increases in hepatic lipid peroxidation and enzyme cytochrome P450 2E1 expression also improve significantly with BS-induced weight loss.[134]

MUSCULOSKELETAL DISORDERS

Obesity is associated with a range of mobility problems, musculoskeletal pains, osteoarthritis and gout, all of which significantly affect quality of life.[135] For every 2-unit increase (5 kg) in BMI, there is a 36% increase in the risk of developing painful joint conditions such as osteoarthritis.[136] Disease of the musculoskeletal and connective system, such as arthropathies, osteoporosis, and rheumatism, decreased significantly after BS.[10,16,63] There is also sustained improvement in physical function and reduction of pain following BS.[137] Cottam and colleagues[76] reported 85% resolution of degenerative joint disease after stage I SG and 88% resolution or improvement after stage II RYGB.

A review of all studies on BS and joint pain from 1965 to 2009 reported a subjective improvement in, or resolution of, general joint pain, arthralgia, or osteoarthritis ranging from 32% to 100% at 1 year after surgery.[136] Load-bearing joints like ankle, hip, and knee showed significant improvement. Moreover, joint pain improvement usually occurred within the first 6 months and continued to improve throughout the year.[136]

BS before joint surgery has shown favorable outcomes in joint replacement and arthroplasty.[138] Morbidly obese individuals with severe degenerative joint disease, who are considered unsuitable for arthroplasty because of excess weight, should be considered for BS. Total joint arthroplasty after surgical treatment of obesity has an excellent outcome with an acceptable complication rate.[138]

BS thus shows promise in improving mobility, relieving joint pain, and reducing pain medication use, particularly for the load-bearing joints, in morbidly obese patients. It should also be considered before joint replacement and arthroplasty surgery in the morbidly obese.

PSYCHOLOGICAL, NEUROLOGIC, AND SEXUAL DISORDERS

Psychological factors are intimately connected with morbid obesity and food may be used to satisfy certain cravings. Weight loss greatly improves depression caused by obesity.[76,139] A Greek study[140] surveying 59 obese women before and after bariatric procedures found significant reductions in depression (P<.001) and sexual pain levels (P = .014) as well as significant improvements in sexual desire, arousal (P = .001), lubrication (P = .003), satisfaction (P = .012), and total sexual function (P = .003) 1 year after surgery.

Menstrual irregularities are common in morbidly obese women and may lead to anemia. Polycystic ovary syndrome (PCOS) is frequently (30%–70%) associated with obesity, which significantly modifies both clinical and laboratory expression of the syndrome.[141] BS may resolve obesity-associated PCOS.[142] A decrease in hirsutism, total and free testosterone, androstenedione and dehydroepiandrosterone sulfate, and restoration of regular menstrual cycles and/or ovulation paralleled weight loss after BS.[142] Testosterone levels in men also improved after surgery.[143]

Intracranial Hypertension

Morbid obesity is associated with increased intracranial hypertension, which responds well to BS. Ninety-seven percent of patients having BS were found to have resolution of papilledema after surgery, 92% had complete or nearly complete resolution of visual field deficits, and the remaining patient had stabilization of previously progressive vision loss. BS may thus be an effective treatment of increased intracranial hypertension in obese patients, both in symptom resolution and visual outcome.[144]

In addition, migraine may be exacerbated by obesity and there is marked alleviation of symptoms and reduced incidence and severity of migraine headaches after BS.[145]

CANCER

In the United States, approximately 85,000 new cancer cases per year are related to obesity. Recent research has found that, when the BMI increases by 5 kg/m², cancer mortality increases by 10%.[146] The cancer-protective role of metabolic surgery is strongest for obesity-related tumors in women; however, the underlying mechanisms may involve both weight-dependent and weight-independent effects. These effects include the improvement of insulin resistance with attenuation of the metabolic syndrome as well as decreased oxidative stress and inflammation and beneficial modulation of sex steroids, gut hormones, cellular energetics, immune system, and adipokines.[147]

After 13 years of follow-up in the SOS study, BS has been shown to significantly decrease the incidence of first cancer in women ($P = .0009$).[148] One proposed mechanism for cancer reduction is that RYGB-induced weight loss modifies the production of cytokines related to natural killer cell function and improves their activity.[149]

SUMMARY

Published data show that BS not only leads to significant and sustained weight loss but also resolves or improves multiple comorbidities associated with morbid obesity. Evidence suggests that the earlier the intervention the better the resolution of comorbidities. Patients with metabolic syndrome and comorbidities associated with morbid obesity should be promptly referred for consideration for BS earlier in the disease process.

REFERENCES

1. Pender JR, Pories WJ. Epidemiology of obesity in the United States. Gastroenterol Clin North Am 2005;34(1):1–7.
2. Busetto L, Pisent C, Rinaldi D, et al. Variation in lipid levels in morbidly obese patients operated with the LAP-BAND adjustable gastric banding system: effects of different levels of weight loss. Obes Surg 2000;10(6):569–77.
3. Kuhlmann HW, Falcone RA, Wolf AM. Cost-effective bariatric surgery in Germany today. Obes Surg 2000;10(6):549–52.
4. Maggard MA, Shugarman LR, Suttorp M, et al. Meta-analysis: surgical treatment of obesity. Ann Intern Med 2005;142(7):547–59.

5. Sjostrom L, Narbro K, Sjostrom CD, et al. Effects of bariatric surgery on mortality in Swedish obese subjects. N Engl J Med 2007;357(8):741–52.

6. Buchwald H, Estok R, Fahrbach K, et al. Trends in mortality in bariatric surgery: a systematic review and meta-analysis. Surgery 2007;142(4):621–32 [discussion: 632–5].

7. Buchwald H, Estok R, Fahrbach K, et al. Weight and type 2 diabetes after bariatric surgery: systematic review and meta-analysis. Am J Med 2009;122(3): 248–56, e5.

8. Dimick JB, Welch HG, Birkmeyer JD. Surgical mortality as an indicator of hospital quality: the problem with small sample size. JAMA 2004;292(7):847–51.

9. Christou NV, Sampalis JS, Liberman M, et al. Surgery decreases long-term mortality, morbidity, and health care use in morbidly obese patients. Ann Surg 2004;240(3):416–23 [discussion: 423–4].

10. Cremieux PY, Ledoux S, Clerici C, et al. The impact of bariatric surgery on co-morbidities and medication use among obese patients. Obes Surg 2010;20(7): 861–70.

11. Mokdad AH, Bowman BA, Ford ES, et al. The continuing epidemics of obesity and diabetes in the United States. JAMA 2001;286(10):1195–200.

12. Bruno G, Landi A. Epidemiology and costs of diabetes. Transplant Proc 2011; 43(1):327–9.

13. Hogan P, Dall T, Nikolov P. Economic costs of diabetes in the US in 2002. Diabetes Care 2003;26(3):917–32.

14. Owens TM. Morbid obesity: the disease and comorbidities. Crit Care Nurs Q 2003;26(2):162–5.

15. Cummings DE, Overduin J, Shannon MH, et al. Hormonal mechanisms of weight loss and diabetes resolution after bariatric surgery. Surg Obes Relat Dis 2005; 1(3):358–68.

16. Sjostrom L, Lindroos AK, Peltonen M, et al. Lifestyle, diabetes, and cardiovascular risk factors 10 years after bariatric surgery. N Engl J Med 2004;351(26): 2683–93.

17. Dixon JB, O'Brien PE, Playfair J, et al. Adjustable gastric banding and conventional therapy for type 2 diabetes: a randomized controlled trial. JAMA 2008; 299(3):316–23.

18. Picot J, Jones J, Colquitt J, et al. The clinical effectiveness and cost-effectiveness of bariatric (weight loss) surgery for obesity: a systematic review and economic evaluation. Health Technol Assess 2009;13(41):1–190, 215–357, iii–iv.

19. Pories W, Swanson M, MacDonald K, et al. Who would have thought it? An operation proves to be the most effective therapy for adult-onset diabetes mellitus. Ann Surg 1995;222(3):339–50 [discussion: 350–2].

20. Pories WJ, Albrecht RJ. Etiology of type II diabetes mellitus: role of the foregut. World J Surg 2001;25(4):527–31.

21. Moon Han S, Kim W, Oh J. Results of laparoscopic sleeve gastrectomy (LSG) at 1 year in morbidly obese Korean patients. Obes Surg 2005;15(10):1469–75.

22. Karamanakos S, Vagenas K, Kalfarentzos F, et al. Weight loss, appetite suppression, and changes in fasting and postprandial ghrelin and peptide-YY levels after Roux-en-Y gastric bypass and sleeve gastrectomy: a prospective, double blind study. Ann Surg 2008;247(3):401–7.

23. Rodieux F, Giusti V, D'Alessio D, et al. Effects of gastric bypass and gastric banding on glucose kinetics and gut hormone release. Obesity (Silver Spring) 2008;16(2):298–305.

24. Bobbioni-Harsch E, Sztajzel J, Barthassat V, et al. Independent evolution of heart autonomic function and insulin sensitivity during weight loss. Obesity (Silver Spring) 2009;17(2):247–53.

25. Shah S, Shah P, Todkar J, et al. Prospective controlled study of effect of laparoscopic sleeve gastrectomy on small bowel transit time and gastric emptying half-time in morbidly obese patients with type 2 diabetes mellitus. Surg Obes Relat Dis 2010;6(2):152–7.

26. Woelnerhanssen B, Peterli R, Steinert RE, et al. Effects of postbariatric surgery weight loss on adipokines and metabolic parameters: comparison of laparoscopic Roux-en-Y gastric bypass and laparoscopic sleeve gastrectomy-a prospective randomized trial. Surg Obes Relat Dis 2011. [Epub ahead of print].

27. Bose M, Teixeira J, Olivan B, et al. Weight loss and incretin responsiveness improve glucose control independently after gastric bypass surgery. J Diabetes 2010;2(1):47–55.

28. Ballantyne GH, Wasielewski A, Saunders JK. The surgical treatment of type II diabetes mellitus: changes in HOMA insulin resistance in the first year following laparoscopic Roux-en-Y gastric bypass (LRYGB) and laparoscopic adjustable gastric banding (LAGB). Obes Surg 2009;19(9):1297–303.

29. Abbatini F, Rizzello M, Casella G, et al. Long-term effects of laparoscopic sleeve gastrectomy, gastric bypass, and adjustable gastric banding on type 2 diabetes. Surg Endosc 2010;24(5):1005–10.

30. Kashyap SR, Daud S, Kelly KR, et al. Acute effects of gastric bypass versus gastric restrictive surgery on beta-cell function and insulinotropic hormones in severely obese patients with type 2 diabetes. Int J Obes (Lond) 2010;34(3):462–71.

31. Scerif M, Goldstone AP, Korbonits M. Ghrelin in obesity and endocrine diseases. Mol Cell Endocrinol 2011;340(1):15–25.

32. Rao RS, Kini S. GIP and bariatric surgery. Obes Surg 2011;21(2):244–52.

33. Tharakan G, Tan T, Bloom S. Emerging therapies in the treatment of 'diabesity': beyond GLP-1. Trends Pharmacol Sci 2011;32(1):8–15.

34. Valderas J, Irribarra V, Boza C, et al. Medical and surgical treatments for obesity have opposite effects on peptide YY and appetite: a prospective study controlled for weight loss. J Clin Endocrinol Metab 2010;95(3):1069–75.

35. Drucker DJ. Glucagon-like peptide-1 and the islet beta-cell: augmentation of cell proliferation and inhibition of apoptosis. Endocrinology 2003;144(12):5145–8.

36. Xu G, Stoffers DA, Habener JF, et al. Exendin-4 stimulates both beta-cell replication and neogenesis, resulting in increased beta-cell mass and improved glucose tolerance in diabetic rats. Diabetes 1999;48(12):2270–6.

37. Murphy KG, Bloom SR. Gut hormones and the regulation of energy homeostasis. Nature 2006;444(7121):854–9.

38. Alam ML, Van der Schueren BJ, Ahren B, et al. Gastric bypass surgery, but not caloric restriction, decreases dipeptidyl peptidase-4 activity in obese patients with type 2 diabetes. Diabetes Obes Metab 2011;13(4):378–81.

39. Rubino F, Forgione A, Cummings DE, et al. The mechanism of diabetes control after gastrointestinal bypass surgery reveals a role of the proximal small intestine in the pathophysiology of type 2 diabetes. Ann Surg 2006;244(5):741–9.

40. Speck M, Cho YM, Asadi A, et al. Duodenal-jejunal bypass protects GK Rats from beta-cell loss and aggravation of hyperglycemia and increases enteroendocrine cells co-expressing GIP and GLP-1. Am J Physiol Endocrinol Metab 2011;300(5):E923–32.

41. Ferzli GS, Dominique E, Ciaglia M, et al. Clinical improvement after duodenoje-junal bypass for nonobese type 2 diabetes despite minimal improvement in gly-cemic homeostasis. World J Surg 2009;33(5):972–9.
42. Lee HC, Kim MK, Kwon HS, et al. Early changes in incretin secretion after lapa-roscopic duodenal-jejunal bypass surgery in type 2 diabetic patients. Obes Surg 2010;20(11):1530–5.
43. Agren G, Narbro K, Naslund I, et al. Long-term effects of weight loss on phar-maceutical costs in obese subjects. A report from the SOS intervention study. Int J Obes Relat Metab Disord 2002;26(2):184–92.
44. Potteiger CE, Paragi PR, Inverso NA, et al. Bariatric surgery: shedding the monetary weight of prescription costs in the managed care arena. Obes Surg 2004;14(6):725–30.
45. Segal JB, Clark JM, Shore AD, et al. Prompt reduction in use of medications for comorbid conditions after bariatric surgery. Obes Surg 2009;19(12):1646–56.
46. Fried M, Ribaric G, Buchwald JN, et al. Metabolic surgery for the treatment of type 2 diabetes in patients with BMI <35 kg/m^2: an integrative review of early studies. Obes Surg 2010;20(6):776–90.
47. Carbonell A, Wolfe L, Meador J, et al. Does diabetes affect weight loss after gastric bypass? Surg Obes Relat Dis 2008;4(3):441–4.
48. Maciejewski ML, Livingston EH, Kahwati LC, et al. Discontinuation of diabetes and lipid-lowering medications after bariatric surgery at Veterans Affairs medical centers. Surg Obes Relat Dis 2010;6(6):601–7.
49. Prachand V, Ward M, Alverdy J. Duodenal switch provides superior resolution of metabolic comorbidities independent of weight loss in the super-obese (BMI > or = 50 kg/m^2) compared with gastric bypass. J Gastrointest Surg 2010;14(2): 211–20.
50. MacDonald KJ, Long S, Swanson M, et al. The gastric bypass operation reduces the progression and mortality of non-insulin-dependent diabetes melli-tus. J Gastrointest Surg 1997;1(3):213–20 [discussion: 220].
51. Flum D, Dellinger E. Impact of gastric bypass operation on survival: a popula-tion-based analysis. J Am Coll Surg 2004;199(4):543–51.
52. Mingrone G, Castagneto M. Bariatric surgery: unstressing or boosting the beta-cell? Diabetes Obes Metab 2009;11(Suppl 4):130–42.
53. Abellán P, Cámara R, Merino-Torres J, et al. Severe hypoglycemia after gastric bypass surgery for morbid obesity. Diabetes Res Clin Pract 2008;79(1):e7–9.
54. Hinojosa M, Varela J, Smith B, et al. Resolution of systemic hypertension after laparoscopic gastric bypass. J Gastrointest Surg 2009;13(4):793–7.
55. Varela JE, Hinojosa M, Nguyen N. Correlations between intra-abdominal pres-sure and obesity-related co-morbidities. Surg Obes Relat Dis 2009;5(5): 524–8.
56. Ruano M, Silvestre V, Castro R, et al. Morbid obesity, hypertensive disease and the renin-angiotensin-aldosterone axis. Obes Surg 2005;15(5):670–6.
57. Chowbey PK, Dhawan K, Khullar R, et al. Laparoscopic sleeve gastrectomy: an Indian experience-surgical technique and early results. Obes Surg 2010;20(10): 1340–7.
58. Dunkle-Blatter SE, St Jean MR, Whitehead C, et al. Outcomes among elderly bariatric patients at a high-volume center. Surg Obes Relat Dis 2007;3(2): 163–9 [discussion: 169–70].
59. Pajecki D, Dalcanalle L, Souza de Oliveira C, et al. Follow-up of Roux-en-Y gastric bypass patients at 5 or more years postoperatively. Obes Surg 2007; 17(5):601–7.

60. Carlin A, Yager K, Rao D. Vitamin D depletion impairs hypertension resolution after Roux-en-Y gastric bypass. Am J Surg 2008;195(3):349–52 [discussion: 352].

61. Vogel JA, Franklin BA, Zalesin KC, et al. Reduction in predicted coronary heart disease risk after substantial weight reduction after bariatric surgery. Am J Cardiol 2007;99(2):222–6.

62. Sjostrom CD, Peltonen M, Wedel H, et al. Differentiated long-term effects of intentional weight loss on diabetes and hypertension. Hypertension 2000;36(1):20–5.

63. Magee CJ, Barry J, Arumugasamy M, et al. Laparoscopic sleeve gastrectomy for high-risk patients: weight loss and comorbidity improvement-short-term results. Obes Surg 2011;21(5):547–50.

64. Omana J, Nguyen S, Herron D, et al. Comparison of comorbidity resolution and improvement between laparoscopic sleeve gastrectomy and laparoscopic adjustable gastric banding. Surg Endosc 2010;24(10):2513–7.

65. Cunneen SA. Review of meta-analytic comparisons of bariatric surgery with a focus on laparoscopic adjustable gastric banding. Surg Obes Relat Dis 2008;4(Suppl 3):S47–55.

66. Kasalicky M, Michalsky D, Housova J, et al. Laparoscopic sleeve gastrectomy without an over-sewing of the staple line. Obes Surg 2008;18(10):1257–62.

67. Lakdawala M, Bhasker A, Mulchandani D, et al. Comparison between the results of laparoscopic sleeve gastrectomy and laparoscopic Roux-en-Y gastric bypass in the Indian population: a retrospective 1 year study. Obes Surg 2010;20(1):1–6.

68. Benaiges D, Goday A, Ramon JM, et al. Laparoscopic sleeve gastrectomy and laparoscopic gastric bypass are equally effective for reduction of cardiovascular risk in severely obese patients at 1 year follow up. Surg Obes Relat Dis 2011. [Epub ahead of print].

69. Fernstrom JD, Courcoulas AP, Houck PR, et al. Long-term changes in blood pressure in extremely obese patients who have undergone bariatric surgery. Arch Surg 2006;141(3):276–83.

70. Sugerman H, Wolfe L, Sica D, et al. Diabetes and hypertension in severe obesity and effects of gastric bypass-induced weight loss. Ann Surg 2003;237(6):751–6 [discussion: 757–8].

71. Schauer P, Burguera B, Ikramuddin S, et al. Effect of laparoscopic Roux-en Y gastric bypass on type 2 diabetes mellitus. Ann Surg 2003;238(4):467–84 [discussion: 484–5].

72. Dixon JB, O'Brien PE. Lipid profile in the severely obese: changes with weight loss after lap-band surgery. Obes Res 2002;10(9):903–10.

73. Jamal M, Wegner R, Heitshusen D, et al. Resolution of hyperlipidemia follows surgical weight loss in patients undergoing Roux-en-Y gastric bypass surgery: a 6-year analysis of data. Surg Obes Relat Dis 2010;7(4):473–9.

74. Wood PD, Stefanick ML, Dreon DM, et al. Changes in plasma lipids and lipoproteins in overweight men during weight loss through dieting as compared with exercise. N Engl J Med 1988;319(18):1173–9.

75. Rossner S, Bjorvell H. Early and late effects of weight loss on lipoprotein metabolism in severe obesity. Atherosclerosis 1987;64(2–3):125–30.

76. Cottam D, Qureshi FG, Mattar SG, et al. Laparoscopic sleeve gastrectomy as an initial weight-loss procedure for high-risk patients with morbid obesity. Surg Endosc 2006;20(6):859–63.

77. Scopinaro N, Marinari GM, Camerini GB, et al. Specific effects of biliopancreatic diversion on the major components of metabolic syndrome: a long-term follow-up study. Diabetes Care 2005;28(10):2406–11.

78. Donadelli SP, Salgado W Jr, Marchini JS, et al. Change in predicted 10-year cardiovascular risk following Roux-en-Y Gastric bypass surgery: who benefits? Obes Surg 2011;21(5):569–73.
79. Pontiroli AE, Gniuli D, Mingrone G. Early effects of gastric banding (LGB) and of biliopancreatic diversion (BPD) on insulin sensitivity and on glucose and insulin response after OGTT. Obes Surg 2010;20(4):474–9.
80. Cossu ML, Noya G, Tonolo GC, et al. Duodenal switch without gastric resection: results and observations after 6 years. Obes Surg 2004;14(10):1354–9.
81. Lakhani M, Fein S. Effects of obesity and subsequent weight reduction on left ventricular function. Cardiol Rev 2011;19(1):1–4.
82. Karason K, Wallentin I, Larsson B, et al. Effects of obesity and weight loss on left ventricular mass and relative wall thickness: survey and intervention study. BMJ 1997;315(7113):912–6.
83. Jhaveri RR, Pond KK, Hauser TH, et al. Cardiac remodeling after substantial weight loss: a prospective cardiac magnetic resonance study after bariatric surgery. Surg Obes Relat Dis 2009;5(6):648–52.
84. Cunha Lde C, da Cunha CL, de Souza AM, et al. Evolutive echocardiographic study of the structural and functional heart alterations in obese individuals after bariatric surgery. Arq Bras Cardiol 2006;87(5):615–22.
85. Garza CA, Pellikka PA, Somers VK, et al. Structural and functional changes in left and right ventricles after major weight loss following bariatric surgery for morbid obesity. Am J Cardiol 2010;105(4):550–6.
86. Algahim MF, Lux TR, Leichman JG, et al. Progressive regression of left ventricular hypertrophy two years after bariatric surgery. Am J Med 2010;123(6): 549–55.
87. McCloskey C, Ramani G, Mathier M, et al. Bariatric surgery improves cardiac function in morbidly obese patients with severe cardiomyopathy. Surg Obes Relat Dis 2007;3(5):503–7.
88. Nerla R, Tarzia P, Sestito A, et al. Effect of bariatric surgery on peripheral flow-mediated dilation and coronary microvascular function. Nutr Metab Cardiovasc Dis 2010. [Epub ahead of print].
89. Bezante GP, Scopinaro A, Papadia F, et al. Biliopancreatic diversion reduces QT interval and dispersion in severely obese patients. Obesity (Silver Spring) 2007; 15(6):1448–54.
90. Perry CD, Hutter MM, Smith DB, et al. Survival and changes in comorbidities after bariatric surgery. Ann Surg 2008;247(1):21–7.
91. Delling L, Karason K, Olbers T, et al. Feasibility of bariatric surgery as a strategy for secondary prevention in cardiovascular disease: a report from the Swedish obese subjects trial. J Obes 2010;2010. pii: 102341.
92. Anagnostis P, Athyros VG, Adamidou F, et al. Vitamin D and cardiovascular disease: a novel agent for reducing cardiovascular risk? Curr Vasc Pharmacol 2010;8(5):720–30.
93. Habib P, Scrocco J, Terek M, et al. Effects of bariatric surgery on inflammatory, functional and structural markers of coronary atherosclerosis. Am J Cardiol 2009;104(9):1251–5.
94. Wang Y, Zhang C. Bariatric surgery to correct morbid obesity also ameliorates atherosclerosis in patients with type 2 diabetes mellitus. Am J Biomed Sci 2009; 1(1):56–69.
95. Sturm W, Tschoner A, Engl J, et al. Effect of bariatric surgery on both functional and structural measures of premature atherosclerosis. Eur Heart J 2009;30(16): 2038–43.

96. Tschoner A, Sturm W, Ress C, et al. Effect of weight loss on serum pigment epithelium-derived factor levels. Eur J Clin Invest 2011;41(9):937–42.

97. Sledzinski T, Sledzinski M, Smolenski RT, et al. Increased serum nitric oxide concentration after bariatric surgery–a potential mechanism for cardiovascular benefit. Obes Surg 2010;20(2):204–10.

98. Sareli AE, Cantor CR, Williams NN, et al. Obstructive sleep apnea in patients undergoing bariatric surgery–a tertiary center experience. Obes Surg 2011; 21(3):316–27.

99. Olejniczak PW, Fisch BJ. Sleep disorders. Med Clin North Am 2003;87(4): 803–33.

100. Sharkey KM, Machan JT, Tosi C, et al. Predicting obstructive sleep apnea among women candidates for bariatric surgery. J Womens Health (Larchmt) 2010;19(10):1833–41.

101. Pallayova M, Steele KE, Magnuson TH, et al. Sleep apnea determines soluble TNF-alpha receptor 2 response to massive weight loss. Obes Surg 2011; 21(9):1413–23.

102. Sammour T, Hill A, Singh P, et al. Laparoscopic sleeve gastrectomy as a single-stage bariatric procedure. Obes Surg 2010;20(3):271–5.

103. Todkar J, Shah S, Shah P, et al. Long-term effects of laparoscopic sleeve gastrectomy in morbidly obese subjects with type 2 diabetes mellitus. Surg Obes Relat Dis 2010;6(2):142–5.

104. Lima Filho JA, Ganem EM, de Cerqueira BG. Reevaluation of the airways of obese patients undergone bariatric surgery after reduction in body mass index. Rev Bras Anestesiol 2011;61(1):31–40.

105. Lettieri CJ, Eliasson AH, Greenburg DL. Persistence of obstructive sleep apnea after surgical weight loss. J Clin Sleep Med 2008;4(4):333–8.

106. Reddy RC, Baptist AP, Fan Z, et al. The effects of bariatric surgery on asthma severity. Obes Surg 2011;21(2):200–6.

107. Ritz E, Koleganova N, Piecha G. Is there an obesity-metabolic syndrome related glomerulopathy? Curr Opin Nephrol Hypertens 2011;20(1):44–9.

108. Chagnac A, Weinstein T, Herman M, et al. The effects of weight loss on renal function in patients with severe obesity. J Am Soc Nephrol 2003;14(6):1480–6.

109. Serra A, Granada ML, Romero R, et al. The effect of bariatric surgery on adipo-cytokines, renal parameters and other cardiovascular risk factors in severe and very severe obesity: 1-year follow-up. Clin Nutr 2006;25(3):400–8.

110. Navarro-Diaz M, Serra A, Romero R, et al. Effect of drastic weight loss after bari-atric surgery on renal parameters in extremely obese patients: long-term follow-up. J Am Soc Nephrol 2006;17(12 Suppl 3):S213–7.

111. Fox CS, Larson MG, Leip EP, et al. Predictors of new-onset kidney disease in a community-based population. JAMA 2004;291(7):844–50.

112. Ribstein J, Halimi JM, du Cailar G, et al. Renal characteristics and effect of angiotensin suppression in oral contraceptive users. Hypertension 1999;33(1): 90–5.

113. Agrawal V, Khan I, Rai B, et al. The effect of weight loss after bariatric surgery on albuminuria. Clin Nephrol 2008;70(3):194–202.

114. Saliba J, Kasim NR, Tamboli RA, et al. Roux-en-Y gastric bypass reverses renal glomerular but not tubular abnormalities in excessively obese diabetics. Surgery 2010;147(2):282–7.

115. Alexander JW, Goodman HR, Hawver LR, et al. Improvement and stabilization of chronic kidney disease after gastric bypass. Surg Obes Relat Dis 2009;5(2): 237–41.

116. Cuda S, Chung M, Denunzio T, et al. Reduction of proteinuria after gastric bypass surgery: case presentation and management. Surg Obes Relat Dis 2005;1(1):64–6.
117. Soto F, Higa-Sansone G, Copley J, et al. Renal failure, glomerulonephritis and morbid obesity: improvement after rapid weight loss following laparoscopic gastric bypass. Obes Surg 2005;15(1):137–40.
118. Agnani S, Vachharajani VT, Gupta R, et al. Does treating obesity stabilize chronic kidney disease? BMC Nephrol 2005;6(1):7.
119. Tafti BA, Haghdoost M, Alvarez L, et al. Recovery of renal function in a dialysis-dependent patient following gastric bypass surgery. Obes Surg 2009;19(9): 1335–9.
120. Currie A, Chetwood A, Ahmed AR. Bariatric surgery and renal function. Obes Surg 2011;21(4):528–39.
121. Thakar C, Kharat V, Blanck S, et al. Acute kidney injury after gastric bypass surgery. Clin J Am Soc Nephrol 2007;2(3):426–30.
122. Modanlou KA, Muthyala U, Xiao H, et al. Bariatric surgery among kidney transplant candidates and recipients: analysis of the United States Renal Data System and literature review. Transplantation 2009;87(8):1167–73.
123. Jacobson BC, Somers SC, Fuchs CS, et al. Body-mass index and symptoms of gastroesophageal reflux in women. N Engl J Med 2006;354(22):2340–8.
124. El-Serag HB, Ergun GA, Pandolfino J, et al. Obesity increases oesophageal acid exposure. Gut 2007;56(6):749–55.
125. Schneider JM, Brucher BL, Kuper M, et al. Multichannel intraluminal impedance measurement of gastroesophageal reflux in patients with different stages of morbid obesity. Obes Surg 2009;19(11):1522–9.
126. de Jong JR, Besselink MG, van Ramshorst B, et al. Effects of adjustable gastric banding on gastroesophageal reflux and esophageal motility: a systematic review. Obes Rev 2010;11(4):297–305.
127. Himpens J, Dapri G, Cadière G. A prospective randomized study between laparoscopic gastric banding and laparoscopic isolated sleeve gastrectomy: results after 1 and 3 years. Obes Surg 2006;16(11):1450–6.
128. Miguel GP, Azevedo JL, de Souza PH, et al. Erosive esophagitis after bariatric surgery: banded vertical gastrectomy versus banded Roux-en-Y gastric bypass. Obes Surg 2011;21(2):167–72.
129. Lazoura O, Zacharoulis D, Triantafyllidis G, et al. Symptoms of gastroesophageal reflux following laparoscopic sleeve gastrectomy are related to the final shape of the sleeve as depicted by radiology. Obes Surg 2011;21(3):295–9.
130. Foster A, Laws H, Gonzalez Q, et al. Gastrointestinal symptomatic outcome after laparoscopic Roux-en-Y gastric bypass. J Gastrointest Surg 2003;7(6): 750–3.
131. Perry Y, Courcoulas A, Fernando H, et al. Laparoscopic Roux-en-Y gastric bypass for recalcitrant gastroesophageal reflux disease in morbidly obese patients. JSLS 2004;8(1):19–23.
132. Weiner RA. Surgical treatment of non-alcoholic steatohepatitis and non-alcoholic fatty liver disease. Dig Dis 2010;28(1):274–9.
133. de Andrade AR, Cotrim HP, Alves E, et al. Nonalcoholic fatty liver disease in severely obese individuals: the influence of bariatric surgery. Ann Hepatol 2008;7(4):364–8.
134. Bell LN, Temm CJ, Saxena R, et al. Bariatric surgery-induced weight loss reduces hepatic lipid peroxidation levels and affects hepatic cytochrome P-450 protein content. Ann Surg 2010;251(6):1041–8.

135. Han TS, Tijhuis MA, Lean ME, et al. Quality of life in relation to overweight and body fat distribution. Am J Public Health 1998;88(12):1814–20.
136. Vincent HK, Ben-David K, Cendan J, et al. Effects of bariatric surgery on joint pain: a review of emerging evidence. Surg Obes Relat Dis 2010;6(4):451–60.
137. Kral JG, Sjostrom LV, Sullivan MB. Assessment of quality of life before and after surgery for severe obesity. Am J Clin Nutr 1992;55(2 Suppl):611S–4S.
138. Parvizi J, Trousdale RT, Sarr MG. Total joint arthroplasty in patients surgically treated for morbid obesity. J Arthroplasty 2000;15(8):1003–8.
139. Holzwarth R, Huber D, Majkrzak A, et al. Outcome of gastric bypass patients. Obes Surg 2002;12(2):261–4.
140. Assimakopoulos K, Karaivazoglou K, Panayiotopoulos S, et al. Bariatric surgery is associated with reduced depressive symptoms and better sexual function in obese female patients: a one-year follow-up study. Obes Surg 2011;21(3): 362–6.
141. Vrbikova J, Hainer V. Obesity and polycystic ovary syndrome. Obes Facts 2009; 2(1):26–35.
142. Escobar-Morreale HF, Botella-Carretero JI, Alvarez-Blasco F, et al. The polycystic ovary syndrome associated with morbid obesity may resolve after weight loss induced by bariatric surgery. J Clin Endocrinol Metab 2005;90(12):6364–9.
143. Strohmayer E, Via MA, Yanagisawa R. Metabolic management following bariatric surgery. Mt Sinai J Med 2010;77(5):431–45.
144. Fridley J, Foroozan R, Sherman V, et al. Bariatric surgery for the treatment of idiopathic intracranial hypertension. J Neurosurg 2011;114(1):34–9.
145. Bond DS, Vithiananthan S, Nash JM, et al. Improvement of migraine headaches in severely obese patients after bariatric surgery. Neurology 2011;76(13): 1135–8.
146. Basen-Engquist K, Chang M. Obesity and cancer risk: recent review and evidence. Curr Oncol Rep 2011;13(1):71–6.
147. Ashrafian H, Ahmed K, Rowland SP, et al. Metabolic surgery and cancer: protective effects of bariatric procedures. Cancer 2011;117(9):1788–99.
148. Sjostrom L, Gummesson A, Sjostrom CD, et al. Effects of bariatric surgery on cancer incidence in obese patients in Sweden (Swedish Obese Subjects Study): a prospective, controlled intervention trial. Lancet Oncol 2009;10(7): 653–62.
149. Moulin CM, Marguti I, Peron JP, et al. Bariatric surgery reverses natural killer (NK) cell activity and NK-related cytokine synthesis impairment induced by morbid obesity. Obes Surg 2011;21(1):112–8.

Bariatric Surgery Outcomes

Kristoffel R. Dumon, MD[a], Kenric M. Murayama, MD[b],*

KEYWORDS

• Bariatric surgery • Outcomes • Obesity

Obesity is a global health problem and the exponential increase in obesity worldwide has brought into sharp focus the lack of effective methods for treating or preventing the disease. The projections of the World Health Organization indicated that, globally in 2005, approximately 1.6 billion adults (age >15 years) were overweight and at least 400 million adults were obese.[1] In the United States, obesity, defined by a body mass index (BMI, calculated as weight in kilograms divided by the square of height in meters) of 30 kg/m^2 or more, affects more than one-third of adults (>72 million people). This statistic includes 33.3% of men and 35.3% of women. Morbid obesity (BMI >40 kg/m^2) affects approximately 15 million individuals, 4.7% of the US population.[2] Obesity is associated with an increased risk of death, and morbid obesity carries a significant risk of life-threatening complications such as heart disease, diabetes, and high blood pressure. Bariatric surgery is recognized as the only effective treatment of morbid obesity.[3] The number of bariatric operations in the United States. increased from 13,386 in 1998 to 220,000 in 2008.[4,5] The estimated number of bariatric operations performed in the United States in 2008 was more than 13 times the number performed in 1992. Despite this increase, only 1% of the eligible morbidly obese population are treated with bariatric surgery.[6,7]

IMPORTANCE OF OUTCOMES: UNDERSTANDING ASSOCIATED RISKS AND ENSURING BEST PATIENT OUTCOMES

With the increasing number of bariatric surgical procedures being performed, outcome assessment is of even greater importance. We reviewed the risks including death, short-term and long-term complications, and potential benefits, such as impact on comorbid conditions, quality of life (QoL), and life expectancy. We recognize that the outcome data used for the initial meta-analysis reviews for bariatric surgery have limitations: many published data are reported in case studies and case series

[a] Department of Surgery, Perelman School of Medicine, University of Pennsylvania, 3400 Spruce Street, 4 Silverstein, Philadelphia, PA 19104, USA
[b] Department of Surgery, Perelman School of Medicine, Penn Presbyterian Medical Center, University of Pennsylvania, 51 North 39th Street, W-266, Philadelphia, PA 19104, USA
* Corresponding author.
E-mail address: kenric.murayama@uphs.upenn.edu

Surg Clin N Am 91 (2011) 1313–1338
doi:10.1016/j.suc.2011.08.014
0039-6109/11/$ – see front matter © 2011 Elsevier Inc. All rights reserved.

involving a single surgeon or institution. Also, surgical components such as pouch size and limb length as well as the type of surgical procedure performed vary over time among surgeons and surgical centers. Furthermore, parameters used to define diagnosis, improvement, resolution, or cure of selected comorbid diseases have not been standardized. Follow-up and reporting are often incomplete, which may predispose some studies to selection bias. Another major limitation in reporting outcomes for bariatric surgery is that some of the data used for review and analysis originated from procedures not commonly performed. Procedures such as horizontal gastroplasty and vertical banded gastroplasty are no longer performed. In addition, although the Roux-en-Y gastric bypass (RYGB) is the most commonly performed operation in the United States, newer procedures like laparoscopic adjustable gastric banding (LAGB) and laparoscopic sleeve gastrectomy (LSG) have gained acceptance. Because of its recent introduction, results of LSG are frequently not included in the available comparative reviews.

Worldwide, a total of 344,000 bariatric procedures are performed annually; RYGB, both laparoscopic and open, is the most common (47%), followed by LAGB (42%), LSG (5%), and biliopancreatic diversion with or without duodenal switch (BPD/DS) (2%).[8] In the United States, based on the 2010 data of approximately 58,000 procedures documented in the Bariatric Outcomes Longitudinal Database (BOLD), the most commonly performed bariatric operation was RYGB (54.7%), followed by LAGB (39.6%), LSG (2.3%), and BPD/DS (0.9%). Most of these procedures are performed laparoscopically, except for the BPD/DS, which is primarily performed with an open approach.[9]

The National Institutes of Health recently initiated the Longitudinal Assessment of Bariatric Surgery (LABS) as a 3-year, multicenter prospective study to better define the outcomes of bariatric surgery and a similar case distribution was found. Results of the LABS study show that of the 4776 patients who had a primary bariatric procedure, RYGB was performed in 3412 patients (71.4%) and 87.2% were performed laparoscopically. LAGB was performed in 1198 patients (25.1%), and 166 patients underwent other procedures (3.4%).[10] As expected, there continues to be a trend to replace open surgery with the laparoscopic approach. In 2006, laparoscopic procedures represented 83.18% of all bariatric procedures and by 2008 they represented 88.93% of all bariatric procedures.[11]

In addition, the importance of best practices in weight-loss surgery and the delivery of comprehensive perioperative care are now becoming apparent.[12–14] The American College of Surgeons and the American Society for Metabolic and Bariatric Surgery have established criteria for accreditation of bariatric surgical centers.[15] The percentage of procedures performed in high-volume centers (>100 procedures annually) increased from 39% in 1997 to 77% in 2003,[16] a factor known to influence patient outcomes.[17] Recently, this relationship between surgeon volume and patient outcome was further strengthened by the results of the LABS study, which showed that the patient's risk of experiencing an adverse outcome after RYGB decreased significantly with the increase in surgeon RYGB volume.[18]

Mortality of Bariatric Surgery

The reported operative (30-day) mortality for bariatric surgery ranges from 0.1% to 2%.[7,19,20] In evaluating this wide range in mortality, several factors need to be considered: (1) the skill of the bariatric surgeon; (2) the available facilities of the institution in which the surgery is performed; (3) the volume of procedures being performed and the stage in the learning curve of the surgeon and the institution; (4) type of surgery (RYGB, LAGB, LSG, BPD/DS); (5) patient selection with respect to age, gender, race, and body habitus; and (6) the presence of significant comorbidities such as diabetes, hyperlipidemia, hypertension, and obstructive sleep apnea.[7]

In a comprehensive meta-analysis, Buchwald and colleagues[7] reported early and late mortality after bariatric surgery (**Table 1**). The study evaluated the results of the less than 30-day mortality and 30-day to 2-year mortality in 85,048 patients who underwent bariatric surgery from 478 treatment groups in 361 studies, published from January 1, 1990 to April 30, 2006. Total early mortality (30 days) was 0.28% (95% confidence interval [CI], 0.22–0.34). Total late mortality (30-day to 2-year) was 0.35% (95% CI, 0.12–0.58). Mortality was lowest for laparoscopic procedures (0.5% early and late combined). In the open RYGB procedures, the early mortality was 0.44% and the late mortality was 0.69%. A notable exception was seen with BPD/DS procedures. The investigators report 0.76% mortality for open BPD/DS and 1.11% for laparoscopic BPD/DS. Revisional surgery was associated with higher mortality (up to 1.65%). Subgroup analyses of 30-day mortality show a higher mortality for male, superobese, and elderly patients (>65 years).[7]

More recent data reported a 30-day mortality not exceeding 0.3%. In 2007, federal government data from the Agency for Healthcare Research and Quality and clinical studies reported significant improvements in safety of bariatric surgery.[21] In addition, a privately funded study analyzing the risk-adjusted, in-hospital complication rates associated with bariatric surgery programs affiliated with hospitals in 19 states where data are publicly available suggests a reduction in mortality over the last few years.[11] The study analyzed 190,502 bariatric surgery discharges from 2006 to 2008. Over this 3-year study period (2006–2008), 130 patients receiving bariatric surgery died during their hospital stay (early mortality of 0.068%). The study indicated that outcomes for bariatric surgery are improving, with the mortality for 2008 (0.062%) being more than 25% lower than the rate for 2006 (0.086%).[11]

In addition, the first report of BOLD data registered 78 deaths out of 57,918 bariatric surgical procedures and noted a 30-day mortality of 0.09%.[9]

The large Swedish Obesity Study (SOS) reported a mortality of 0.25% in the surgery cohort, with 5 of 2010 patient deaths within 90 days of surgery (**Table 2**).[22] Similarly, the LABS study assessed the overall risk of death and other adverse outcomes after bariatric surgery. The results of this prospective, multicenter, observational study of 30-day outcomes in consecutive patients undergoing bariatric surgical procedures at 10 clinical sites in the United States from 2005 to 2007 showed that the overall mortality of bariatric surgery was 0.3% (15 deaths out of 4610 patients).[10] None of the 1198 patients who had undergone LAGB died, whereas 0.2% of the 2975 patients who had undergone laparoscopic RYGB and 2.1% of the 437 patients who had undergone open RYGB died. Patients who underwent open RYGB in that study had a higher BMI and more severe coexisting conditions. The study also reports a composite end point of 30-day major adverse outcomes (including death; venous thromboembolism; percutaneous, endoscopic, or operative reintervention; and failure to be discharged from the hospital). A total of 4.3% of patients had at least 1 major adverse outcome. A history of deep vein thrombosis or pulmonary embolus, a diagnosis of obstructive sleep apnea, and impaired functional status were each independently associated with an increased risk of adverse outcomes. Extreme high and low values of BMI were also associated with an increased risk of adverse events, whereas age, sex, race, ethnic group, and other coexisting conditions were not.

Overall, these studies indicate that improved mortality is secondary to laparoscopic approaches, better anesthesia, and better monitoring and oversight. Lower mortality is observed in healthier patients with lower BMI who have operations performed by an experienced surgeon at a higher-volume center. The higher mortality has been

Table 1
Mortality of bariatric surgery

	All Procedures Combined	Gastric Banding		Gastric Bypass		Vertical Banded Gastroplasty		BPD/DS	
		Open Surgery	Laparoscopic Surgery	Open Surgery	Laparoscopic Surgery	Open Surgery	Laparoscopic Surgery	Open Surgery	Laparoscopic Surgery
n	85048	1319	17644	9727	19677	7768	1652	5588	539
Death within 30 days (range)	0.28 (0.22–0.34)	0.18 (0.00–0.49)	0.06 (0.01–0.11)	0.44 (0.25–0.64)	0.16 (0.09–0.23)	0.33 (0.15–0.51)	0.21 (0.00–0.48)	0.76 (0.29–1.23)	1.11 (0.00–2.70)
Death 30 d–2 y (range)	0.35 (0.12–0.58)	0.00 (0.00–3.93)	0.00 (0.00–0.08)	0.69 (0.03–1.35)	0.09 (0.00–0.18)	0.23 (0.00–0.86)	0.00 (0.00–0.86)	0.85 (0.00–1.97)	—

Data from Buchwald H, Estok R, Fahrbach K, et al. Trends in mortality in bariatric surgery: a systematic review and meta-analysis. Surgery 2007;142(4):621–32 [discussion: 632–5].

Table 2 Early mortality (%) of bariatric surgery				
Year	Study	N	Early Mortality	Time Period (d)
2007	Buchwald et al[7]	85,048	0.28	30
2007	SOS[22]	2010	0.25	90
2009	LABS[10]	4610	0.30	30
2010	BOLD[9]	57,918	0.09	30
2010	HG[11]	190,502	0.07	In hospital

Abbreviations: BOLD, Bariatric Outcomes Longitudinal Database; HG, Health Grades; LABS, Longitudinal Assessment of Bariatric Surgery; SOS, Swedish Obese Subjects Study.

correlated with visceral obesity, male sex, BMI greater than 50 kg/m^2, diabetes mellitus, sleep apnea, and older patients, particularly if the operation is performed at a lower-volume center.[7,10,23]

Weight Loss: Comparing Bariatric Surgery with Nonsurgical Therapies

In recent years, bariatric surgery has been the topic of several large meta-analyses and systematic literature reviews. A 2009 health technology assessment[24] and 2009 Cochrane Database review[25] focused on the clinical efficacy and cost-effectiveness of weight-loss surgeries. In 2004, Buchwald and colleagues[19] analyzed data from 136 studies involving more than 22,000 patients to determine the impact of bariatric procedures on weight and comorbid conditions. Maggard and colleagues[26] conducted a similar meta-analysis in 2005, reviewing 147 studies to evaluate the effect of weight-loss surgeries on morbidity and mortality. The SOS study,[22] a large, nonrandomized intervention trial comparing weight-loss outcomes in a group of more than 4000 surgical and nonsurgical subjects, recently reported 10-year data. **Table 3** compares weight-loss data between medical treatment and bariatric surgery. Comparing results among various analyses can be challenging because of differences in how individual studies report data. Also, it can be argued that weight loss, conventionally expressed as percent excess weight loss (EWL), is likely to be the least important measure of bariatric surgical outcomes. But EWL is highly correlated with recognized risk factors and with patient satisfaction. Bariatric surgery led to a statistically significant reduction in weight in all studies. In the 2 randomized controlled trials that reported outcomes at 2 years, mean percent initial weight loss in the surgical groups was 20% and 21.6%, whereas the nonsurgical groups had lost only 1.4% and 5.5%, respectively, of their initial weight.[6,27] In the 2 cohort studies reporting outcomes at 2 years, percent weight change ranged from a weight loss of 16% to 28.6% in the surgical groups, but the medical groups had gained weight, with percent

Table 3 Weight loss: comparing bariatric surgery with nonsurgical therapies						
Author	Year	Study	Outcome (y)	Medical	LAGB	RYGB
Dixon et al[6]	2008	RCT	EWL 2	4.3	62.5	
O'Brien et al[27]	2006	RCT	EWL 2	21.8	87.2	
Buddeberg et al[28]	2006	Cohort	EWL 3.2	11.5	36	52
SOS[22]	2007	Cohort	TWL 10	1.5	14	25

Abbreviations: Cohort, cohort study; EWL, excess weight loss at 2 and at 3.2 y; RCT, randomized controlled trial; SOS: Swedish Obese Subjects Study; TWL, total body weight loss at 10 y.

weight change ranging from 0.1% to 0.5%.[24,25,28] The study by O'Brien and colleagues[3,27] of 80 adults with mild to moderate obesity (BMI 30–35 kg/m²) who were randomized to an intensive medical program versus placement of an LAGB showed a mean EWL in the surgical groups of 87.2% versus 21.6% in the medical group after 2 years (**Fig. 1**). The large, prospective, cohort in the SOS study found that weight loss was still apparent 10 years after surgery, showing 25% of total body weight loss in surgical subjects compared with 1.5% for the nonsurgical patients (**Fig. 2**).[22,24] Based on the 2009 Cochrane Database and the 2009 Health Technology Assessment, it is clear that bariatric surgery is a more effective intervention for weight loss than nonsurgical options.[24,25]

Buchwald and colleagues[19] conducted a systematic review and meta-analysis of open and laparoscopic bariatric surgery outcomes reported in the clinical literature from 1990 to 2003 focusing on weight loss, operative mortality, and comorbidity outcomes. In comparing the different surgical procedures, Buchwald and colleagues showed that mean EWL (and 95% CI) after BPD was 70.1% (66.3%–75.9%), gastric bypass 61.6% (56.7%–66.5%), vertical banded gastroplasty 68.2% (61.5%–74.8%), and adjustable gastric banding 47.5% (40.7%–54.2%). These estimates have been widely used as clinical benchmarks in the field. In 2009 Garb and colleagues[5] conducted a meta-analysis of 28 studies that reported bariatric surgery weight loss outcomes in the literature from 2003 to 2007 involving 7383 patients. This study showed similar outcomes in terms of percent EWL to those reported by Buchwald and colleagues. Specifically, Garb and colleagues reported a composite EWL of 49.4% for LAGB versus the estimate of 47.5% by Buchwald and colleagues and a composite EWL of 62.6% for laparoscopic RYGB versus 61.6% reported by Buchwald and colleagues The superior EWL with laparoscopic RYGB persisted at all 3 postsurgical time points examined (1, 2, and >3 years). Specifically, for LAGB, EWL was 42.6% at 1 year, 50.3% at 2 years, and 55.2% at more than 3 years after surgery and for RYGB, this was 61.5% at 1 year, 69.7% at 2 years, and 71.2% at more than 3 years after surgery. Although patient retention in clinical reports is high at 1 year for studies involving both

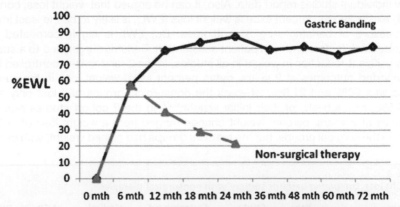

Fig. 1. Weight loss, expressed as percent of percent EWL (%EWL) in a randomized, controlled trial (RCT) of gastric banding versus optimal nonsurgical therapy in mild to moderately obese patients (data derived from continued follow-up of gastric banding patients from the RCT). The gastric banding group show durability of the weight loss at 6-year follow-up. (*Data from* O'Brien PE. Bariatric surgery: mechanisms, indications and outcomes. J Gastroenterol Hepatol 2010;25(8):1358–65; and O'Brien PE, Dixon JB, Laurie C, et al. Treatment of mild to moderate obesity with laparoscopic adjustable gastric banding or an intensive medical program: a randomized trial. Ann Intern Med 2006;144(9):625–33.)

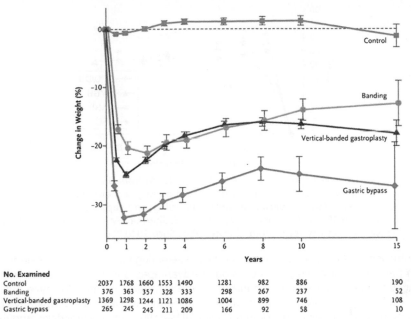

No. Examined									
Control	2037	1768	1660	1553	1490	1281	982	886	190
Banding	376	363	357	328	333	298	267	237	52
Vertical-banded gastroplasty	1369	1298	1244	1121	1086	1004	899	746	108
Gastric bypass	265	245	245	211	209	166	92	58	10

Fig. 2. Mean percent weight change during a 15-year period in the control group and surgery group, according to the method of bariatric surgery as reported in SOS (error bars = 95% C.I.). (*From* Sjostrom L, Narbro K, Sjostrom CD, et al. Effects of bariatric surgery on mortality in Swedish obese subjects. N Engl J Med 2007;357(8):747; with permission.)

types of surgery, more than 50% of patients were lost to follow-up at 2 years, and more than 80% were lost at more than 3 years. Despite these concerns, this meta-analysis provides further support of the superiority of laparoscopic RYGB when compared with LAGB in terms of percent EWL reported in earlier studies. For LSG, early, nonrandomized data suggest that LSG is efficacious. Average weight loss results from 15 published studies (940 patients) indicate EWL of 59.8% at 1 year, 64.7% at 2 years, and 66.0%, results comparable to the EWL with laparoscopic RYGB. However, data are not mature enough to clarify if weight loss after LSG is durable (**Fig. 3**).

Comparison Between Bariatric Procedures

Obesity surgery has evolved over the past 50 years. Many surgical techniques have been described and abandoned, but numerous different techniques are still in use.[29] RYGB, LAGB, and BPD/DS are validated procedures that may be performed laparoscopically. LSG is a promising procedure that over the last few years has generated significant interest and needs to be added to the list of available operations. Although all of the operations do result in successful weight loss, they differ in terms of morbidity and mortality, magnitude and maintenance of weight loss, rate of resolution of comorbidities, and side effect profile.[30] We have summarized these data in **Tables 4** and **5** and **Fig. 4**. Although BPD/DS, RYGB, and LAGB are all are superior to nonsurgical therapy, the relative effectiveness of these procedures has not been fully compared and available data are rarely randomized or controlled and often compare nonequivalent cohorts. Thus, in comparing these data, there are currently no large-scale head-to-head randomized trials comparing surgical procedures. No consensus exists as to which procedure offers the best option overall, and there are

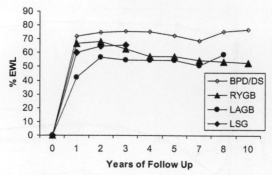

Fig. 3. EWL at 1, 2, 3 years for LAGB, LSG, and RYGB. (*Data from* Garb J, Welch G, Zagarins S, et al. Bariatric surgery for the treatment of morbid obesity: a meta-analysis of weight loss outcomes for laparoscopic adjustable gastric banding and laparoscopic gastric bypass. Obes Surg 2009;19(10):1447–55; and Shi X, Karmali S, Sharma AM, et al. A review of laparoscopic sleeve gastrectomy for morbid obesity. Obes Surg 2010;20(8):1171–7.)

no established criteria or algorithms to assist in selecting the appropriate operation for each patient. All of these procedures have advantages and disadvantages, with no clear evidence of one being recognized as the standard of care. We have outlined the relative strength and weakness of each procedure in **Table 6**. Comparative data find that procedures with more dramatic clinical benefits carry greater risks, and those offering greater safety and flexibility are associated with less reliable efficacy (**Table 7**).[3,30] As outlined in **Table 8**, O'Brien[3] has developed a relative risk score for each type of weight-loss approach. Despite the lack of consensus, it is clear that obesity surgery today offers the only effective long-term treatment option for the severely obese patient.[23]

Laparoscopic RYGB

Outcomes
Numerous studies, including several prospective randomized controlled trials,[31–38] a large prospective case-controlled cohort study,[39] numerous case series, and 4 meta-analyses[19,25,26,40] compare laparoscopic RYGB (LRYGB) with open RYGB as well as with medical weight management and other surgical procedures.[30]

Table 4 Surgical procedures compared			
Outcomes	LAGB	LRYGB	LSG
Number of cases	3374	3195	940
Operative time (min)	77.5	64.8	100.4
Hospital stay (d)	1.7	4.2	4.4
% EWL (1 y)	37.8	62.8	59.8
% EWL (2 y)	45.0	54.4	64.7
%EWL (3 y)	55.0	66.0	66.0
Comorbidity resolution (%)	41–59	65–84	45–95.5
Complications (%)	6.50	9.50	12.1
Mortality (%)	0.47	0.56	0.3

Data from Shi X, Karmali S, Sharma AM, et al. A review of laparoscopic sleeve gastrectomy for morbid obesity. Obes Surg 2010;20(8):1171–7.

Table 5
Surgical procedures compared mortality and morbidity

Operation	30-Day Mortality (%)	Overall Complications (%)	Major Complications (%)
LAGB	0.05–0.4	9	0.2
RYGB	0.5–1.1	23	2
Laparoscopic BPD/DS	2.5–7.6	25	5
LSG	0.3	11.2	4.7

Data from Refs.[7,30,73]

Patients who undergo LRYGB typically experience an EWL of 60% to 70%, with 75% control of comorbidities.[19,25,26,39] In general, these outcomes are better than those for banding procedures, which have an EWL of 45% to 50% and less predictable improvement of comorbidities, but not so good as the outcomes for BPD/DS, which has an EWL of 70% to 80% and excellent control of comorbidities (**Table 9**).[19,30] Open and LRYGB have similar efficacy and in case series[40] and prospective randomized trials,[32–34,37] there are no significant differences in weight loss for up to 3 years of follow-up evaluation. RYGB is more effective than medical therapy in terms of weight loss and resolution of comorbidities. Some studies indicate that morbidly obese patients using behavioral and medical weight management alone may gain weight over the 5 years to 10 years.[25,39] Patients undergoing RYGB have a lower 5-year mortality than nonsurgical patients (0.68% vs 6.17%) despite a 0.4% perioperative mortality.[41]

Complications

The mortality after RYGB ranges from 0.3% in case series to 1% in controlled trials, and the rate of preventable and nonpreventable adverse surgical events is 18.7%.[26] The mortality in a review of selected LRYGB series ranged from 0.5% to 1.1%.[42]

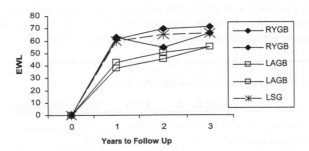

Year	Author	n	Procedure	1 Year	2 Years	3 Years
					Excess weight loss	
2009	Garb	7383	RYGB	61.5	69.7	71.2
2010	Shi	3195	RYGB	62.8	54.4	66.0
2009	Garb	7383	LAGB	42.6	50.3	55.2
2010	Shi	3374	LAGB	37.8	45.0	55.0
2010	Shi	940	LSG	59.8	64.7	66.0

Fig. 4. Surgical procedures compared percentage of EWL.

Table 6
Comparison of qualities of different bariatric procedures

Procedure	LAGB	RYGB	BPD	LSG
Objective				
Least perioperative risk	■■■	■■	■	■■
Most effective durable weight loss	■	■■	■■■	?
Best comorbidity resolution	■	■■	■■■	■■
Most reversible	■■■	■	■	■
Best procedure for avoiding reoperation because of				
Technical complications: early	■■■	■■	■	■■
Technical complications: late	■	■■	■■	■■■
Metabolic complications: late	■■■	■■	■	■■■
Least chance of inadequate weight loss	■	■■	■■■	?
Subjective				
Fewest outpatient visits required	■	■■■	■■	■■■
Fewest unintended metabolic complications of poor follow-up	■■■	■■	■	■■■
Durable weight loss despite poor patient compliance	■	■■	■■■	?

■ to ■■■, worst to best in category.
Data from Refs.[3,30,73]

The most frequently reported perioperative complications associated with LRYGB are wound infection (2.98%), anastomotic leak (2.05%), gastrointestinal tract hemorrhage (1.93%), bowel obstruction (1.73%), and pulmonary embolus (0.41%), whereas the most frequently reported late complications are stomal stenosis (4.73%), bowel obstruction (3.15%), and incisional hernia (0.47%).[30,43] The safety of LRYGB has been compared with that of open RYGB, and results show that laparoscopic patients have a reduced incidence of iatrogenic injury to the spleen requiring splenectomy, wound infection, incisional hernia, and perioperative mortality, but higher rates of bowel obstruction, intestinal hemorrhage, and stomal stenoses.[43]

Table 7
Comparison of attributes of the principal bariatric procedures

Attribute	Gastric Band	RYGB	Sleeve Gastrectomy	BPD ± DS
Safe	+++	++	++	+
Effective	++	++	++	+++
Durable	+++	+++	?	+++
Side effects	+	++	+	++
Reversible easily	Yes	No	No	No
Minimally invasive	+++	++	++	+
Controllable/adjustable	Yes	No	No	No
Low revision rate	+	+	?	+
Requires follow-up	+++	++	+	++

+ to +++, worst to best in category.
Data from O'Brien PE. Bariatric surgery: mechanisms, indications and outcomes. J Gastroenterol Hepatol 2010;25(8):1358–65.

Table 8
Weight-loss approaches and their relative risks, side effects, invasiveness, and costs

Ranking by Risk	Approach	Risk Score
1.	Lifestyle changes: eat less, more activity and exercise, modify behavior	1
2.	Drugs and low-energy diets	2
3.	Endoscopic approaches (eg, intragastric balloon)	4
4.	Gastric banding	5
5.	Sleeve gastrectomy	7
6.	RYGB	8
7.	Open BPD	9
8.	Laparoscopic BPD	10

Data from O'Brien PE. Bariatric surgery: mechanisms, indications and outcomes. J Gastroenterol Hepatol 2010;25(8):1358–65.

LAGB

Various types of LAGB exist, although only the LAP-BAND (Allergan Inc, Irvine, CA) and the REALIZE (Ethicon Endo-Surgery Inc, Cincinnati, OH) adjustable gastric band currently have US Food and Drug Administration (FDA) approval for use in the United States. The equivalence between the 2 FDA-approved devices in the United States has been shown,[44] but comparative trials with other devices do not exist. Recently, the LAP-BAND system has received approval for placement in patients with class I obesity (BMI 30–34.9 kg/m^2) who have major obesity-related comorbidities.[30]

Outcomes

LAGB is effective at producing weight loss, with patients losing approximately 50% of their excess body weight.[19,45] This weight loss occurs in a gradual manner, with approximately 35% EWL by 6 months, 40% by 12 months, and 50% by 24 months. This percentage seems to remain stable after 3 to 8 years based on the few studies providing a follow-up period of this length.[46–49] However, as many as 25% of LAGB patients fail to lose 50% of their excess body weight by 5 years.[19,50] The short-term (12-month) weight loss with LAGB is inferior to that with RYGB[51] and this difference persists: a randomized controlled trial found that EWL at 5 years was 47.5% with LAGB versus 66.6% with RYGB.[52] However, life-threatening complications occur less frequently with LAGB than with LRYGB.

Table 9
Improvement of comorbidities after bariatric surgery

Operation	Diabetes Resolved (%)	Hypercholesterolemia Improved (%)	Hypertension Resolved (%)	Sleep Apnea Resolved (%)
AGB	47.8	71.1	38.4	94.6
RGB	83.8	93.6	75.4	86.6
BPD ± DS	97.9	99.5	81.3	95.2
LSG	77.2	61.0	71.7	83.6

Data from Refs.[7,30,73]

LAGB has beneficial effects on the comorbidities of obesity. Type 2 diabetes is improved in up to 90% of patients as a result of increased insulin sensitivity and increased pancreatic β-cell function,[53] and diabetic medications are eliminated for 64% of patients.[54,55] After LAGB, resolution of type 2 diabetes is a result of weight loss and, therefore, is slower to occur than after RYGB or BPD/DS, in which the diabetes may resolve almost immediately.[53,56] Symptoms of gastroesophageal reflux disease may be eliminated for up to 89% of patients at 12 months, even for those with large hiatus hernias,[57,58] but with the side effect of impaired lower esophageal sphincter relaxation and possible altered esophageal motility.[59] The rate of obstructive sleep apnea decreases from 33% to 2% for LAGB patients.[60] Major QoL improvements are seen after LAGB, with significant improvement of all subscales of the Medical Outcomes Study Short Form 36 general QoL questionnaire, particularly in areas of bodily pain, general health perception, and mental health perception.[61–63]

LAGB has been compared with intensive pharmacotherapy, behavioral modification, diet modification, and exercise among patients with class I obesity (BMI of 30–35 kg/m^2). In this population, LAGB is seen to be more effective in reducing weight, resolving metabolic derangements, and improving QoL.[27,30]

Complications

Among all bariatric operations, early mortality is the lowest for LAGB. Case series and systematic reviews show early mortality after LAGB at 0.05% to 0.4%,[26,64] compared with 0.5% to 1.1% for LRYGB,[42] 0.5% to 1.0% for open RYGB,[19,26] 1.1%[26] for open BPD/DS, and 2.5% to 7.6% for laparoscopic BPD/DS.[65–67]

Regarding relative morbidity, comparative data are few. Overall complications and major complications were less common with LAGB than with LRYGB or laparoscopic BPD/DS in a single-center experience.[68] LAGB placement by the perigastric approach[63] is associated with higher complication rates: gastrointestinal perforation (1%) and other visceral injury (1%). Band-related complications such as slippage/pouch dilation (24%), esophageal dilation (8%), and stoma obstruction (14%) accumulated over a 5-year follow-up period. Port-site complications including pain, port displacement, and leak were found in about 7% of patients and the mean explantation or major revision rate by 9 years was 33%.[30]

In contrast, the pars flaccida technique for band placement[63] is associated with fewer complications, with reduced slippage/pouch dilation (7%), esophageal dilation (1%), and stoma obstruction (2%) at 1 year. Because of the reduction of band-specific complications, the pars flaccida technique has been widely adopted.[69,70] In 1 series in which only the pars flaccida technique was used with a 7-year follow-up period, the slippage/pouch dilation incidence was 12%; however, the cumulative reoperation rate was 32%.[70]

LSG

LSG is an emerging treatment modality for the surgical management of morbid obesity. LSG may induce weight loss by restrictive and endocrine mechanisms. A systematic review of the literature analyzing the clinical outcomes of LSG suggests that LSG is efficacious in the management of morbid obesity and may offer certain advantages when compared with the existing options of LAGB and laparoscopic RYGB. These advantages include technical ease, lack of an intestinal anastomosis, normal intestinal absorption, no risk of internal hernias, no implantation of a foreign body, and pylorus preservation, which prevents dumping syndrome. In addition, LSG is considered by some to be the most appropriate option in extremely obese patients.[71]

Outcomes

For LSG, the reported EWL ranges from 33% to 90%, with follow-up between 6 months and 36 months. Comorbidity resolution 12 to 24 months after LSG has been reported in 365 patients. The data show rates of resolution and improvement of diabetes, hypertension, hyperlipidemia, degenerative joint disease, gastroesophageal reflux, peripheral edema, sleep apnea, and depression after LSG ranging from 45% to 95.3%. These results are comparable with other restrictive procedures. One randomized trial was published that compared LSG with LAGB; results showed LSG to be at least as effective and durable as gastric banding at 1 and 3 years after surgery.[72,73] Medium-term clinical outcomes for LSG will emerge in the near future; however, long-term (>10 years) weight loss and comorbidity resolution data for LSG will remain undefined for several years.

Complications

As with other procedures for bariatric surgery, perioperative risk for LSG appeared to be low even in patients considered high risk. The overall reported mortality for LSG was 0.3%. Published complication rates ranged from 0% to 29% (average 11.2%). The most important major complications associated with LSG include staple line leak (1.17%) and postoperative hemorrhage (3.57%). Early nonrandomized data suggest that LSG is efficacious in the surgical management of morbid obesity; however, it is not clear if weight loss after LSG is durable long-term (beyond 3–5 years) and, therefore, the need for revisional surgery after LSG is still uncertain.[72]

Laparoscopic BPD/DS

Outcomes

BPD/DS leads to dramatic weight loss during the first 12 postoperative months, which then continues at a slower rate over the next 6 months. Weight loss is durable up to at least 5 years postoperatively. Up to 95% of patients with a BMI less than 50 kg/m^2, and 70% of those with a BMI exceeding 50 kg/m^2, achieve more than 50% EWL.[74,75] Current data suggest that the weight loss effect of BPD/DS is greater and more durable than that of LAGB (see **Table 6**).[46,76] Some therefore argue that BPD/DS and RYGB may be superior to LAGB for patients with a BMI of 50 kg/m^2 or greater.[77] As with all bariatric operations, weight may be regained over time,[78] highlighting the importance of long-term follow-up and assessment.

The BPD/DS procedure has a dramatic impact on comorbidities (see **Table 9**). In a recent meta-analysis BPD/DS was found to induce more weight loss and to lead to greater improvement of diabetes, hyperlipidemia, hypercholesterolemia, hypertriglyceridemia, and obstructive sleep apnea than any other type of bariatric procedure.[19] At least 90% of patients with type 2 diabetes cease diabetic medications by 12 to 36 months.[74,79] Between 50% and 80% of hypertensive patients are cured, with another 10% experiencing improvement.[80] Up to 98% of patients with obstructive sleep apnea experience resolution.[76,81] Despite the favorable reports of BPD/DS for the treatment of morbid obesity, it has been slow to gain widespread acceptance because of perioperative risks and long-term nutrition problems. BPD/DS currently accounts for only 0.9% of procedures performed in the United States.[9,30]

Complications

The reported 30-day mortality for open BPD/DS is 0.76% and 1.11% for laparoscopic BPD/DS.[7] Earlier reports for laparoscopic BPD/DS series indicate a 30-day mortality ranging from 2.6% to 7.6%.[65,66] Major complications, which occur in up to 25% of cases, may include early occurrence of anastomotic leak, duodenal stump leak, intra-abdominal infection, hemorrhage, and venous thromboembolism.[67,82–84]

Reported late complications include bowel obstruction, incarceration, or anastomotic stricture.[68]

The performance of a sleeve gastrectomy as part of the BPD/DS allows patients two-thirds of their preoperative dietary volume without specific food intolerances; however, diarrhea is a not infrequent chronic complication of BPD/DS. A common channel length of 50 cm is associated with reports of diarrhea in most patients,[85] whereas a length of 100 cm is not.[83] Because of fat malabsorption resulting from BPD/DS, supplementation of fat-soluble vitamins is recommended. Deficiency of these vitamins is more likely with a shorter common channel. Iron deficiency is common, with 6% of patients experiencing serious iron deficiency anemia (hemoglobin <10 mg/dL),[86] and replacement of iron should be based on surveillance of biochemical and hematologic markers of deficiency. Calcium and vitamin D malabsorption also are common and manifest as secondary hyperparathyroidism.[86,87] Supplements do not prevent the development of secondary hyperparathyroidism and an increase in bone resorption is known to occur irrespective of parathormone levels, suggesting a phenomenon of bone reshaping parallel to the loss of weight.[88] Cholelithiasis postoperatively occurs in 6%[89] to 25%[90] of patients. Some surgeons advocate routine cholecystectomy given the alteration in endoscopic accessibility to the biliary tract, whereas others argue for delayed cholecystectomy only if symptoms develop because cholecystitis occurs uncommonly after BPD/DS.[91]

INFLUENCE OF PATIENT CHARACTERISTICS ON EARLY COMPLICATIONS

In evaluating different bariatric surgical procedures, one has to consider that more than half of the patients undergoing surgery have multiple coexisting conditions at the time of surgery. The risk of developing general complications including venous thromboembolism (1%), pulmonary or respiratory insufficiency (<1%), hemorrhage (1%), abdominal reoperation (2.6%), endoscopic interventions (1.1%), and wound infection (2%) is influenced by both patient characteristics and selection of the surgical procedure. Recent high-quality studies indicate that, overall, these complications occur in about 4.1% of bariatric surgery patients.[10,23] Occurrence is influenced by procedure type, with 1.0% of patients undergoing placement of am LAGB, 4.8% of those who underwent LRYGB, and 7.8% of those who underwent open RYGB developing one of these complications. Also, patient characteristics such as a history of deep vein thrombosis or pulmonary embolus, a diagnosis of obstructive sleep apnea, and impaired functional status and both extremely high and low values of BMI are each independently associated with an increased risk of developing a major complication, whereas age, sex, race, ethnic group, and other coexisting conditions are not.[10] Therefore, both improvement of surgical techniques (eg, addition of laparoscopy) and optimization of patient management strategies aimed at lowering complications (eg, decreasing pulmonary complications, reducing medical errors, preventing iatrogenic hypotension, and reducing wound infections) have been instrumental in decreasing these rates.[12,23,43,92] The overall risk of death and other adverse outcomes after bariatric surgery is low and varies considerably according to patient characteristics. In helping patients make appropriate choices, short-term safety should be considered in conjunction with both the long-term effects of bariatric surgery and the risks associated with being morbidly obese.

COMPARATIVE EFFECTIVENESS STUDIES

Most of our knowledge about the comparative effectiveness of various weigh-loss operations has come from observational research that has often been of limited duration of follow-up. Consequently, there is no strong evidence to recommend any of the different bariatric procedures over the others, and the numbers of studies that directly compare the different surgical weight-loss strategies remain limited. We therefore focused on a select number of recent studies that address this topic (**Table 10**).

RYGB Versus AGB

Multiple retrospective studies have reported on the outcomes of LRYGB versus LAGB, but there are few prospective, randomized trials comparing the outcomes of LRYGB versus LAGB. In a randomized trial, Nguyen and colleagues[93] evaluated the outcomes, convalescence, QoL, and costs of LRYGB versus LAGB. In this study, 111 patients underwent LRYGB and 86 patients underwent LAGB. The study concluded that LRYGB and LAGB are both safe and effective approaches for the treatment of morbid obesity. There were no early deaths in either group. Compared with LAGB, operative blood loss was higher and the mean operative time and length of stay were longer in the LRYGB group. LRYGB was associated with more perioperative and late complications and a higher 30-day readmission rate. The 30-day complication rate was 21.6% for LRYGB versus 7.0% for LAGB; however, there were no life-threatening complications such as leaks or sepsis. The most frequent late complication in the LRYGB group was stricture (14.3%). The 1-year mortality was 0.9% for the LRYGB group and 0% for

Table 10
Comparative effectiveness studies: RYGB, AGB, LSG

RYGB vs AGB		
	RYGB	**AGB**
Early Complications (%)	13–22	1.6–7.0
Late Complications (%)	36.2	27.4
Mortality (%)	0.0–0.9	0.0–0.0
%EWL (4–5 y)	68–93	45–59
Treatment Failure (%)	0–6	17–46
Comorbidity Resolution	++++	++
QoL Improvement	++	++
CV Risk Improvement	+++	++
CV Mortality Reduction	+++	++
RYGB vs LSG		
	RYGB	**LSG**
Early Complications (%)	9–20	4–6.5
Late Complications	—	—
Mortality (%)	0.0	0.0
%EWL (1 y)	64–86	59–79
Comorbidity Resolution	++++	+++
Lipid Improvement	+++	++
Metabolic Syndrome	+++	++
LSG vs AGB		
	LSG	**AGB**
%EWL (1 y)	50.6	40.3
Comorbidity Resolution	+++	++

+ to +++, worst to best in category.

the LAGB group. LRYGB resulted in better weight loss at medium-term and long-term follow-up. The percent EWL at 4 years was 68 ± 19% in the LRYGB group compared with 45 ± 28% in the LAGB group (P<.05). Also, there was a wide variation in weight loss after LAGB. Treatment failure, defined as losing less than 20% of excess weight or conversion to another bariatric operation for failure of weight loss, occurred in 16.7% of the patients who underwent LAGB and in 0% of those who underwent LRYGB, with male gender being a predictive factor for poor weight loss after LAGB. At 1 year after surgery, QoL improved in both groups to that of US norms. The total cost was higher for LRYGB compared with LAGB procedure.

In a 5-year follow-up study, Boza and colleagues[94] compared LRYGB (n = 91) versus LAGB (n = 62). The mean operative time was 150 ± 58 minutes for LRYGB and 73 ± 23 minutes for LAGB (P<.05). In the LRYGB group the conversion rate was 8% and the reoperation rate was 4.3% versus 0% for the LAGB group. Early post-operative complications were observed in 12 patients for the LRYGB group and 1 patient after LAGB (P = .014). Late complications developed in 33 patients after LRYGB and in 17 patients after LAGB (P = not significant [NS]). The investigators observed a greater percentage of EWL at 1 and 5 years after LRYGB compared with LAGB. The percentage of EWL at 5 years postoperatively was 92.9% ± 25.6% for LRYGB compared with 59.1% ± 46.8% (P<.001) for LAGB. Surgical failure, defined as percentage of EWL less than 50%, was seen in more than 40% of the patients with LAGB, with a 24.1% reoperation rate at 5-year follow-up. In contrast, at 5 years, only 6% for LRYGB showed surgical failure.

Two recent studies have compared the short-term and long-term effects of LRYGB and LAGB on cardiovascular risk factors.[95,96] From a short-term perspective, Wood-ard and colleagues[95] reported 1-year improvements in biochemical cardiovascular risk factors in both LRYGB and LAGB. At 12 months postoperatively, LRYGB patients had lost 77% of their excess weight and had significant improvements in biochemical cardiovascular risk factors such as total cholesterol, low-density lipoprotein, high-density lipoprotein (HDL), triglyceride (Trig), Trig/HDL, C-reactive protein, fasting insulin, and hemoglobin (Hgb) A1C. LAGB patients lost 47.6% of their excess weight and also had significant improvements in biochemical cardiovascular risk factors such as Trig, Trig/HDL, and Hgb A1C. The investigators concluded that improvements in a greater number of biochemical cardiovascular risk factors are seen in the LRYGB group. The values indicate a significantly better improvement of the risk profile in LRYGB versus LAGB patients.

From a long-term perspective, a meta-analytical study performed by Pontiroli and Morabito[96] showed that bariatric surgery reduces long-term mortality. Although both LAGB and RYGB reduce mortality, there is a greater effect of LRYGB on cardio-vascular mortality.

RYGB Versus LSG

Initial results suggest that LSG is safe and effective. Case series indicate that weight loss and resolution of comorbidities after LSG are comparable with those with LRYGB, but there are only a few studies directly comparing LRYGB to LSG.

In a multicenter, retrospective study of 400 patients, Chouillard and colleagues[97] analyzed the weight loss, resolution of comorbidities, and complications of both LSG and LRYGB using a case-control study design. The postoperative complications, the percentage of EWL, and the resolution of comorbidities in each group were compared at 6, 12, and 18 months postoperatively. The study indicates that LRYGB was associated with a greater short-term morbidity. The morbidity was significantly greater in the LRYGB group (20.5%) compared with the LSG group (6.5%; P<.05).

The percentage of EWL at 1 year was 58% for the LSG and 64% for LRYGB (P = NS). The overall remission of type 2 diabetes was significantly better in the LRYGB group compared with LSG (P<.05). At 18 months, 86% of those with diabetes in the LRYGB group were without any medication compared with only 62% of previously diabetic patients in the LSG group (P<.05). The resolution of other comorbidities such as hypertension and sleep apnea was comparable in both groups.

Similarly, in a prospective study of 117 patients, Leyba and colleagues[98] reported on the short-term outcome of LSG compared with LRYGB. These investigators reported a shorter operative time (82 minutes) for LSG compared with LRYGB (98 minutes). The major complication rate was 4.7% for LSG and 9.3% for LRYGB (P = NS). The EWL at 1 year was 86% for LRYGB and 78.8% for LSG (P = NS) Resolution of comorbidities was seen in 40% for LSG and 64.7% of LRYGB (P = NS). The study concluded that in the short-term, both techniques are comparable regarding safety and effectiveness, with no clear distinction between both procedures.

In a case-control study of 22 patients, comparing LRYGB and LSG, Iannelli and colleagues[99] studied inflammation, insulin resistance, lipid disturbances, and metabolic syndrome. In this detailed study, patients undergoing LRYGB reported a significantly higher level of improvement of lipid profiles, with a stronger impact on systemic low-grade inflammation and less metabolic syndrome than those with LSG at 1-year follow-up.

LSG Versus AGB

Comparative studies of LSG and LAGB are rare. In the first retrospective review of 123 patients, Omana and colleagues[100] compared the rates for resolution and improvement of common comorbidities between LSG and laparoscopic AGB. The comorbid conditions included were type 2 diabetes mellitus, hypertension, hyperlipidemias, degenerative joint disease, gastroesophageal reflux disease, obstructive sleep apnea, and asthma. The overall percent EWLs were 50.6% for LSG and 40.3% for LAGB (P = .03) at 1-year follow-up. Compared with LAGB, LSG showed a greater impact on resolution of 3 significant comorbidities: improvement of type 2 diabetes mellitus (100% vs 46%), hypertension (78% vs 48%), and hyperlipidemia (87% vs 50%). The investigators observed a similar rate of resolution or improvement for the other comorbidities studied.

IMPROVEMENT OF LIFE EXPECTANCY/LONG-TERM SURVIVAL ADVANTAGE

The results of a recent meta-analysis, as well as outcomes of an increasing number of carefully conducted studies, report decreased mortality in patients who have undergone bariatric surgery compared with those who have not.[17,22,41,96,101–105] The meta-analysis conducted by Pontiroli and Morabito[96] indicated that bariatric surgery reduces risk of mortality and cardiovascular mortality when compared with participants not undergoing surgery. Both RYGB and LAGB seem to reduce mortality risk. Most studies indicate that the reduced mortality is specifically caused by decreases in myocardial infarction, diabetes mellitus, and cancer-related deaths.

In 2007, the SOS study, the first prospective controlled study designed specifically to assess mortality, reported a 25% mortality decrease in bariatric surgery patients at 10 years compared with a well-matched control population.[22] The University of Utah study,[101] published simultaneously with the SOS study, found a 40% decrease in mortality after RYGB compared with a matched nonsurgical cohort at 2 years with significant decreases in cancer, diabetes mellitus, and myocardial infarction deaths. The results of these 2 studies were supported by earlier findings of Flum and

Dellinger[17] in their report of a retrospective cohort study of more than 66,000 patients who had undergone RYGB in the state of Washington. At 15-year follow-up, the surgical cohort had 27% fewer deaths than the cohort of obese subjects who did not undergo bariatric surgery.[17] The McGill Bariatric Cohort Study, an observational 2-cohort study, noted an 89% reduction in mortality in patients who underwent surgery for obesity compared with a matched cohort of severely obese patients at 5 years. This study also noted a significant decrease in treatment of cancer in the surgical group.[41] An Australian cohort study on LAGB reported a reduction in the relative risk of death in the surgical group. Surgical patients had a 72% lower hazard of death than the community controls.[105] Similarly, Busetto and colleagues[104] found that LAGB patients have a lower risk of death than matched cohorts who did not have surgery. Other studies, using different types of databases, also suggest that mortality is reduced after surgery.[106,107] MacDonald and colleagues[102] found that the mortality in patients who underwent bariatric surgery was 9% (n = 154) compared with 28% (n = 78) in those who did not. In a similar study, Sowenimo and colleagues[103] found an 81% reduction in mortality for bariatric surgery patients versus those who did not have surgery when compared at 4 years.

QOL

Obesity results in physical and psychosocial comorbidities as well as poor QoL and, in general, QoL and psychosocial functioning improve after bariatric surgery.[108] However, the results are mixed, with some studies indicating no improvement or a reversion to baseline levels of psychosocial distress.[109] The variability in results may be representative of methodologic issues, such as differences in assessment measures, outcome variables studied, or time frame used for follow-up. In a recent study, Mohos and colleagues[110] compared QoL parameters after LRYGB and LSG. The results of the study indicate a relatively high score of the QoL in both groups of patients. RYGB was associated with a trend toward a better QoL without reaching statistical significance compared with LSG. Similarly, a study by Campos and colleagues[111] indicates a better QoL after LRYGB versus LAGB. In this study, comparing the complications and 1-year outcomes of LRYGB and LAGB in 200 pair-matched morbidly obese patients, the investigators found that QoL measures were better in the LRYGB group. Further research designed to address these methodologic issues is needed to more fully elucidate psychosocial outcome of bariatric surgery. However, it seems that at least in the short-term, bariatric surgery may improve QoL and psychosocial outcome in a substantial proportion of patients.[112]

HEALTH CARE COST IMPACT

The cost-effectiveness of bariatric surgery is an important outcome measure that requires additional study. Current statistical studies estimate that more than 9% of all US health care dollars spent are for the treatment of medical conditions either caused or exacerbated by obesity. According to a statistical review by the Rand Corporation, 20% of health care dollars spent by people aged 50 to 69 years will be obesity-related by the year 2020, up 50% from 2000. To date, investigators have used national, state, and institutional databases to estimate the following variables: surgical hospital costs and charges,[113,114] pharmaceutical costs,[115] health care use claims,[115,116] and cost per quality-adjusted life year (QALY).[24] Overall, bariatric surgery patients can expect to stay in the hospital, on average, 2.22 days but average lengths of stay varies by state.[11] Overall, bariatric surgery patients are charged, on average, $38,254 for a laparoscopic procedure, whereas the average charge for an open procedure (eg, gastric bypass or malabsorptive) is $38,323. The question to be answered is whether these bariatric surgical procedures are worth their cost. Although definitive conclusions cannot be made, many studies suggest that surgical obesity treatment decreases the use of medications for diabetes and cardiovascular disease, the frequency of outpatient visits, and long-term direct health care costs and seems to be worth the costs of the intervention.[117] Some claim that the improvement/cure of obesity-associated conditions with bariatric surgery reduces the requirement for visits to the physician's office or the hospital, which translates to a reduction in health care costs.[118,119] In comparing the return on investment analysis for treating patients after bariatric surgery with morbidly obese patients treated conventionally over a 5-year period, the return on investment averages 3.5 years for bariatric surgery.[120] Similar cost savings with bariatric surgery were reported by Cremieux and colleagues,[121] who concluded that downstream savings associated with bariatric surgery are estimated to offset the initial costs in 2 to 4 years. Similarly, in a review to assess the cost-effectiveness of bariatric surgery for obesity, bariatric surgery was cost-effective compared with nonsurgical treatment. However, there are concerns that the estimates used for some studies may be not generalizable because of methodological shortcomings and the modeling assumptions made.[24] In an alternative economic model, surgical management was more costly than nonsurgical management, but resulted in improved outcomes. In this model for morbid obesity, incremental cost-effectiveness ratios ranged between $3200 and $6400 per QALY gained.[24]

In contrast, other studies identified a significant high complication rate during the 6 months after surgery, resulting in costly readmissions and emergency department visits in nearly 40% of patients.[113] Future health and economic outcome studies will need to assess all aspects of preoperative, perioperative, and postoperative care.[122] The advancement of less invasive surgical techniques along with shorter duration of hospital stay will likely have additional cost benefits.

SUMMARY

Bariatric surgery is an effective treatment of patients with morbid obesity. Current evidence, including the results of randomized controlled studies, documents that bariatric surgery produces durable weight loss. It leads to long-term remission of type 2 diabetes in up to 80% and has beneficial effects on other comorbidities. Obesity surgery leads to a significant reduction in mortality in the long-term. Although the severely obese present with serious surgical risks, bariatric surgery is performed safely with a 0.35% 90-day mortality in Centers of Excellence throughout the United States (similar to the complication rates after cholecystectomy).[123] RYGB, adjustable gastric banding, and BPD/DS are validated procedures that may be performed laparoscopically. LSG also is a promising procedure. Comparing procedures remains difficult, but data suggest that procedures with more dramatic clinical benefits carry greater risks, and those offering greater safety and flexibility are associated with less reliable efficacy. Currently, the choice of operation should be driven by patient and surgeon preferences, as well as by considerations regarding the relative importance placed on the desired outcome.[30] Future studies are needed to better understand the economic impact and risk benefit according to the underlying procedure and impact on improvement of comorbid conditions and QoL.

REFERENCES

1. World Health Organization. Overweight and Obesity. Factsheet no. 311. Geneva (Switzerland): World Health Organization; 2006.

2. Flegal KM, Carroll MD, Ogden CL, et al. Prevalence and trends in obesity among US adults, 1999-2008. JAMA 2010;303(3):235–41.
3. O'Brien PE. Bariatric surgery: mechanisms, indications and outcomes. J Gastroenterol Hepatol 2010;25(8):1358–65.
4. American Society for Metabolic and Bariatric Surgery (ASMBS) Fact sheet. Available at: http://www.asbs.org/Newsite07/media/asmbs_fs_surgery.pdf. Accessed March 27, 2011.
5. Garb J, Welch G, Zagarins S, et al. Bariatric surgery for the treatment of morbid obesity: a meta-analysis of weight loss outcomes for laparoscopic adjustable gastric banding and laparoscopic gastric bypass. Obes Surg 2009;19(10): 1447–55.
6. Dixon JB, O'Brien PE, Playfair J, et al. Adjustable gastric banding and conventional therapy for type 2 diabetes: a randomized controlled trial. JAMA 2008; 299(3):316–23.
7. Buchwald H, Estok R, Fahrbach K, et al. Trends in mortality in bariatric surgery: a systematic review and meta-analysis. Surgery 2007;142(4):621–32 [discussion: 632–5].
8. Buchwald H, Oien DM. Metabolic/bariatric surgery Worldwide 2008. Obes Surg 2009;19(12):1605–11.
9. DeMaria EJ, Pate V, Warthen M, et al. Baseline data from American Society for Metabolic and Bariatric Surgery-designated Bariatric Surgery Centers of Excellence using the Bariatric Outcomes Longitudinal Database. Surg Obes Relat Dis 2010;6(4):347–55.
10. Flum DR, Belle SH, King WC, et al. Perioperative safety in the longitudinal assessment of bariatric surgery. N Engl J Med 2009;361(5):445–54.
11. Nicholas C, May R. HealthGrades Fifth Annual Bariatric Surgery Trends in American Hospitals Study. Golden (CO): Health Grades, Inc; 2010.
12. Blackburn GL, Hutter MM, Harvey AM, et al. Expert panel on weight loss surgery: executive report update. Obesity (Silver Spring) 2009;17(5):842–62.
13. Kelly J, Tarnoff M, Shikora S, et al. Best practice recommendations for surgical care in weight loss surgery. Obes Res 2005;13(2):227–33.
14. Lehman Center Weight Loss Surgery Expert Panel. Commonwealth of Massachusetts Betsy Lehman Center for Patient Safety and Medical Error Reduction Expert Panel on Weight Loss Surgery: executive report. Obes Res 2005;13(2): 205–26.
15. Kushner RF, Noble CA. Long-term outcome of bariatric surgery: an interim analysis. Mayo Clin Proc 2006;81(Suppl 10):S46–51.
16. Birkmeyer NJ, Wei Y, Goldfaden A, et al. Characteristics of hospitals performing bariatric surgery. JAMA 2006;295(3):282–4.
17. Flum DR, Dellinger EP. Impact of gastric bypass operation on survival: a population-based analysis. J Am Coll Surg 2004;199(4):543–51.
18. Smith MD, Patterson E, Wahed AS, et al. Relationship between surgeon volume and adverse outcomes after RYGB in Longitudinal Assessment of Bariatric Surgery (LABS) study. Surg Obes Relat Dis 2010;6(2):118–25.
19. Buchwald H, Avidor Y, Braunwald E, et al. Bariatric surgery: a systematic review and meta-analysis. JAMA 2004;292(14):1724–37.
20. Buchwald H. Bariatric surgery for morbid obesity: health implications for patients, health professionals, and third-party payers. J Am Coll Surg 2005; 200(4):593–604.
21. Statistical Brief #23. Bariatric Surgery Utilization and Outcomes in 1998 and 2004. Rockville (MD): Agency for Healthcare Research and Quality (AHRQ); 2007.

22. Sjostrom L, Narbro K, Sjostrom CD, et al. Effects of bariatric surgery on mortality in Swedish obese subjects. N Engl J Med 2007;357(8):741–52.
23. Poirier P, Cornier MA, Mazzone T, et al. Bariatric surgery and cardiovascular risk factors: a scientific statement from the American Heart Association. Circulation 2011;123(15):1683–701.
24. Picot J, Jones J, Colquitt JL, et al. The clinical effectiveness and cost-effectiveness of bariatric (weight loss) surgery for obesity: a systematic review and economic evaluation. Health Technol Assess 2009;13(41):1–190, 215–357, iii–iv.
25. Colquitt JL, Picot J, Loveman E, et al. Surgery for obesity. Cochrane Database Syst Rev 2009;2:CD003641.
26. Maggard MA, Shugarman LR, Suttorp M, et al. Meta-analysis: surgical treatment of obesity. Ann Intern Med 2005;142(7):547–59.
27. O'Brien PE, Dixon JB, Laurie C, et al. Treatment of mild to moderate obesity with laparoscopic adjustable gastric banding or an intensive medical program: a randomized trial. Ann Intern Med 2006;144(9):625–33.
28. Buddeberg-Fischer B, Klaghofer R, Krug L, et al. Physical and psychosocial outcome in morbidly obese patients with and without bariatric surgery: a 4 1/2-year follow-up. Obes Surg 2006;16(3):321–30.
29. Buchwald H, Buchwald JN. Evolution of operative procedures for the management of morbid obesity 1950–2000. Obes Surg 2002;12(5):705–17.
30. Farrell TM, Haggerty SP, Overby DW, et al. Clinical application of laparoscopic bariatric surgery: an evidence-based review. Surg Endosc 2009;23(5):930–49.
31. Inabnet WB, Quinn T, Gagner M, et al. Laparoscopic Roux-en-Y gastric bypass in patients with BMI <50: a prospective randomized trial comparing short and long limb lengths. Obes Surg 2005;15(1):51–7.
32. Westling A, Gustavsson S. Laparoscopic vs open Roux-en-Y gastric bypass: a prospective, randomized trial. Obes Surg 2001;11(3):284–92.
33. Nguyen NT, Goldman C, Rosenquist CJ, et al. Laparoscopic versus open gastric bypass: a randomized study of outcomes, quality of life, and costs. Ann Surg 2001;234(3):279–89 [discussion: 289–91].
34. Lujan JA, Frutos MD, Hernandez Q, et al. Laparoscopic versus open gastric bypass in the treatment of morbid obesity: a randomized prospective study. Ann Surg 2004;239(4):433–7.
35. Lee WJ, Huang MT, Yu PJ, et al. Laparoscopic vertical banded gastroplasty and laparoscopic gastric bypass: a comparison. Obes Surg 2004;14(5):626–34.
36. Olbers T, Fagevik-Olsen M, Maleckas A, et al. Randomized clinical trial of laparoscopic Roux-en-Y gastric bypass versus laparoscopic vertical banded gastroplasty for obesity. Br J Surg 2005;92(5):557–62.
37. Puzziferri N, Austrheim-Smith IT, Wolfe BM, et al. Three-year follow-up of a prospective randomized trial comparing laparoscopic versus open gastric bypass. Ann Surg 2006;243(2):181–8.
38. Olbers T, Bjorkman S, Lindroos A, et al. Body composition, dietary intake, and energy expenditure after laparoscopic Roux-en-Y gastric bypass and laparoscopic vertical banded gastroplasty: a randomized clinical trial. Ann Surg 2006;244(5):715–22.
39. Sjostrom L, Lindroos AK, Peltonen M, et al. Lifestyle, diabetes, and cardiovascular risk factors 10 years after bariatric surgery. N Engl J Med 2004;351(26): 2683–93.
40. Shekelle PG, Morton SC, Maglione M, et al. Pharmacological and surgical treatment of obesity. Evid Rep Technol Assess (Summ) 2004;(103):1–6.

41. Christou NV, Sampalis JS, Liberman M, et al. Surgery decreases long-term mortality, morbidity, and health care use in morbidly obese patients. Ann Surg 2004;240(3):416–23 [discussion: 423–4].

42. Nguyen NT, Wilson SE. Complications of antiobesity surgery. Nat Clin Pract Gastroenterol Hepatol 2007;4(3):138–47.

43. Podnos YD, Jimenez JC, Wilson SE, et al. Complications after laparoscopic gastric bypass: a review of 3464 cases. Arch Surg 2003;138(9):957–61.

44. Suter M, Giusti V, Worreth M, et al. Laparoscopic gastric banding: a prospective, randomized study comparing the Lapband and the SAGB: early results. Ann Surg 2005;241(1):55–62.

45. Galvani C, Gorodner M, Moser F, et al. Laparoscopic adjustable gastric band versus laparoscopic Roux-en-Y gastric bypass: ends justify the means? Surg Endosc 2006;20(6):934–41.

46. O'Brien PE, McPhail T, Chaston TB, et al. Systematic review of medium-term weight loss after bariatric operations. Obes Surg 2006;16(8):1032–40.

47. O'Brien PE, Brown WA, Smith A, et al. Prospective study of a laparoscopically placed, adjustable gastric band in the treatment of morbid obesity. Br J Surg 1999;86(1):113–8.

48. Angrisani L, Alkilani M, Basso N, et al. Laparoscopic Italian experience with the Lap-Band. Obes Surg 2001;11(3):307–10.

49. DeMaria EJ, Sugerman HJ, Meador JG, et al. High failure rate after laparoscopic adjustable silicone gastric banding for treatment of morbid obesity. Ann Surg 2001;233(6):809–18.

50. Angrisani L, Di Lorenzo N, Favretti F, et al. The Italian Group for LAP-BAND: predictive value of initial body mass index for weight loss after 5 years of follow-up. Surg Endosc 2004;18(10):1524–7.

51. O'Brien PE. Outcomes of laparoscopic adjustable gastric banding. In: Sugerman HJ, Nguyen NT, editors. Management of morbid obesity. New York: Taylor & Francis; 2006. p. 181–90.

52. Angrisani L, Lorenzo M, Borrelli V. Laparoscopic adjustable gastric banding versus Roux-en-Y gastric bypass: 5-year results of a prospective randomized trial. Surg Obes Relat Dis 2007;3(2):127–32 [discussion: 132–3].

53. Dixon JB, Dixon AF, O'Brien PE. Improvements in insulin sensitivity and beta-cell function (HOMA) with weight loss in the severely obese. Homeostatic model assessment. Diabet Med 2003;20(2):127–34.

54. Dixon JB, O'Brien PE. Health outcomes of severely obese type 2 diabetic subjects 1 year after laparoscopic adjustable gastric banding. Diabetes Care 2002;25(2):358–63.

55. Abu-Abeid S, Keidar A, Szold A. Resolution of chronic medical conditions after laparoscopic adjustable silicone gastric banding for the treatment of morbid obesity in the elderly. Surg Endosc 2001;15(2):132–4.

56. Rubino F, Gagner M. Potential of surgery for curing type 2 diabetes mellitus. Ann Surg 2002;236(5):554–9.

57. Dixon JB, O'Brien PE. Gastroesophageal reflux in obesity: the effect of lap-band placement. Obes Surg 1999;9(6):527–31.

58. Angrisani L, Iovino P, Lorenzo M, et al. Treatment of morbid obesity and gastroesophageal reflux with hiatal hernia by Lap-Band. Obes Surg 1999;9(4):396–8.

59. Weiss HG, Nehoda H, Labeck B, et al. Treatment of morbid obesity with laparoscopic adjustable gastric banding affects esophageal motility. Am J Surg 2000;180(6):479–82.

60. Dixon JB, Schachter LM, O'Brien PE. Sleep disturbance and obesity: changes following surgically induced weight loss. Arch Intern Med 2001;161(1):102–6.
61. Horchner R, Tuinebreijer MW, Kelder PH. Quality-of-life assessment of morbidly obese patients who have undergone a Lap-Band operation: 2-year follow-up study. Is the MOS SF-36 a useful instrument to measure quality of life in morbidly obese patients? Obes Surg 2001;11(2):212–8 [discussion: 219].
62. Weiner R, Datz M, Wagner D, et al. Quality-of-life outcome after laparoscopic adjustable gastric banding for morbid obesity. Obes Surg 1999;9(6):539–45.
63. Martin LF, Smits GJ, Greenstein RJ. Treating morbid obesity with laparoscopic adjustable gastric banding. Am J Surg 2007;194(3):333–43 [discussion: 344–8].
64. Chapman AE, Kiroff G, Game P, et al. Laparoscopic adjustable gastric banding in the treatment of obesity: a systematic literature review. Surgery 2004;135(3): 326–51.
65. Paiva D, Bernardes L, Suretti L. Laparoscopic biliopancreatic diversion: technique and initial results. Obes Surg 2002;12(3):358–61.
66. Kim WW, Gagner M, Kini S, et al. Laparoscopic vs. open biliopancreatic diversion with duodenal switch: a comparative study. J Gastrointest Surg 2003;7(4): 552–7.
67. Ren CJ, Patterson E, Gagner M. Early results of laparoscopic biliopancreatic diversion with duodenal switch: a case series of 40 consecutive patients. Obes Surg 2000;10(6):514–23 [discussion: 524].
68. Parikh MS, Laker S, Weiner M, et al. Objective comparison of complications resulting from laparoscopic bariatric procedures. J Am Coll Surg 2006;202(2): 252–61.
69. Favretti F, Segato G, Ashton D, et al. Laparoscopic adjustable gastric banding in 1,791 consecutive obese patients: 12-year results. Obes Surg 2007;17(2): 168–75.
70. Balsiger BM, Ernst D, Giachino D, et al. Prospective evaluation and 7-year follow-up of Swedish adjustable gastric banding in adults with extreme obesity. J Gastrointest Surg 2007;11(11):1470–6 [discussion: 1446–77].
71. Cottam D, Qureshi FG, Mattar SG, et al. Laparoscopic sleeve gastrectomy as an initial weight-loss procedure for high-risk patients with morbid obesity. Surg Endosc 2006;20(6):859–63.
72. Himpens J, Dobbeleir J, Peeters G. Long-term results of laparoscopic sleeve gastrectomy for obesity. Ann Surg 2010;252(2):319–24.
73. Shi X, Karmali S, Sharma AM, et al. A review of laparoscopic sleeve gastrectomy for morbid obesity. Obes Surg 2010;20(8):1171–7.
74. Gagner M, Matteotti R. Laparoscopic biliopancreatic diversion with duodenal switch. Surg Clin North Am 2005;85(1):141–9, x–xi.
75. Anthone GJ. The duodenal switch operation for morbid obesity. Surg Clin North Am 2005;85(4):819–33, viii.
76. Dolan K, Hatzifotis M, Newbury L, et al. A comparison of laparoscopic adjustable gastric banding and biliopancreatic diversion in superobesity. Obes Surg 2004;14(2):165–9.
77. Bowne WB, Julliard K, Castro AE, et al. Laparoscopic gastric bypass is superior to adjustable gastric band in super morbidly obese patients: a prospective, comparative analysis. Arch Surg 2006;141(7):683–9.
78. Biron S, Hould FS, Lebel S, et al. Twenty years of biliopancreatic diversion: what is the goal of the surgery? Obes Surg 2004;14(2):160–4.
79. Marinari GM, Papadia FS, Briatore L, et al. Type 2 diabetes and weight loss following biliopancreatic diversion for obesity. Obes Surg 2006;16(11):1440–4.

80. Adami G, Murelli F, Carlini F, et al. Long-term effect of biliopancreatic diversion on blood pressure in hypertensive obese patients. Am J Hypertens 2005;18(6):780–4.
81. Simard B, Turcotte H, Marceau P, et al. Asthma and sleep apnea in patients with morbid obesity: outcome after bariatric surgery. Obes Surg 2004;14(10):1381–8.
82. Scopinaro N, Gianetta E, Civalleri D, et al. Two years of clinical experience with biliopancreatic bypass for obesity. Am J Clin Nutr 1980;33(Suppl 2):506–14.
83. Marceau P, Biron S, Bourque RA, et al. Biliopancreatic diversion with a new type of gastrectomy. Obes Surg 1993;3(1):29–35.
84. Hess DS, Hess DW, Oakley RS. The biliopancreatic diversion with the duodenal switch: results beyond 10 years. Obes Surg 2005;15(3):408–16.
85. Dolan K, Hatzifotis M, Newbury L, et al. A clinical and nutritional comparison of biliopancreatic diversion with and without duodenal switch. Ann Surg 2004; 240(1):51–6.
86. Marceau P, Hould FS, Lebel S, et al. Malabsorptive obesity surgery. Surg Clin North Am 2001;81(5):1113–27.
87. Chapin BL, LeMar HJ Jr, Knodel DH, et al. Secondary hyperparathyroidism following biliopancreatic diversion. Arch Surg 1996;131(10):1048–52 [discussion: 1053].
88. Moreiro J, Ruiz O, Perez G, et al. Parathyroid hormone and bone marker levels in patients with morbid obesity before and after biliopancreatic diversion. Obes Surg 2007;17(3):348–54.
89. Michielson D, Van Hee R, Hendrickx L. Complications of biliopancreatic diversion surgery as proposed by Scopinaro in the treatment of morbid obesity. Obes Surg 1996;6(5):416–20.
90. Scopinaro N, Gianetta E, Civalleri D, et al. Bilio-pancreatic bypass for obesity: II. Initial experience in man. Br J Surg 1979;66(9):618–20.
91. Bardaro SJ, Gagner M, Consten E, et al. Routine cholecystectomy during laparoscopic biliopancreatic diversion with duodenal switch is not necessary. Surg Obes Relat Dis 2007;3(5):549–53.
92. Nguyen NT, Paya M, Stevens CM, et al. The relationship between hospital volume and outcome in bariatric surgery at academic medical centers. Ann Surg 2004;240(4):586–93 [discussion: 593–4].
93. Nguyen NT, Slone JA, Nguyen XM, et al. A prospective randomized trial of laparoscopic gastric bypass versus laparoscopic adjustable gastric banding for the treatment of morbid obesity: outcomes, quality of life, and costs. Ann Surg 2009; 250(4):631–41.
94. Boza C, Gamboa C, Awruch D, et al. Laparoscopic Roux-en-Y gastric bypass versus laparoscopic adjustable gastric banding: five years of follow-up. Surg Obes Relat Dis 2010;6(5):470–5.
95. Woodard GA, Peraza J, Bravo S, et al. One year improvements in cardiovascular risk factors: a comparative trial of laparoscopic Roux-en-Y gastric bypass vs. adjustable gastric banding. Obes Surg 2010;20(5):578–82.
96. Pontiroli AE, Morabito A. Long-term prevention of mortality in morbid obesity through bariatric surgery. a systematic review and meta-analysis of trials performed with gastric banding and gastric bypass. Ann Surg 2011;253(3):484–7.
97. Chouillard EK, Karaa A, Elkhoury M, et al. Laparoscopic Roux-en-Y gastric bypass versus laparoscopic sleeve gastrectomy for morbid obesity: case-control study. Surg Obes Relat Dis 2011;7(4):500–5.
98. Leyba JL, Aulestia SN, Llopis SN. Laparoscopic Roux-en-Y gastric bypass versus laparoscopic sleeve gastrectomy for the treatment of morbid obesity. A prospective study of 117 patients. Obes Surg 2011;21(2):212–6.

99. Iannelli A, Anty R, Schneck AS, et al. Inflammation, insulin resistance, lipid distur-
    bances, anthropometrics, and metabolic syndrome in morbidly obese patients:
    a case control study comparing laparoscopic Roux-en-Y gastric bypass and
    laparoscopic sleeve gastrectomy. Surgery 2011;149(3):364–70.
100. Omana JJ, Nguyen SQ, Herron D, et al. Comparison of comorbidity resolution
    and improvement between laparoscopic sleeve gastrectomy and laparoscopic
    adjustable gastric banding. Surg Endosc 2010;24(10):2513–7.
101. Adams TD, Gress RE, Smith SC, et al. Long-term mortality after gastric bypass
    surgery. N Engl J Med 2007;357(8):753–61.
102. MacDonald KG Jr, Long SD, Swanson MS, et al. The gastric bypass operation
    reduces the progression and mortality of non-insulin-dependent diabetes melli-
    tus. J Gastrointest Surg 1997;1(3):213–20 [discussion: 220].
103. Sowemimo OA, Yood SM, Courtney J, et al. Natural history of morbid
    obesity without surgical intervention. Surg Obes Relat Dis 2007;3(1):73–7
    [discussion: 77].
104. Busetto L, Mirabelli D, Petroni ML, et al. Comparative long-term mortality after
    laparoscopic adjustable gastric banding versus nonsurgical controls. Surg
    Obes Relat Dis 2007;3(5):496–502 [discussion: 502].
105. Peeters A, O'Brien PE, Laurie C, et al. Substantial intentional weight loss and
    mortality in the severely obese. Ann Surg 2007;246(6):1028–33.
106. Kral JG. Studies show reduction in mortality after bariatric surgery. Surg Obes
    Relat Dis 2006;2(5):564.
107. Naslund I. [Weight reduction reduces overmortality caused by severe obesity.
    Six studies yield sustainable evidence]. Lakartidningen 2008;105(20):1486–8
    [in Swedish].
108. Herpertz S, Kielmann R, Wolf AM, et al. Does obesity surgery improve psycho-
    social functioning? A systematic review. Int J Obes Relat Metab Disord 2003;
    27(11):1300–14.
109. van Hout GC, Boekestein P, Fortuin FA, et al. Psychosocial functioning following
    bariatric surgery. Obes Surg 2006;16(6):787–94.
110. Mohos E, Schmaldienst E, Prager M. Quality of life parameters, weight change and
    improvement of co-morbidities after laparoscopic Roux Y gastric bypass and lapa-
    roscopic gastric sleeve resection–comparative study. Obes Surg 2011;21(3):
    288–94.
111. Campos GM, Rabl C, Roll GR, et al. Better weight loss, resolution of diabetes,
    and quality of life for laparoscopic gastric bypass vs banding: results of a 2-
    cohort pair-matched study. Arch Surg 2011;146(2):149–55.
112. Elder KA, Wolfe BM. Bariatric surgery: a review of procedures and outcomes.
    Gastroenterology 2007;132(6):2253–71.
113. Encinosa WE, Bernard DM, Chen CC, et al. Healthcare utilization and outcomes
    after bariatric surgery. Med Care 2006;44(8):706–12.
114. Livingston EH. Hospital costs associated with bariatric procedures in the United
    States. Am J Surg 2005;190(5):816–20.
115. Potteiger CE, Paragi PR, Inverso NA, et al. Bariatric surgery: shedding the
    monetary weight of prescription costs in the managed care arena. Obes Surg
    2004;14(6):725–30.
116. Agren G, Narbro K, Naslund I, et al. Long-term effects of weight loss on phar-
    maceutical costs in obese subjects. A report from the SOS intervention study.
    Int J Obes Relat Metab Disord 2002;26(2):184–92.
117. Salem L, Jensen CC, Flum DR. Are bariatric surgical outcomes worth their cost?
    A systematic review. J Am Coll Surg 2005;200(2):270–8.

118. Craig BM, Tseng DS. Cost-effectiveness of gastric bypass for severe obesity. Am J Med 2002;113(6):491–8.
119. Hodo DM, Waller JL, Martindale RG, et al. Medication use after bariatric surgery in a managed care cohort. Surg Obes Relat Dis 2008;4(5):601–7.
120. Sampalis JS, Liberman M, Auger S, et al. The impact of weight reduction surgery on health-care costs in morbidly obese patients. Obes Surg 2004; 14(7):939–47.
121. Cremieux PY, Buchwald H, Shikora SA, et al. A study on the economic impact of bariatric surgery. Am J Manag Care 2008;14(9):589–96.
122. Courcoulas AP, Flum DR. Filling the gaps in bariatric surgical research. JAMA 2005;294(15):1957–60.
123. Pories WJ. Bariatric surgery: risks and rewards. J Clin Endocrinol Metab 2008; 93(11 Suppl 1):S89–96.

Adolescent Bariatric Surgery

Anna R. Ibele, MD[a,b], Samer G. Mattar, MD[c],*

KEYWORDS

• Bariatric surgery • Obesity • Adolescent • Pediatric
• Outcomes • Complications

DEMOGRAPHICS OF CHILDHOOD OBESITY

The so-called obesity epidemic among adults in the United States has been well documented. Based on data from the American Heart Association, between 2003 and 2006, 36.8% of African American men and 52.9% of African American women were obese, indicated by a body mass index (BMI) of 30 kg/m^2 or greater. For Caucasians, 32.3% of men and 32.7% of women fell into this category, and for Hispanics 26.8% of men and 41.9% of women had a BMI of 30 kg/m^2 or greater.[1] The American Academy of Pediatrics (AAP) classifies children with a BMI between 85th and 95th percentile as overweight, based on 1973 norms for age and gender. The AAP defines pediatric obesity as a BMI greater than the 95th percentile based on these norms.[2] Over the past 30 years, the United States has seen an almost threefold increase in the incidence of children who fall into the category of overweight as defined by the AAP criteria. Among children aged 2 to 19 years, 12 million (>20% of the pediatric population) are currently considered obese.[3]

The factors that may be driving this epidemiologic surge in overweight and obesity rates have come under intense research. Several groups have shown that children of lower socioeconomic status and minority status are disproportionately affected by this epidemic.[3–5] The effects of socioeconomic status and culture on childhood obesity are complex and multifaceted. Over the past 30 years, economic forces have resulted in an increase in the incidence of dual-earner households, and with this change in household dynamics, families are increasingly relying on the availability of fast food or processed food for daily consumption. These industrially prepared foods have

Disclosures: Dr Ibele has no disclosures. Dr Mattar has received honorariums from Covidien and Ethicon Endosurgery.
a Minimally Invasive and Bariatric Surgery, Department of Surgery, Indiana University School of Medicine, 545 Barnhill Drive, Emerson Hall 203, Indianapolis, IN 46202, USA
b Division of Pediatric Surgery, Department of Surgery, University of Louisville, 315 East Broadway, Suite 565, Louisville, KY 40202, USA
c Indiana University Health Bariatrics and Weight Loss, Indiana University School of Medicine, 6640 Intech Boulevard # 10-300, Indianapolis, IN 46278-2011, USA
* Corresponding author.
E-mail address: smattar@iupui.edu

Surg Clin N Am 91 (2011) 1339–1351
doi:10.1016/j.suc.2011.08.005
0039-6109/11/$ – see front matter © 2011 Elsevier Inc. All rights reserved.

surgical.theclinics.com

become ubiquitous in our society and are often more affordable than other, more nutritious home-prepared meals. Furthermore, many public school systems have been offering meals that are of high caloric and low nutritional value. Many educational systems have entered into attractive contracts with beverage companies in exchange for much-needed financial support. Schools have also been reducing structured physical education programs from their high school and junior high school curriculums. Because of the lack of adequate supervision, many families do not allow prolonged outdoor activities, and therefore entertainment often is provided in the form of "electronic babysitters," or technology, such as television and video games, which have largely replaced afterschool physical activity.[6–10]

HEALTH IMPACT OF CHILDHOOD OBESITY

Dietary and lifestyle choices that result in childhood obesity are difficult to reverse and have life-long implications. Morbid obesity is typically associated with numerous life-threatening medical conditions, and adolescents are not immune. As the prevalence of obesity increases in adolescents, a parallel rise occurs in the prevalence of obesity-related comorbidities, such as diabetes, nonalcoholic fatty liver disease, obstructive sleep apnea, and metabolic syndrome with resultant cardiovascular complications.

The incidence of diabetes is rapidly rising, representing a potential for serious complications in the future. Type 2 diabetes mellitus (DM) is a metabolic disease that is difficult to control, and for which various therapies, including insulin, promote additional weight gain through their anabolic effects, thereby furthering a dangerous cycle. Furthermore, the incidence of diabetes-related complications, such as retinopathy, renal disease, and small vessel disease, is directly related to the duration of the disease, therefore adding an important incentive for early treatment. In 1992, type 2 DM was a rare occurrence in most pediatric centers. By 1994, it represented up to 16% of new cases, and by 1999 the incidence of new diagnoses ranged between 8% and 45%, depending on geographic location.[11]

Nonalcoholic fatty liver disease (NAFLD), has also been rising at an alarming rate in adolescents. This progressive disease advances through a spectrum of severity that includes steatohepatitis and ends with liver cirrhosis. NAFLD is rapidly becoming the most common indication for liver transplantation among young adults. A recent study found that 23% of 127 obese 12th graders in the United States had elevation in alanine transaminase attributable to NAFLD.[12] NAFLD was found to be present in 43% of a group of 181 obese adolescents in Brazil, and this was found to correlate with degree of visceral body fat and insulin resistance.[13]

Obstructive sleep apnea (OSA) has been shown to be an independent risk factor for cardiovascular disease in adults and is associated with left ventricular hypertrophy and abnormal ventricular geometry in children.[14] OSA has been shown to correlate with severity of obesity in adults.[15] Marcus and colleagues[16] reported that 36% of obese children and adolescents had abnormal polysomnograms, and they also showed a positive correlation between the degree of obesity and the severity of OSA.

Based on a 17-year cohort study following obese adolescents, Freedman and colleagues[17] extrapolated that 77% of children who are obese at age 15 to 17 years will be obese adults. Because the cardiovascular complications of metabolic syndrome result from many years of exposure, the early onset of obesity portends significant risk for cardiovascular disease later in life. Becque and colleagues[18] found that among 36 children presenting for a supervised weight loss program, 35 had four or more serious cardiovascular risk factors. Bibbins-Domingo and colleagues found that the incidence of coronary artery disease in young adults is expected to increase by 5% to 10% within the next 10 years ,which will lead to more than 100,000 excess cases of coronary artery disease attributable to increased obesity in teenagers and young adults.[19]

Important behavioral consequences are also associated with obesity in the teenage years. Adolescents with obesity are more likely to be bullied and, according to surveys, are typically viewed by teachers and fellow students as lazy and often experience discrimination at the hands of their educators.[20] Attention deficit hyperactivity disorder and depression are found at increased rates in obese adolescents compared with peers who are not overweight, and obese children are at greater risk of not completing their education.[21] One recent adolescent socialization study surveyed children on their views regarding peer relationships and found that obese children had an average of 3.4% fewer friendship nominations (ie, when one child in a survey names the other child as a friend) than did their nonoverweight peers. Obese adolescents were also more likely to receive zero friendship nominations.[22] In a retrospective review of psychological data collected on the first 40 adolescents presenting for laparoscopic adjustable gastric band at an adolescent bariatric clinic in Chicago, 32% were found to be clinically depressed, 13% had current suicidal ideation, 15% had previously attempted suicide, 50% reported bullying, and 10% had dropped out of school.[23]

BEHAVIORAL AND MEDICAL THERAPY

The obesity crisis in children has recently reached national prominence as a result of heightened political attention, including high-profile campaigns such as Michelle Obama's "Let's Move" task force on childhood obesity. Politicians, educators, pediatricians, and sociologists have called for reforms in the home, the fast food industry, grocery stores, and the public school system, but changing this complex social and medical problem is difficult and expensive, and much work remains. Although preventative strategies and anticipatory guidance are emphasized in the primary care community, solving the problem of how to help children who are already obese is even more complicated. The mainstay of primary care physicians is to institute and reinforce behavior and dietary modification, but many have found it difficult to council at-risk patients and their families and get them to adhere to these programs. Epstein and colleagues[24] published a 10-year experience of children who were counseled on behavioral and dietary approaches to weight loss, finding that at the end of the study period, 34% of children had experienced 20% excess weight loss (EWL) and 30% were no longer obese. The majority opinion in the primary care literature is that the best programs for dietary and behavioral modification are multidisciplinary school-based programs for adolescents that incorporate behavioral counseling, dietary counseling, nutrition education, scheduled physical activity, and parent training.

However, these multicomponent school-based programs are costly and difficult to initiate and maintain. Therefore, many health care providers have considered other solutions, such as medical management combined with lifestyle changes. Few drugs are approved by the U.S. Food and Drug Administration (FDA) to facilitate weight loss in adolescents. Sibutramine is a serotonin and norepinephrine reuptake inhibitor that causes satiety. It was approved for children aged 16 and older, and in one large, randomized, controlled, prospective series, resulted in a mean weight loss of 7.8 kg in the study group compared with 3.2 kg in the placebo group ($P = .001$) at 6 months.[25] Unfortunately, because of serious cardiac complications that have occurred in adults, the FDA recently prohibited the marketing and sale of this drug.

Orlistat is a reversible inhibitor of pancreatic and gastric lipase that leads to a significant reduction in the absorption of fat-based components of the diet. It is approved by the FDA for children aged 12 and older and, in a meta-analysis of randomized controlled clinical trials, was found to result in a loss of BMI of 0.6 kg/m² at 54 weeks.[26] Patients on orlistat must be kept under surveillance because fat malabsorption may also reduce the absorption of fat-soluble vitamins (A, D, E, and K) and, by extension, can contribute to various forms of metabolic bone disease.

Other drugs that have been studied, but are not FDA-approved, include metformin, topiramate, and ramonabant. Metformin is a biguanide antidiabetic drug that suppresses hepatic glucose production and decreases insulin resistance, causing abdominal fat loss in patients who also have insulin resistance, but it can result in troublesome hypoglycemia. Topiramate is an antiseizure medication that causes weight loss via an unknown mechanism. Side effects include drowsiness and impaired cognition, and it is not approved for weight loss in adolescents. Rimonabant is a cannabinoid receptor antagonist that is not approved in the United States because of increased risk for depression and suicide.[27]

INDICATIONS FOR BARIATRIC SURGERY

The National Institutes of Health (NIH) published criteria for bariatric surgery for adults that are widely followed by physicians and insurance providers (**Box 1**).[28] However, the appropriate referral criteria for adolescents have been widely debated among the surgical community.

In 2009, the International Pediatric Endosurgery Group (IPEG) published a series of guidelines that advocate surgery for adolescents with a BMI greater than 35 kg/m² with type 2 DM, moderate OSA, or pseudotumor cerebri, or patients with a BMI of 40 kg/m² or greater with one of several other comorbidities. In addition, to address concerns about the potential for bariatric surgery to interfere with a child's growth

---

Box 1
Summary 1991 NIH consensus statement for patient selection criteria for bariatric surgery

The patient is an adult (specifically, not an adolescent)

The patient's BMI is:

- Greater than 40 kg/m²
- Between 35 and 40 kg/m², with related comorbidities
- Between 35 and 40 kg/m², with functional limitations because of body size or joint disease

If, after evaluation by a multidisciplinary team, the patient is judged to:

- Have a low probability of success with nonoperative weight-loss measures
- Be well informed about the long- and short-term risks and benefits of surgery
- Be highly motivated to lose weight through surgery
- Have an acceptable operative risk
- Be willing to undergo lifelong medical surveillance

Data from Gastrointestinal Surgery for Severe Obesity. National Institutes of Health Consensus Development Conference Statement, March 25–27, 1991. U.S. Department of Health & Human Services. National Institutes of Health Web site. Available at: http://consensus.nih.gov/1991/1991GISurgeryObesity084html.htm. Accessed August 25, 2011; with permission.

and development, candidates should have attained or nearly attained 95% of their anticipated adult stature as measured with bone age. Patients should also be able and willing to adhere to postoperative nutritional guidelines, have the intellectual maturity for decision making, and be able to provide informed consent for their surgical management and long-term care (**Box 2**).[29]

Although many bariatric and pediatric surgeons accept these criteria, the opinions of many pediatricians and family physicians differ drastically regarding patient referral and eligibility. Woolford and colleagues[30] surveyed 275 pediatricians and 375 family physicians regarding indications for bariatric surgery in adolescents, and 48% of

---

Box 2
IPEG guidelines for adolescent bariatric surgery

Adolescents being considered for bariatric surgery should:

- Be very severely obese (BMI $\geq$35 kg/m^2) with serious obesity-related comorbidities

OR

- Be morbidly obese (BMI $\geq$40 kg/m^2) with less-serious obesity-related comorbidities

AND

- Have attained or, depending on the severity of comorbidity, nearly attained adult stature

- Have at least 6 months of failed organized conventional attempts at weight management

- Shown commitment to comprehensive pediatric psychological evaluation both before and after surgery and agree to avoid pregnancy for at least 1-year postoperatively

- Be capable of and willing to adhere to nutritional guidelines postoperatively

- Have decisional capacity and provide informed assent for surgical management

Serious comorbid conditions:

- Type 2 DM

- OSA (apnea-hypopnea index [AHI] >5 events per hour)

- Pseudotumor cerebri

Less-serious comorbidities:

- Weight-related arthropathy

- OSA (AHI>5 events per hour)

- Hypertension

- Dyslipidemia

- Venous stasis disease

- Panniculitis

- Urinary Incontinence

- Significant impairment in activity of daily living

- NAFLD (includes steatohepatitis)

- Gastroesophageal reflux

- Severe psychosocial distress

- Significantly impaired quality of life

This Guideline was prepared by the IPEG Guidelines Committee and was reviewed and approved by the Executive Committee of the IPEG, November, 2008.

respondents said that they would never refer an obese adolescent for bariatric surgery. Most of them endorsed a minimum age of 18 years for referral and 99% endorsed participation in a weight management program before surgery. In another study, Igbal and colleagues[31] surveyed 61 primary care physicians on their referral practices of adolescents for bariatric surgery, and found that 42% of respondents had referred an adult or pediatric patient for bariatric surgery and 88% were satisfied with the result of the referral. However, 88% also said that they would never refer a child younger than 13 years for a bariatric procedure, whereas only 44.3% said that they would be somewhat or very likely to refer an adolescent. Reasons cited include unknown long-term effects (n = 51), concern over perioperative risks (n = 44), age alone (n = 37), poor social support for the patient (n = 34), poor patient cognitive function (n = 27), lack of an existing local pediatric bariatric program (n = 21), and the opinion that nonoperative options for weight loss are superior (n = 5). These same respondents said they would consider surgery for significant weight-related comorbidities (n = 45), failure of medical therapy (n = 40), need for durable weight loss (n = 37), and psychosocial issues (n = 37).[31]

The prevalence of these reservations in the primary care community may account for the numerous adult patients who give a history of childhood obesity and chronic comorbidities that have existed since their late teens and early 20s. Although the concerns of the primary care physicians are understandable, delay in referral until adulthood may not be in the patient's best interest. Adult patients who are super morbidly obese (BMI >55 kg/m^2) or super-super morbidly obese and who undergo bariatric surgery do not attain the same nadir BMIs as less-obese patients who undergo these procedures. Inge and colleagues[32] studied this phenomenon in 61 adolescents undergoing gastric bypass. Patients who presented with an initial BMI between 40 and 54.9 experienced a 37.2% decrease in BMI and reached a nadir BMI of 31. Patients who presented with an initial BMI between 65 and 95 also experienced a 37.7% decrease in BMI, nadiring at a BMI of 47 (still morbidly obese). The group concluded that the best results from weight loss surgery occur with timely referral, and that severely obese teenagers should receive early referral for surgical consideration and not be delayed.

OUTCOMES OF BARIATRIC SURGERY IN ADOLESCENTS

The successes of bariatric surgery in adults are well described and extensively published. One recent meta-analysis of 136 studies, incorporating 22,094 patients, describes the results of adult bariatric surgery. The mean percentages of excess weight loss achieved at 1 year with an adjustable gastric band, gastric bypass, and biliopancreatic diversion/duodenal switch were 47%, 62%, and 70%, respectively. Operative mortality was 0.1% for purely restrictive procedures, 0.5% for gastric bypass, and 1.1% for biliopancreatic diversion or duodenal switch. Diabetes completely resolved in 77% of patients, hypertension resolved in 62%, and hyperlipidemia improved in 70%.[33]

Much less is known about the long-term results of bariatric surgery in adolescents. Surgical weight loss procedures were performed for adolescents as early as the 1970s, but initially these were only performed for "extreme cases." In 1974, Randolph and colleagues[34] published a small series on jejunoileal bypass for morbidly obese adolescents, and 10 years after this, Silber and colleagues[35] reviewed medical records and contacted these patients to obtain long-term follow-up. Of 11 patients who underwent jejunoileal bypass between 1972 and 1974, 8 survived at 10-year follow-up. Two patients with Prader-Willi syndrome who were considered to have a very high surgical risk at the time of operation died within a year. A third patient died of liver failure within the first year of follow-up. Patients experienced significant weight loss and reported improved quality of life and psychosocial functioning, but many experienced serious complications, including nephrolithiasis, renal cortical nephropathy, progressive hepatic structural abnormalities, and multiple nutritional deficiencies. These complications are now known to be the long-term sequelae of jejunoileal bypass and led to the demise of the procedure. As a result of this series, few reports of bariatric surgery in adolescents were published for many years.

As safer weight loss operations were developed and as laparoscopic techniques became more widely available, public demand for bariatric surgery increased. By the late 1990s, the number of adolescent bariatric operations performed nationally increased fivefold, and a 2005 review of members of the American Society of Metabolic and Bariatric Surgeons found that 53% of responders had performed bariatric surgery in an obese adolescent, 70% planned to start a regular surgery program for adolescents, and 84% were interested in multicenter studies in this area.[33] In 2003, a survey of the Kids' Inpatient Database, a national database of inpatient stays for children, determined that more than 100 hospitals performed bariatric surgical procedures on adolescents; 87% performed four or fewer adolescent cases annually, and 39% of these cases were performed at centers that performed fewer than 200 total cases annually. The mean age of patients undergoing surgery was 16 years, with a minimum age of 12 years, and a 6% in-hospital overall complication rate was reported.[36]

Adolescent bariatric surgery remains controversial because of concerns about the immediate risks of surgery, the ethical implications of consenting an adolescent for a life-altering procedure, and potential long-term complications associated with these procedures. Uncertainty exists about the efficacy of these operations in young adults and whether young patients will be able to comply with the postoperative dietary and lifestyle regimens necessary to maintain success of bariatric procedures. Many pediatricians are concerned about growth and development and the nutritional implications that restrictive and malabsorptive procedures may have on adolescents. Concerns also exist about family dynamics and the presence of a supportive environment that will foster an adolescent's adherence to the necessary lifestyle changes.

The two most common weight loss operations in adolescents in the United States are the adjustable gastric band and the Roux-en-Y gastric bypass. The band facilitates weight loss through a restrictive device in which a saline-filled chamber is placed around the stomach and can be adjusted to achieve optimal satiety without dysphagia. The gastric bypass works using both a restrictive component (the small gastric pouch) and a malabsorptive component – diversion of enteric contents away from biliopancreatic secretions via the Roux limb. Appetite is suppressed in both operations but to a larger degree with the gastric bypass. The adjustable gastric band is not currently approved by the FDA as a device for implantation in adolescent patients, but data from many participating centers are available from a recently completed FDA study, and approval of the gastric band is pending.

The clinical data currently available on the efficacy and complication rates of these procedures in adolescents are based on several small series, some of which are prospective. O'Brien and colleagues[37] published a prospective randomized trial in which 50 adolescents between ages 14 and 18 years with BMIs greater than 35 kg/m^2 were assigned to medically supervised lifestyle intervention or gastric banding. At 2 years postoperatively, mean percent EWL in the band group was 78.8% versus 13.2% in the lifestyle group. At study entry, 36% of band patients and 40% of lifestyle patients had metabolic syndrome, and at 24 months no band patients had metabolic syndrome compared with 44% of the lifestyle modification patients. Notably, the band group had a 33% reoperative rate at 2 years because of band slippage, pouch dilation, and injury to port site tubing.

Nadler and colleagues[38] published a retrospective review of 53 patients aged 13 to 17 years who underwent placement of a laparoscopic adjustable gastric band as part of an FDA-approved study. Mean percent EWL for these patients was 37.5% at 6 months, 62.7% at 1 year, and 48.5% at 18 months. Two patients experienced band slippage requiring laparoscopic repositioning. Two patients required repair of hiatal hernia, 1 patient developed nephrolithiasis and cholelithiasis, 4 patients developed iron deficiency, and 5 had mild hair loss. A report on the postoperative complications associated with adjustable gastric band is available from a meta-analysis published in 2008, which included six studies with long-term follow-up, encompassing 352 adolescents undergoing laparoscopic adjustable gastric banding. At 3 years postoperatively, 8% of patients required reoperation (28/352) for band slippage, gastric dilation, intragastric band migration, psychological intolerance of the band, hiatal hernia, cholecystitis, and tube damage. Band slippage was the most common complication, occurring in 3% (12/352) patients. Patients also experienced small rates of iron deficiency (8/352) and mild hair loss (5/352).[39]

The available series evaluating the outcomes of gastric bypass in adolescents examine smaller populations. Stanford and colleagues[40] followed the outcomes of four adolescents undergoing laparoscopic Roux-en-Y gastric bypass with an average preoperative BMI of 55 kg/m^2. At a median follow-up of 17 months, patients experienced an average of 87% EWL with an average postoperative BMI of 35 kg/m^2. Adolescents experienced nearly complete resolution of asthma, hypertriglyceridemia, and gastroesophageal reflux. Another series by Strauss and colleagues[41] included 10 children aged 17 years or younger with a follow-up of greater than 1 year after Roux-en-Y gastric bypass. One patient experienced a weight gain of 14 kg at 144 months postoperatively. Of the remaining 9, mean percent EWL was 62% at 60 months. Two patients required cholecystectomy for stone formation, one required exploratory laparotomy for small bowel obstruction, and one required operative repair of an incisional hernia. Five adolescents developed postoperative iron deficiency anemia and three had folate deficiency. The gastric bypass has particularly good rates of diabetes resolution for adolescents. In 2004, Inge and colleagues[42] compared 11 adolescents with type 2 DM undergoing Roux-en-Y gastric bypass with 67 treated medically. At 1 year after surgery or initiation of therapy, BMI decreased by 34% in the bypass group, and these patients experienced an average change in fasting glucose of 81%. Medically managed adolescents had no change in their baseline BMI and no change in diabetic medication use.

In their meta-analysis, Treadwell and colleagues[39] reviewed post–gastric bypass complications in six studies that included a total of 131 patients. No operation-related hospital deaths occurred, but one death occurred in a child 9 months after gastric bypass who contracted severe Clostridium difficile colitis and experienced multisystem organ failure. Shock, pulmonary embolism, postoperative bleeding, severe malnutrition, and bowel obstruction occurred postoperatively, but because of variability in the way these complications were reported, the authors of the meta-analysis were unable to calculate actual incidences. Protein-calorie malnutrition and micronutrient deficiency were also reported, but their overall incidence in adolescents is unclear.

Sleeve gastrectomy recently became of interest to adolescent bariatric surgeons. The procedure involves creating a tubular J-shaped stomach through resection of the greater curve of the stomach alongside a bougie used for calibration. Sleeve gastrectomy also markedly diminishes appetite, but its mode of function remains under investigation. It is believed to work through restriction because of the smaller capacity and less-distensible lesser curve-based pouch and through alterations in the level of ghrelin (a hormone that regulates appetite control and is produced predominantly in the fundus). In adults the procedure typically results in an EWL of 50% to 65%.[43,44] The procedure may be of benefit to adolescents because it does not involve a malabsorptive component or placement of a foreign body, or require any adjustments.

To date, only a few small relevant series have been published. Till and colleagues[45] published a series of four children aged 8 to 17 years with obesity and serious medical comorbidities who underwent sleeve gastrectomy. No postoperative complications occurred, and at mean follow-up of 12 months, mean BMI had decreased from 48.4 to 37.2 kg/m^2. Baltasar and colleagues[46] describe a 10-year-old boy with a BMI of 42 kg/m^2 and Blount disease who was wheelchair-bound and underwent laparoscopic sleeve gastrectomy. At 8 months postoperatively, his BMI decreased from 42 to 28 kg/m^2 and no metabolic complications were detected. Although the procedure shows some promise in the adolescent population, no large clinical series have been published on sleeve gastrectomy for adolescents, and further data on long-term outcomes and complications are needed.

A current multiinstitutional prospective study is the Teen-LABS (Longitudinal Assessment of Bariatric Surgery) program. This study includes prospectively collected data from four high-volume institutions. The goals of the project are to collect outcomes of weight loss, comorbidity resolution, psychosocial status, and complications of 200 obese adults who were obese before 18 years of age and did not receive surgery, and compare them to a group of adolescents who were obese and did undergo a weight loss procedure. Data collection for this study is ongoing.[47]

ETHICAL ISSUES

Understandably, ethical concerns exist regarding weight loss surgery in adolescents. In a commentary summarizing the issues involved, Dr Donna Caniano[48] emphasized the principles of beneficence, nonmaleficence, autonomy, and justice. The surgeon must be assured that the procedure is in the patient's best interest: preoperatively the medical team should confirm that adequate medical and psychological evaluation of the patient is performed, sufficient effort has been made to achieve weight loss through nonsurgical means, and the surgical team and hospital are appropriately experienced and equipped to provide safe perioperative and long-term care.

To preserve patient autonomy, informed consent must take into account that the patient and family may have an overly optimistic view of the results of bariatric surgery because of media reports and advertisements for bariatric procedures. To ensure that families understand the actual risks and benefits of surgery, an extensive preoperative discussion that includes the teenager, parents, and family should be conducted. The bariatric surgeon should pay careful attention to understanding the adolescent's values and behavior patterns and whether the teenager has a habit of not keeping promises and not meeting goals. Informed consent should include disclosure of patient's obesity and the extent of it and a description of the extent of their medical comorbidities and why they are related to their obesity. The adolescent and the parents or guardians should also understand the nature of the proposed operation, the risks and benefits of surgery, and the impact that these could have on their lives and quality of life. Patients and families should understand the actions and behaviors that they will need to continue postoperatively, and the short- and long-term follow-up schedule should be outlined before the procedure. Financial aspects of treatment, complications, and short-and long-term care should also be explained. Caniano[48] also suggests that the family be given data about the outcomes for the surgical team and how these compare with published outcomes.

Additional areas of debate are where bariatric procedures should be performed and who should perform them. Currently, adolescent bariatric surgery is being offered by fellowship-trained adult bariatric and minimally invasive surgeons, fellowship-trained pediatric surgeons, and general surgeons. Surgery is performed either at children's hospitals by pediatric surgeons or at adult hospitals, with adolescents staying on adult inpatient postsurgical wards. Regardless of who is performing these procedures and where they are performed, the authors believe that these operations should only be conducted at centers that adhere to the bariatric Centers of Excellence model. Bariatric surgical programs should be thorough and comprehensive, they should involve extensive preoperative evaluation and counseling by a multidisciplinary team, and the surgeons performing the procedure should have extensive technical experience in the procedure. Having a pediatrician or family physician involved in the preoperative and postoperative management of these teenagers is also very important. In an opinion letter, Spear and colleagues[49] described the ideal adolescent program: it should have an affiliation with a pediatric hospital, specific guidelines for the preoperative evaluation and candidacy of adolescents should be available, and a multidisciplinary team should be involved, which includes a surgeon, pediatrician, dietitian, mental health specialist, exercise therapist, and case manager. The program should offer procedures that are approved in adolescents, and organized comprehensive postoperative care should be provided and involve the surgeon and the patient's primary care provider.

SUMMARY

To conclude, the authors believe that anticipatory guidance, prevention, and behavioral intervention are first-line therapy for adolescent obesity. However, when these fail, bariatric surgery has a role in the obese adolescent patient. Although bariatric surgery has associated risks and recognized complications, the risks and complications of obesity-related comorbidities are definite and life-threatening. When an adolescent is referred for consideration of surgery, extensive preoperative evaluation and counseling should be conducted with the patient and family. No consensus exists regarding the optimal weight loss operation for an adolescent. The authors recommend that these operations be tailored to the adolescent, their medical history, and their needs, just as they are for adult patients. Surgery should be performed by surgeons with technical experience and within institutions that have a high clinical volume and a profound commitment to the bariatric program. Postoperatively, patients and families should receive long-term counseling and care from a multidisciplinary team that includes a pediatrician, nutritionist, psychologist, and social worker.

The problem of adolescent obesity is relevant to all surgeons and physicians, not just those who care for children. The authors know from their collective clinical experience that obesity in childhood is not something patients just "grow out of," and that recognition of this problem and optimizing treatment early can provide patients with healthier and longer lives.

REFERENCES

1. Healthy weight, overweight, and obesity among U.S. adults. National Health and Nutrition Examination Survey, Centers for Disease Control. Available at: http://www.cdc.gov/nchs/data/nhanes/databriefs/adultweight.pdf. Accessed August 25, 2011.

2. Ogden CL Flegal KM. Changes in terminology for childhood overweight and obesity. Available at: http://www.cdc.gov/nchs/data/nhsr/nhsr025.pdf. Accessed August 25, 2011.
3. Prevalence of overweight among children and adolescents, United States 1999–2002. Available at: http://www.cdc.gov/nchs/products/pubs/pubd/hestats/overwght99.htm. Accessed August 25, 2011.
4. Ogden CL, Flegal KM, Carroll MD, et al. Prevalence and trends in overweight among US children and adolescents 1999-2000. JAMA 2002;288:1728–32.
5. Hedley AA, Ogden CL, Johnson CL, et al. Prevalence of overweight and obesity among US children, adolescents and adults, 1999-2002. JAMA 2004;291: 2847–50.
6. Centers for Disease Control and Prevention. Participation in high school physical education—United States, 1991–2003. MMWR Morb Mortal Wkly Rep 2004;53: 844–7.
7. Kinsey JD. Food and families' socioeconomic status. J Nutr 1994;124(Suppl 9): 1878S–85S.
8. Kautiainen S, Koivusilta L, Lintonen T, et al. Use of information and communication technology and prevalence of overweight and obesity among adolescents. Int J Obes 2005;29:925–33.
9. Fulton JE, Wang X, Yore MM, et al. Television viewing, computer use, and BMI among U.S. children and adolescents. J Phys Act Health 2009;6(Suppl 1): S28–35.
10. Duffey KJ, Gordon-Larsen P, Steffen LM, et al. Regular consumption from fast food establishments relative to other restaurants is differentially associated with metabolic outcomes in young adults. J Nutr 2009;139:2113–8.
11. Fontaine KR, Barofsky I. Type 2 diabetes mellitus in children and youth: a new epidemic. J Pediatr Endocrinol Metab 2002;15:737–44.
12. Schwimmer JB, McGreal N, Deutsch R, et al. Influence of gender, race, and ethnicity on suspected fatty liver in obese adolescents. Pediatrics 2005;115: e561–5.
13. Dâmaso AR, do Prado WL, de Piano A, et al. Relationship between nonalcoholic fatty liver disease prevalence and visceral fat in obese adolescents. Dig Liver Dis 2008;40:132–9.
14. Amin RS, Kimball TR, Bean JA, et al. Left ventricular hypertrophy and abnormal ventricular geometry in children and adolescents with obstructive sleep apnea. Am J Respir Crit Care Med 2002;15:1395–9.
15. Gami AS, Caples SM, Somers VK. Obesity and obstructive sleep apnea. Endocrinol Metab Clin North Am 2003;32:869–94.
16. Marcus CL, Curtis S, Koerner CB, et al. Evaluation of pulmonary function and polysomnography in obese children and adolescents. Pediatr Pulmonol 1996;21: 176–83.
17. Freedman DS, Khan LK, Dietz WH, et al. Relationship of childhood obesity to coronary heart disease risk factors in adulthood: the Bogalusa Heart Study. Pediatrics 2001;108:712–8.
18. Becque MD, Katch V, Rocchini AP, et al. Coronary risk incidence of obese adolescents: reduction by exercise plus diet intervention. Pediatrics 1988;81:605–12.
19. Bibbins-Domingo K, Coxson P, Pletcher MJ, et al. Adolescent overweight and future adult coronary heart disease. N Engl J Med 2007;357:2371–9.
20. Jassen I, Crain WM, Boyce WF, et al. Associations between over-weight and obesity with bullying behaviors in school-aged children. Pediatrics 2004;113: 1187–94.

21. Agranat-Meged AN, Deitcher C, Goldzweig G, et al. Childhood obesity and attention deficit/hyperactivity disorder: a newly described comorbidity in obese hospitalized children. Int J Eat Disord 2005;37:357-9.
22. Puhl R, Brownell KD. Bias, discrimination and obesity. Obes Res 2001;9:788-805.
23. Duffecy J, Bleil ME, Labott SM, et al. Psychopathology in adolescents presenting for laparoscopic banding. J Adolesc Health 2008;43:623-5.
24. Epstein LH, Valoski A, Wing RR, et al. Ten-year follow-up of behavioral family-based treatment for obese children. JAMA 1990;264:2519-23.
25. Berkowitz RI, Wadden T, Tershakovec AM, et al. Behavior therapy and sibutramine for the treatment of adolescent obesity: a randomized controlled trial. Ann Intern Med 2003;289:1805-12.
26. Chanoine JP, Hampl S, Jensen C, et al. Effect of orlistat on weight and body composition in obese adolescents: a randomized controlled trial. JAMA 2005; 15:2873-83.
27. McGovern L, Johnson JN, Paulo R, et al. Clinical review: treatment of pediatric obesity: a systematic review and meta-analysis of randomized trials. J Clin Endocrinol Metab 2008;93:4600-5.
28. National Institutes of Health Consensus Development Conference Statement on Gastrointestinal Surgery for Severe Obesity, 1991. Available at: http://consensus.nih.gov/1991/1991GISurgeryObesity084html.htm. Accessed August 25, 2011.
29. IPEG Standards and Safety Committee. IPEG guidelines for surgical treatment of extremely obese adolescents. J Laparoendosc Adv Surg Tech A 2009;19(Suppl 1): xiv-xvi.
30. Woolford SJ, Clark SJ, Gebremariam A, et al. To cut or not to cut: physicians' perspectives on referring adolescents for bariatric surgery. Obes Surg 2010; 20:937-42.
31. Iqbal CW, Kumar S, Iqbal AD, et al. Perspectives on pediatric bariatric surgery: identifying barriers to referral. Surg Obes Relat Dis 2009;5:88-93.
32. Inge TH, Jenkins TH, Zeller M, et al. Baseline BMI is a strong predictor of nadir BMI after adolescent gastric bypass. J Pediatr 2010;156:103-8.
33. Buchwald H, Avidor Y, Braunwald E, et al. Bariatric surgery: a systemic review and meta-analysis. JAMA 2004;292:1724-37.
34. Randolph JG, Weintraub WH, Rigg A. Jejunoileal bypass for morbid obesity in adolescents. J Pediatr Surg 1974;9:341-5.
35. Silber T, Randolph J, Robbins S. Long-term morbidity and mortality in morbidly obese adolescents after jejunoileal bypass. J Pediatr 1986;108:318-22.
36. Schilling PL, Davis MM, Albanese CT, et al. National trends in adolescent bariatric surgical procedures and implications for surgical centers of excellence. J Am Coll Surg 2008;206:1-12.
37. O'Brien PE, Sawyer SM, Brown LC, et al. Laparoscopic adjustable gastric banding in severely obese adolescents. A randomized trial. JAMA 2010;303: 512-26.
38. Nadler EP, Youn H, Ginsburg HB, et al. Short-term results in 53 US obese pediatric patients treated with laparoscopic adjustable gastric banding. J Pediatr Surg 2007;42:137-42.
39. Treadwell JR, Sun F, Schoelles K. Systematic review and meta-analysis of bariatric surgery for pediatric obesity. Ann Surg 2008;248:763-76.
40. Stanford A, Glascock JM, Eid GM, et al. Laparoscopic Roux-en-Y gastric bypass in morbidly obese adolescents. J Pediatr Surg 2003;38:430-3.
41. Strauss RS, Bradley LJ, Brolin RE. Gastric bypass surgery in adolescents with morbid obesity. J Pediatr 2001;138:499-504.

42. Inge TH, Garcia V, Daniels S, et al. A multidisciplinary approach to the adolescent bariatric surgical patient. J Pediatr Surg 2004;39:442–7.
43. Bohdjalian A, Langer FB, Shakeri-Leidenmühler S, et al. Sleeve gastrectomy as sole and definitive bariatric procedure: 5-year results for weight loss and ghrelin. Obes Surg 2010;20:535–40.
44. Himpens J, Dapri G, Cadière GB. A prospective randomized study between laparoscopic gastric banding and laparoscopic isolated sleeve gastrectomy: results after 1 and 3 years. Obes Surg 2006;16:1450–6.
45. Till H, Blüher S, Hirsch W, et al. Efficacy of laparoscopic sleeve gastrectomy (LSG) as a stand-alone technique for children with morbid obesity. Obes Surg 2008;18:1047–9.
46. Baltasar A, Serra C, Bou R, et al. Sleeve gastrectomy in a 10-year-old child. Obes Surg 2008;18:733–6.
47. Inge TH, Zeller M, Harmon C, et al. Teen-longitudinal assessment of bariatric surgery: methodological features of the first prospective multicenter study of adolescent bariatric surgery. J Pediatr Surg 2007;42:1969–71.
48. Caniano DA. Ethical issues in pediatric bariatric surgery. Semin Pediatr Surg 2009;18:186–92.
49. Spear BA, Barlow SE, Ervin C, et al. Recommendations for treatment of child and adolescent overweight and obesity. Pediatrics 2007;120:S254–88.

Revisional Bariatric Surgery

Todd Andrew Kellogg, MD

KEYWORDS

• Bariatric surgery • Revision • Reoperation

OVERVIEW

With the increasing number of bariatric procedures being performed annually, it is expected that the incidence of revisions will increase. The overall incidence of surgical revision after a primary bariatric operation is 5% to 50%. The lowest rate of revision is associated with the biliopancreatic diversion (BPD) with duodenal switch (BPD-DS) procedure and is 5%.[1,2] The Roux-en-Y gastric bypass (RYGB) fails to produce adequate durable weight loss in 15% to 25%, with revision estimates of 10% to 20%.[3,4] The incidence of revision after vertical banded gastroplasty (VBG) is 25% to 54%.[5–7] The laparoscopic adjustable gastric band (AGB) has the highest rate of revision at 40% to 50%,[8] although recent studies suggest that this rate is decreasing.[9–11]

A distinction should be made between inadequate weight loss or weight regain and need for revision (ie, not all failures need to be revised). There are various indications for revising a primary bariatric operation. The most common indication is failure of the primary operation to provide adequate durable weight loss, which is generally defined as excess weight loss (EWL) of at least 50%. However, adequacy of weight loss must be judged in the context of the presence or absence of comorbid disease. Before considering whether a particular individual is a candidate for a revision of the primary operation, it is important to determine whether the operation failed the patient or whether the patient failed the operation; whether there is there an anatomic cause for the weight regain or the weight regain is primarily a result of behavioral discrepancies such as large portion sizes, high caloric foods, snacking between meals, and lack of exercise. It is imperative that these issues be determined before considering revisional surgery or there will be repeated failure of the operation to provide weight loss or to control weight regain. It should also be considered and accepted that, as with many other diseases, not everyone can be cured of their obesity; there is a group of nonresponders who are resistant to weight loss despite the surgeon's best efforts.

In the early days of bariatric surgery, it was questioned whether the risk associated with revision of bariatric procedures was worth the benefit.[12,13] There are now

The author has nothing to disclose.
Division of Bariatric and Gastrointestinal Surgery, University of Minnesota, 420 Delaware Street Southeast, MMC 290, Minneapolis, MN 55455, USA
E-mail address: Kell0018@umn.edu

Surg Clin N Am 91 (2011) 1353–1371
doi:10.1016/j.suc.2011.08.004
0039-6109/11/$ – see front matter © 2011 Elsevier Inc. All rights reserved.

surgical.theclinics.com

case-matched[3] and case-controlled[4] studies, as well as multiple retrospective series, that leave little doubt that revisions are effective and that there is a benefit in terms of both weight loss and overall health. As with reoperation in general, the associated morbidity and mortality are higher than with primary bariatric procedures, but are acceptably low if careful selection of patients is coupled with adequate surgeon experience and expertise.[14] Nevertheless, although there are many reports in the literature evaluating outcomes after revision of primary bariatric surgical procedures and suggesting operative strategies for revision, there are no data-driven algorithms for surgical revisions based on randomized controlled trials.

PREOPERATIVE EVALUATION AND TESTING

The need for revision should be based on the suspected cause of the patient's symptoms. Preoperative evaluation and anatomic studies need to be performed to help determine the root cause. Because bariatric procedures are not strictly standardized and there is some variation among surgeons, preoperative evaluation of the anatomy is imperative.

Dietary Intake Diary and Nutrition Counseling

When a patient reports the inability to eat appropriately in terms of food choices or adequate calories, or complains of persistent nausea and vomiting, this history must be verified before considering revision. Nutrition consultation, preferably with a bariatric-specialized registered dietician, is mandatory. A food diary listing the patient's day-to-day dietary history should be kept and reported dietary behaviors investigated. For some patients with weight regain or even persistent nausea and vomiting, dietary modification alone can improve symptoms and correct weight regain. Appetite suppressant medications can be added to curb appetite and therefore augment behavior modification.

Upper Endoscopy

Inspection of the upper gastrointestinal (GI) tract should always be performed before revisional surgery. The usefulness is multiple. Endoscopic review of the anatomy can provide diagnostic information concerning the previous procedure should operative reports not be available. Inspection of the mucosa can determine the sequelae of acid or bile reflux, or the presence of stoma narrowing, marginal ulcers, bleeding, eroded foreign bodies, and other potential problems such as migrated sutures or the presence of a gastrogastric fistula.[15]

Contrast Upper GI Study

A contrast upper GI study is essential. This study provides information that is useful for diagnosis and strategic preoperative planning by providing a road map for the surgeon contemplating revising the upper GI tract. A preoperative upper GI study also provides a comparison for any postoperative studies that may be needed. This study gives a more dynamic view of the upper GI tract and can identify functional narrowing, dilatation, gastrogastric fistula, and may help identify the original operation in cases in which the original operative note is unavailable and the patient cannot recall.

Other Studies

Esophageal manometry is occasionally warranted to determine whether esophageal peristalsis has been affected by the primary bariatric procedure, which can affect the approach to revision, especially when the primary procedure was an AGB.[16] Gastric emptying studies can also be useful to identify functional abnormalities.

Review of Operative Notes

It is imperative that the operative notes from the primary bariatric operation be reviewed. Details of technique as well as reported anatomic variations can substantially affect operative strategy. Essential details include the lengths of bypassed intestines (such as Roux limb and biliopancreatic limb lengths after RYGB), estimates of pouch size, and whether a gastrostomy tube was placed. Important technical aspects to be considered include the details of any foreign body that was placed, for example, AGB type and size and VBG band type. Understanding the anastomotic technique used can guide dissection and potentially affect the operative plan. Anatomic variations deduced on primary operation can be anticipated on revision.

GENERAL OPERATIVE PRINCIPLES OF BARIATRIC REVISIONARY SURGERY

Adhesiolysis

The surgeon should be prepared for challenging adhesiolysis, particularly if the primary operation was performed using an open approach. The need for extensive adhesiolysis is not a contraindication to the laparoscopic approach; magnification can provide an advantage and exposure is often superior. The most difficult adhesions are usually encountered at the gastric lesser curve where structures to be identified include the stomach, liver, pancreas, left gastric artery, and the inferior vena cava. At the angle of His, the proximity of the spleen to the gastric fundus can be challenging if dense adhesions are present in this region. Intraloop small bowel adhesions can be tedious to contend with laparoscopically but otherwise are not usually difficult to manage.

Gastric Stapling

For revision operations involving the stomach, transection of the stomach with linear staplers should always be performed with staple loads with a staple height of 4.5 mm or 4.8 mm because of the increased thickness of the tissues secondary to tissue fibrosis from scarring or chronic tissue inflammation with edema. All staple lines are oversewn using a similar rationale. For operations involving revision of a previously constructed gastrojejunostomy, Roux limb dissection should be completed before constructing the new gastrojejunostomy to ensure Roux limb viability. Whenever there is crossing of staple lines, this area should be carefully inspected and reinforced as needed.

Leak Testing

The anastomotic leak rate is increased when performing anastomoses of previously operated tissues.[14] Therefore, the integrity of any high-risk anastomosis should be verified before concluding the operation. The 2 most common methods of leak testing are methylene blue instillation and gas insufflation, usually via an enteroscope. The methylene blue test is usually performed by instilling dilute methylene blue (1 ampule in 250 mL of sterile water or saline) via a nasogastric tube in a carefully controlled volume adequate to distend the bowel with the bowel distal to the anastomosis occluded either digitally or using a bowel clamp. It is helpful to place a clean white sponge around the anastomosis to assist in detecting leakage. Leak testing using gas insufflation can also be performed via a nasogastric tube. However, this type of testing is best performed using an endoscope. In this technique, the bowel is occluded just distal to the anastomosis. An endoscope is then placed transorally and carefully guided into position near the anastomosis. The anastomosis is flooded with irrigation until covered. Using the endoscope, air or CO_2 is injected, with careful inspection of the area for bubbling. If a leak is found, it is repaired and the leak test repeated. No patient should leave the operating room until the leak test is negative. Several studies have shown a benefit from intraoperative leak testing during primary RYGB, including decreased postoperative leak rates at the gastrojejunal anastomosis.[17–19] One study found that the endoscopic leak test was superior to the orogastric tube technique.[19]

Gastrostomy Tube

As previously discussed, the risk of a gastrojejunal anastomotic leak is increased with revisional procedures. Therefore, placement of a gastrostomy tube with revision to RYGB should always be strongly considered and should always be placed when there is evidence of preoperative malnutrition or when extensive lysis of adhesions involving the gastric remnant is required, which may increase the risk of postoperative gastric remnant distention.

Drains

Intra-abdominal drains are used on a selective basis and should always be used in difficult anastomoses or when a repair is necessary because of a positive intraoperative leak test, which may also increase the likelihood of a controlled fistula if a leak were to develop. Drains are best placed in a dependent area in proximity to, but not in contact with, the at-risk anastomosis.

LAPAROSCOPIC VERSUS OPEN APPROACH

Most bariatric revision procedures involving the upper GI tract can be performed laparoscopically by a skilled and experienced laparoscopic bariatric surgeon even if the primary operation was performed using the open technique.[20,21] The benefits of the laparoscopic approach are identical to those for a primary laparoscopic operation: fewer wound complications, less postoperative pain and narcotic requirement, shorter hospital stay, and earlier return to work.[22] From a technical perspective, laparoscopy affords increased visibility and magnification of tissues. Although cost-effective as a primary procedure,[23] to date, no data are available to determine whether revisions performed laparoscopically are cost-effective compared with the open approach.

Revisions involving the small bowel can be difficult after a primary open procedure because of multiple adhesions of the small bowel and mesentery that can severely limit its mobility. Although, with time and effort, nearly all cases can be completed laparoscopically, it needs to be decided whether the benefits outweigh an extreme effort. The decision whether to proceed with a laparoscopic or open approach should be made according to the skill and experience of the surgeon and good judgment on a case-by-case basis.

REVISION OF RYGB
General Operative Strategy in Revisional Bariatric Surgery

Whether performed open or laparoscopically, the operative strategy is the same. The first step is lysis of adhesions, which may be extensive. If the gastrojejunostomy is to be revised, the upper abdomen is entered. Adhesions of the greater omentum are typically encountered first. Also commonly encountered here is adhered transverse colon and associated epiploic fat. After adhesions to the abdominal wall are taken down in all directions, a retractor system is placed to provide exposure and thereby allow further dissection in the upper abdominal compartment. The undersurface of the left lateral segment of the liver will be adhered to the anterior surface of the gastric pouch, and these structures should be separated. Complete dissection and exposure of the gastric pouch and remnant is performed. Several variations in the gastrojejunal arrangement are possible and nothing should be assumed if the operative report is unavailable and findings on preoperative testing are ambiguous. Possibilities include a loop gastric bypass, horizontally partitioned gastric pouch with Roux-en-Y small bowel reconstruction, and vertical pouch with or without banding. Patients are sometimes referred for revision with no records and only an understanding that they had a stomach stapling in the 1970s or 1980s. In the author's experience, this generic term does not suggest the likelihood of one procedure type versus another.

With revision of the gastrojejunostomy, the entire Roux limb (or jejunal loop in the case of a loop gastric bypass) must be exposed, freed of adhesions, and the gastrojejunostomy skeletonized. To provide adequate Roux limb length, the Roux limb mesentery must be carefully dissected to avoid injury and consequent Roux limb ischemia. If the gastrojejunostomy is to be revised, available gastric pouch tissue is limited, and the indication for revision does not include abnormalities at the gastrojejunostomy (eg, marginal ulcers or stricture), it is then feasible to resect the jejunum off the stomach with a linear cutting stapler without resecting gastric tissue. However, in most cases, the gastric pouch is enlarged and the previous gastrojejunal anastomosis is resected with pouch revision by downsizing.

Construction of the gastrojejunal anastomosis should proceed as per the surgeon's preferred technique. The author prefers a partially linearly stapled, partially hand-sewn technique using a 10-mm endoscope as a stent during construction. With revisions, care should be taken to avoid a particularly small stoma, because increased edema and fibrosis can occur, thereby potentially increasing the risk of short-term and long-term stricture. In the case of a loop gastric bypass, continuity of the alimentary limb can be reestablished with an end-to-end anastomosis, and a Roux-en-Y small bowel reconstruction is then performed with a biliopancreatic limb length of at least 40 cm and a Roux limb length of 75 cm to 150 cm.[24]

CONVERSION OF LOOP GASTRIC BYPASS TO ROUX-EN-Y
Indications

At present, gastric bypass for morbid obesity is universally performed using Roux-en-Y small bowel reconstruction. However, this was not always the case. The loop gastric bypass was typically constructed with a large gastric pouch constructed by a horizontally stapled partition, which can be an important factor in weight regain. Moreover, patients with loop gastrojejunostomy anatomy are at increased risk for developing several issues including marginal ulcerations, stricture of the gastrojejunal stoma, poor gastric pouch emptying, and bile reflux. When symptomatic, any of these conditions is an indication for conversion to RYGB.

Management Options and Outcomes

The entire jejunal loop must be exposed and the gastrojejunostomy skeletonized. The gastrojejunal anastomosis is resected with revision of the gastric pouch. If the biliopancreatic limb has adequate length, a jejunojejunostomy can be constructed directly with the distal end. Alternatively, continuity of the jejunum can be reestablished with an end-to-end anastomosis, and a Roux-en-Y small bowel reconstruction is then performed with a biliopancreatic limb length of at least 40 cm (to prevent bile reflux) and a Roux limb length of 75 cm to 150 cm. The gastric pouch is divided to create a new, smaller 15-mL to 30-mL lesser curvature-based pouch. As discussed earlier, this should be done using 4.5-mm or 4.8-mm staple loads and all staple lines oversewn. A proximal gastric resection may be necessary if it appears on inspection that this portion of the stomach has become devascularized or if it simply appears unhealthy and potentially compromised. Potential pitfalls include devascularization of the Roux limb during dissection and adhesiolysis; construction of a Roux limb that is too short, resulting in bile reflux; and leaving a pouch that is too large to provide additional weight loss and that could result in symptoms of gastroesophageal reflux disease (GERD).

Few studies have been performed evaluating outcome after conversion of a loop gastric bypass to a RYGB. Weight loss is expected, particularly if the gastric pouch size has been substantially reduced. Marginal ulcers can recur, especially if preoperative risk factors have not been eliminated. The Roux-en-Y reconstruction eliminates bile reflux in nearly all cases.[25]

REVISION OF PROXIMAL RYGB
Indications

The incidence of weight regain or failure to lose adequate weight after a primary proximal RYGB is about 15% to 25%.[26–28] When a patient presents with weight gain after a proximal RYGB the cause of failure must be determined. Patients in whom an anatomic cause for the weight gain is identified are generally candidates for revision. Exceptions may be patients with a strong behavioral component to the weight gain that contributed significantly to the anatomic changes.

Management Options and Outcomes

Adding restriction

It remains controversial whether increasing restriction is appropriate for patients with inadequate initial weight loss or weight regain after initial RYGB. Changes in the upper GI anatomy can occur that suggest a benefit from alteration through revision. A gastro-gastric fistula after gastric partitioning is an anatomic finding that can result in weight regain as well as severe GERD; in this case, repair is indicated and is performed by dividing the stomach just proximal to the previous staple line. Care should be taken not to cross staple lines or create a gastric chamber that cannot drain.

In theory, a large pouch or large stoma could be responsible for weight regain after RYGB. When a loss of satiety is reported and a large pouch with a large gastrojejunal stoma is found on preoperative work-up, revision of the pouch and gastrojejunostomy is a reasonable surgical option. If the gastric pouch and stoma have enlarged substantially, the entire gastrojejunostomy complex can be revised, effectively decreasing the size of both. Other strategies include gastrojejunostomy revision with banding of the pouch near the stoma, which is also referred to as pouch stabilization (ie, the Fobi pouch). Placement of an AGB around the pouch has the advantage of providing additional adjustable gastric restriction without the added risk associated with revision of the anastomosis. When placing an AGB after divided RYGB, gastrogastric fixation of the AGB using the gastric remnant is the general technique adopted to prevent postoperative slippage.[29]

Historically, there has been little direct evidence that RYGB revision involving various strategies of adding gastric restriction results in superior weight loss.[12,13,30]

Moreover, MacLean and colleagues[31] showed that stoma size does not necessarily correlate with initial weight loss or weight regain. However, more recently, others have reported long-term data that support gastric pouch stabilization as a technique to improve weight loss with RYGB.[32,33]

Parikh and colleagues[34] recently published short-term data on revising patients with suboptimal weight loss after RYGB by adding restriction through performing a laparoscopic sleeve resection of the gastrojejunal complex with a bougie in place. At an average follow-up of 12 months, there was no difference in preoperative and postoperative body mass index (BMI) or EWL in patients undergoing sleeve resection with or without added malabsorption by lengthening the Roux limb, although the extent of added malabsorption by Roux limb lengthening was not reported.[34]

Although not extensively studied, RYGB failure treated by AGB placement has had promising initial results. The largest series to date was reported by Bessler and colleagues[29] and consisted of 22 patients with follow-up of up to 5 years. Beginning with a mean BMI at revision of 44.8 ($\pm$ 6.34) kg/m^2, patients experienced a loss of 27%, 47.3%, 42.3%, 43%, and 47% of their excess weight at 1, 2, 3, 4, and 5 years following AGB placement, respectively. Three major complications occurred requiring reoperation. No band erosions were documented. The next largest study assessing AGB placement after RYGB consisted of 11 patients with a mean EWL after RYGB of 38% ($\pm$ 9%) and mean BMI of 43.4 kg/m^2. The average follow-up after laparoscopic AGB placement was 13 months (range 2–32 months). Postrevision mean BMI was 37.1 kg/m^2 and these patients undergoing laparoscopic AGB after failed RYGB had an additional mean 20.8% EWL leading to an overall EWL of 59% for both procedures. Thirty-day morbidity and mortality were nil.[35]

ADDING MALABSORPTION
Conversion to Distal RYGB

Malabsorption can be added to a proximal RYGB by increasing the length of either the Roux or biliopancreatic limb. In a patient with weight gain after having undergone a proximal or short Roux limb (<150 cm) gastric bypass who, on work-up, has normal gastric bypass gastrojejunostomy anatomy (ie, a gastric pouch estimated to be less than 30 mL and a stoma less than 15 mm), conversion to a distal (long-limb) RYGB can be considered. From a technical perspective, this procedure is usually straightforward because the more difficult dissection in the upper abdomen is unnecessary. The length of the Roux limb is measured to ensure that it correlates with the operative note. The biliopancreatic limb is measured from the ligament of Treitz. The end-to-side jejunojejunostomy is skeletonized so that all staple or suture lines are clearly visible. At this point, there are 2 possible ways to proceed. The biliopancreatic limb can be removed from the Roux limb without compromising the Roux limb by using a linear cutting stapler placed just adjacent to the previous staple or suture line. Any tissue that would be rendered nonviable is left on the end of the biliopancreatic limb and can be removed with a second firing before constructing the jejunojejunostomy. It should be verified that the Roux limb lumen is not compromised after this maneuver. The benefit of this operative technique is that only 1 anastomosis needs to be constructed as opposed to 2. Alternatively, the distal Roux limb, distal biliopancreatic limb, and proximal common channel at the jejunojejunostomy can each be transected, which then requires construction of a functional end-to-end jejunojejunostomy to restore continuity of the alimentary limb.

Although the approaches vary, construction of a distal RYGB in general requires measuring the common channel distally to proximally, beginning at the ileocecal valve.

The common channel length is critical; typically this length is 75 to 150 cm. A length less than 75 cm has an unacceptably high risk of protein malnutrition.[36] An ileojejunostomy is then constructed; the author prefers a side-to-side functional end-to-side linearly stapled technique.

In one of the first published studies examining the effect of converting a failed proximal RYGB to a distal RYGB, Sugerman and colleagues[37] examined the records of 27 patients in whom the Roux limb was lengthened from 40 cm to 145 cm with a common channel length of 50 cm in the first 5 patients and 150 cm in the last 22 patients. The biliopancreatic limb was not measured and the gastrojejunostomy was not revised. All 5 patients with a 50-cm common channel developed severe nutritional deficiencies including protein-calorie malnutrition that required revision. Two of these patients died of liver failure. Of the 22 patients with a 150-cm common channel, 3 required common channel lengthening because of malnutrition. All patients had at least 1 nutrition-related blood test abnormality and 4 (18%) required either total parenteral nutrition (TPN) or percutaneous enteric feeding. The EWL was 69% at 5 years after adding malabsorption, with nearly universal resolution of comorbid disease after the first year.

Fobi and colleagues[38] retrospectively reported a series of 65 patients who failed proximal banded RYGB and who were revised to distal RYGB. Indications for revision included failure to lose more than 40% EWL with the primary procedure (21%), BMI greater than 35 kg/m^2 (23%), weight regain of at least 14 kg (21%), patient request for revision during another concomitant operation to maximize weight loss even though BMI was less than 35 kg/m^2 (24%), and band removal required (9%). The strategy used for enhancing the malabsorptive component of the RYGB was to move the Roux limb distally halfway down the common channel, effectively reducing the alimentary limb length by 50%. Three percent of patients developed intractable diarrhea. Fifteen patients (23%) developed protein malnutrition as defined by a serum albumin less than 3 g/dL. All protein-malnourished patients were treated with oral supplements and nutrition counseling. In addition, 8 required percutaneous gastrostomy feedings, 6 required TPN, and 6 patients (9.2%) required reoperation to lengthen the common channel. After revision, the mean weight and BMI loss were 20 kg and 7 kg/m^2. The final mean BMI was 34.6 kg/m^2 for the group.

Brolin and Cody[39] converted 54 patients to a long-limb RYGB who had inadequate weight loss after short-limb RYGB or gastric restrictive operation using an open approach. In each case of RYGB revision, the gastrojejunostomy was revised to enhance gastric restriction. The Roux limb was reanastomosed to the distal ileum at a point 75 to 100 cm from the ileocecal valve. Perioperative complications occurred in 18.5%. There were 9 nonmetabolic late complications and there was a high incidence of anemia in these patients. Metabolic sequelae of conversion to distal RYGB included macronutrient and micronutrient deficiencies; protein malnutrition was present in 7.4%. Mean weight/BMI losses were 37 kg and 13.1 kg/m^2 respectively, with 47.9% of patients losing at least 50% of their excess weight at 1 year after surgery. There was no difference in percent EWL between patients who had revisions of purely restrictive operations and those who had revision of gastric bypass.

Conversion of RYGB to BPD-DS

When gastric bypass fails, some clinicians advocate conversion to duodenal switch. In theory, this conversion should provide an additional 15% to 20% EWL even in the case of a successful RYGB. Revision to BPD-DS is a complicated procedure that requires 3 or 4 bowel anastomoses: gastrogastrostomy, duodenoileostomy, ileoileostomy (a jejunojejunostomy is also necessary to reconnect the alimentary limb if the

RYGB jejunojejunostomy was completely resected). Technically challenging in any case, this procedure can be done open or laparoscopically in 1 or 2 stages.

A controversial indication for conversion of RYGB to BPD-DS is reactive hypoglycemia. If compliance with a low-carbohydrate diet is not successful, this procedure can be considered because it reestablishes the pylorus and thus slows the emptying of carbohydrates into the small bowel, resulting in amelioration of the reactive hypoglycemic response.[40]

Only 3 studies have been published on conversion of RYGB to BPD-DS. In a recently reported study, 41 patients underwent open conversion of their original bariatric operation to a duodenal switch with omentopexy and feeding jejunostomy, including 32 patients who originally underwent RYGB. The average EWL following surgical reintervention was 54% in 25 patients at 6 months, 59% in 15 patients at 1 year, and 77% in 5 patients at 2 years. The incidence of major complications was 32%, including a gastrogastrostomy leak rate of 20%. There were no deaths.[41]

One of the first reports of RYGB conversion to BPD-DS included 47 patients who underwent open revisions to BPD-DS (26 primary RYGB and 5 patients who had initial VBG later revised to a RYGB) and were presenting for their second revision. Three-fourths of patients underwent revision to BPD-DS for either weight regain or inadequate loss (46%) or significant dumping syndrome (28%).The postoperative leak rate was 8.5% and half of these occurred in patients who had first undergone VBG followed by RYGB, with BPD-DS as a second revision. One-half of the leaks occurred at the gastrogastrostomy and one-half were located at the site of the sleeve gastrectomy (SG) proximal to the gastrogastrostomy. At an average follow-up of 30 months, the average BMI decreased from 48.9 to 29.2 kg/m^2 with an EWL of 67% and an average weight loss of 48 kg. All patients had resolution of the primary problem that led to revision.[42]

To date, the largest reported series of laparoscopic conversion of RYGB to BPD-DS comes from Gagner and associates.[43] They reported data for 12 patients who experienced weight regain or inadequate weight loss, 4 of whom had undergone a revision before conversion. The average BMI before conversion was 41 kg/m^2. Seven (58%) underwent conversion to BPD-DS in 1 stage. A circular stapler was used for the gastrogastrostomy in most cases. At 11 months after surgery, average BMI decreased by 10 kg/m^2 and EWL was 63% with resolution of comorbid disease in all cases. One-third developed strictures at the gastrogastrostomy site. There were no leaks or deaths.

REVISION AFTER FAILED RESTRICTIVE PROCEDURES
Revision of VBG

Indications
The main issues that develop after VBG that require considering surgical revision are weight regain secondary to maladaptive eating or weight gain caused by staple line breakdown with or without the development of severe GERD and esophagitis.[44]

A thorough dietary history often reveals the same story from patient to patient; those with maladaptive eating prefer foods that disintegrate easily. For example, in his practice, the author has noted that Cheetos is a food nearly universally consumed by these patients. Healthy foods such as fresh vegetables, fruits, and meats are not well tolerated and therefore have been slowly eliminated from the diet. Malnutrition can ensue. Upper endoscopy can be diagnostic, showing esophagitis, a dilated esophagus, and a gastrogastric fistula to the lower stomach. Contrast upper GI study verifies the presence of a gastrogastric fistula and dilated esophagus and can provide direct evidence of delayed pouch emptying and esophageal reflux. On distention with contrast, relative pouch size can be estimated and this information used for operative planning.

Management options and operative strategies

VBG band removal with or without gastrogastrostomy In a patient with maladaptive eating caused by pouch outlet narrowing or partial obstruction who has not regained significant weight or who requests a reversal of the VBG, simple ring removal is generally sufficient to resolve these symptoms; without the ring in place, the opening from the pouch to the lower stomach quickly dilates and, although rarely required, postoperative endoscopic dilation is effective without the ring in place. If persistent and severe vomiting from pouch outlet obstruction is a key symptom and preoperative studies support the diagnosis of gastric outlet obstruction, a gastrogastrostomy should be strongly considered. The need for gastrogastrostomy can be assessed using intraoperative upper endoscopy. If the area where the ring was located is very narrow and fibrotic, then gastrogastrostomy is recommended. All patients undergoing simple band removal with or without gastrogastrostomy should be advised that any lost weight will almost certainly be regained.

Conversion of VBG to RYGB Most cases of VBG conversion to RYGB can be handled laparoscopically by an appropriately skilled surgeon. Five ports are generally needed to complete the operation laparoscopically. After abdominal entry, lysis of adhesions is performed throughout the abdomen. Most of the adhesions will be located in the upper abdomen. Omentum and transverse colon can be adhered to the anterior abdominal wall in the region of the patient's previous incision. When these have been lysed, attention is turned to the adhesions of the undersurface of the left lateral segment of the liver and the stomach lesser curvature. The caudate lobe of the liver is an important landmark and is identified early. The position of the left gastric artery is noted. A gastroscope is often helpful in guiding dissection of the stomach and verifying the location of the band, staple line, and gastroesophageal junction.

The location of the gastroplasty band is often revealed by the presence of dense adhesions in this area. Silastic bands can generally be visualized or are palpable and can be fairly easily removed by incising the overlying peritonealized tissue, lifting the band off the stomach, and incising the associated suture. Complete band removal should be verified by measuring the removed segments. Polypropylene bands are incorporated to a large extent into the gastric tissue and therefore are much more difficult to remove. In this case, the options are (1) removal and oversewing of the gastric tissue, (2) leaving the band in place, and (3) removing the band and associated portion of the stomach en bloc.

The anterior surface of the stomach is cleared of adhered tissues until the gastroplasty staple line is identified. This usually appears as a clef in the gastric surface extending from the position of the ring to the angle of His. The staple line is skeletonized to precisely determine its position. A retrogastric tunnel is made proximal to the gastroplasty staple line; this may be made easier by mobilizing the greater curvature of the stomach by dividing several proximal short gastric vessels. Once this tunnel is made, a gastric pouch can be constructed using multiple firings of a triple linear cutting stapler with staples that are at least 4.5 mm in staple height. Ideally, the new staple line should be placed just proximal and adjacent to the gastroplasty staple line. If this will result in a pouch that is too large (>30 mL), then the pouch is made to be the appropriate size with resection of the proximal gastric remnant to include the VBG staple line because 2 parallel staple lines separated by a gap of tissue can result in ischemia of this intervening tissue or a chamber with no outlet.

The jejunojejunostomy can be performed before or after completion of the gastrojejunostomy. If a VBG is the only previous abdominal operation, there will be few adhesions involving the inframesocolic abdomen. The jejunojejunostomy is then constructed as in a primary RYGB.[24]

An antecolic or retrocolic Roux limb gastrojejunostomy is then constructed. The surgeon should be aware that, depending on the indication for revision, the gastric tissues are often inflamed, edematous, and fibrotic compared with a primary RYGB, and, on this basis, adjustments in technique need to be considered. All staple lines are oversewn. A remnant gastrostomy tube and intraperitoneal drain should always be considered and is used on a selective basis by the author.

Endoscopic removal has been reported in cases in which the band has eroded into the gastric lumen, although the risk of leak with this approach may be substantial.[45]

VBG revision outcomes

There have been multiple retrospective reviews of both open and laparoscopic approaches that provide evidence for outcome analysis. As with other revisional procedures, the morbidity and mortality with revision of VBG are higher than after primary procedures.[13,46–50] VBG revision has more associated morbidity than conversion to RYGB. Complication rates are in the range of 10% to 40%, with mortality typically 2% or less.[51–55] More recent studies have confirmed these findings and have also shown that conversion of VBG to RYGB resulted in better weight loss than revision of the gastroplasty.[56] Sugerman and colleagues[57] showed that, 1 year after VBG conversion to RYGB, the percentage of EWL was no different from that of a primary RYGB.

Most patients undergoing VBG revision have resolution of VBG-related symptoms, including open reversal of VBG by gastrogastrostomy, which resulted in 89% symptom improvement[58] and conversion of VBG to RYGB, which was associated with 100% symptom improvement.[59]

There is some evidence that weight loss after VBG conversion to RYGB depends on the indication for revision. In a study of 101 patients, Schouten and colleagues[59] found that patients undergoing revision for the indication of recurrent obesity had a significant decrease in BMI after conversion of VBG to RYGB. Patients with excessive weight loss after VBG experienced a slight weight gain, whereas those undergoing revision strictly for maladaptive eating were weight stable after conversion.

Many small reports in the literature address laparoscopic conversion of VBG to RYGB and echo the findings of the open literature. To date, the largest published report is a retrospective analysis of 105 patients laparoscopically converted from VBG to RYGB. The overall (both early and late) complication rate was 38%. With an average follow-up of 31 months, the median EWL was 47% and median decrease in BMI was 8 kg/m^2. Patient symptoms including GERD improved or completely resolved in 95% and all patients had resolution or improvement in dysphagia. Patient comorbid disease, including type 2 diabetes mellitus, obstructive sleep apnea, and hypertension, all improved substantially and similarly to improvements seen with primary RYGB.[60]

Revision After AGB

Indications

Failure of adequate weight loss after adjustable gastric banding has been reported to occur in 40% to 50% of patients in the United States.[8,61] AGB failure can have several different causes and the indication for revision dictates the approach to revision. Patients with failure caused by purely technical problems with the band, including hardware failure or slippage, may benefit from simple band replacement, especially if the original band can be replaced with a next-generation band. However, if the indication is a esophageal motility issue, inadequate weight loss, GERD, or psychological band intolerance, patients are generally better served by conversion to another weight loss procedure.[62–64]

When considering failed AGB, the question of which revision procedure to perform in what circumstances has not been clearly answered; much conjecture is present in the literature but no hard data. However, for patients with inadequate weight loss, there are several studies suggesting that conversion to RYGB is superior to rebanding.[63,65–67]

Management options and operative strategies

AGB removal Simple AGB removal technically is the easiest of the procedures. However, this intervention invariably leads to weight regain and return of obesity.[62,63] The band tubing is followed to the stomach to identify the band. Once the AGB is identified, the overlying peritonealized tissue is incised, which directly exposes the band. The AGB is dissected free, elevated, and transected with either laparoscopic scissors or the ultrasonic shears. Once divided, it is generally easy to pull the AGB off the stomach. Although isolated AGB removal can be performed, in general, it is preferable to restore normal upper gastric anatomy by taking down the gastrogastric sutures and associated adhesions. A safe way to accomplish this is to follow the tract formed by the chronic tissue reaction to the band, using it as a guide to take down the gastrogastric sutures. It has been shown that AGB that have eroded can be safely removed endoscopically, although this practice is not yet universal.[68]

AGB replacement Replacement of the AGB is a reasonable option if the patient has had a good result with the AGB and is being considered for revision based on considerations other than inadequate weight loss or complications of the AGB that would preclude AGB replacement, such a recurrent prolapsed, erosion, or general intolerance with insolvable nausea and vomiting. Careful patient selection is imperative to avoid recurrent complications or recurrent weight loss failure.[64] Substantial additional weight loss should not be expected with AGB replacement.[63]

Some clinicians recommend replacing the band by forming a de novo retrogastroesophageal tunnel either above or below the previously placed tract.[69] This approach avoids adhesions and, if there was an element of prolapse or slippage, this approach can serve to better secure the newly placed band and avoid this complication in the future. Although there are exceptions depending on the indication for replacement, it is generally preferable that normal anatomy be restored before replacing the band to ensure that pouch volume, precise positioning, and band fixation are optimized.

AGB conversion to SG Conversion to SG, another restrictive procedure, is a reasonable choice if the patient has had a reasonable weight loss with the AGB and requires revision for other considerations. Other factors that can affect this decision include persistent technical failures, patient compliance issues with adjustments, and anatomic changes that preclude AGB replacement.

It is imperative that normal anatomy be restored before SG. Once this has been accomplished, the stomach is laid out in its normal position. In performing an SG, larger linear staple height loads (eg, 4.5 mm or 4.8 mm) should be considered for the sleeve resection because of increased thickness of the normally thinner tissue of the gastric fundus.

A few small retrospective studies have examined short-term outcomes after AGB conversion to SG. The largest series examined the short-term outcome of 41 patients. The complication rate was 19.5% and included a gastric leak rate of 5.7%. There was 1 death. EWL was 41.6% at 2years. Two patients required conversion to BPD-DS for poor weight loss.[70] Another study retrospectively examined 36 patients, all revised to SG for insufficient weight loss. The complication rate for this series was 12.2% and included 1 leak. At a mean follow-up of 13.4 months, EWL was 42.7%. Six patients required eventual conversion to BPD-DS, BPD, or RYGB.[71]

AGB conversion to RYGB AGB conversion to RYGB is appropriate for patients with inadequate weight loss, GERD, esophageal dysmotility, and possibly psychological band intolerance (although these patients must be approached with caution).[63] As with other AGB revisions, normal gastric anatomy should be restored before constructing the gastric pouch to ensure that the gastric pouch size is optimized. It is usually prudent to modify the lesser curve and retrocardia dissection to avoid AGB-related fibrotic tissues. Cautious dissection at the angle of His is necessary because adhesions in this area cannot be avoided.

In an analysis of several studies that examined revision of AGB to RYGB, either open or laparoscopically, it was concluded that the operative times are longer than for primary RYGB and even longer with the laparoscopic approach. It was also noted that adhesions and fibrosis led to increased complications including anastomotic leaks. EWL was higher and, in some cases, approached that of a primary RYGB.[62]

One recent study[72] retrospectively analyzed 66 patients who had AGB placed as a primary bariatric procedure. Of these, 47 (71.2%) underwent revision of the AGB and 19 (28.8%) underwent conversion to RYGB. Demographics were similar between the 2 groups. However, patients in the revision group had adequate weight loss with the AGB, whereas those in the conversion group did not. Patients converted to RYGB had an average EWL of 48%, whereas those undergoing AGB revision maintained their weight.

Another early study[66] retrospectively analyzed 70 patients with a median BMI of 45 ($\pm$ 11) kg/m^2 who underwent attempted conversion of AGB to RYGB. Indications for conversion were inadequate weight loss or weight regain after band deflation for gastric pouch dilatation, inadequate weight loss, symptomatic proximal gastric pouch dilatation, intragastric band migration, and psychological band intolerance. Mean operative time was 240 ($\pm$ 40) minutes (range, 210–280 minutes). Mean hospital length of stay was 7.2 days. The early complication rate was 14.3%. Late major complication rate was 8.6%. There was no mortality. Median EWL was 70% ($\pm$ 20%), and 60% of patients achieved a BMI of less than 33 kg/m^2 with mean follow-up of 18 months.

AGB conversion to BPD-DS Another choice of revisional procedure when AGB fails to provide adequate weight loss or is associated with complications is conversion to BPD-DS. In theory, this procedure should result in superior weight loss compared with conversion to either another restrictive procedure or to RYGB. As with most revisions after AGB, and as previously discussed, normal gastric anatomy is restored before SG. The lower gastric and inframesocolic portions of the BPD-DS proceed in the usual manner as in a primary BPD-DS.

There are few studies in the literature reporting on conversion of AGB to BPD-DS. The largest study is a retrospective review of 53 patients who failed to lose adequate weight after AGB. Thirty-two patients underwent laparoscopic conversion to RYGB for a BMI of 43.1 kg/m^2 and 21 underwent conversion to BPD-DS for a BMI of 46.0 kg/m^2. Operative times were an average of 105 minutes longer for BPD-DS and had significantly more associated complications (62%) compared with the RYGB group (12.5%). There were no deaths. At 12 and 18 months after revision, the 2 groups had similar BMIs and the EWL was greater after BPD-DS than after RYGB compared with prerevision weight (66.2% vs 58.8%) and initial weight (73% vs 61.8%), although this difference was not statistically significant.[73]

REVISION AFTER MALABSORPTIVE PROCEDURES
Revision after Biliopancreatic Diversion with Duodenal Switch

Indications

As with all bariatric procedures, the 2 main indications for revision of a malabsorptive operation such as the long-limb gastric bypass or BPD-DS are complications or weight regain/failure to lose adequate weight. The complication requiring revision that is most often associated with malabsorptive procedures is micronutrient and macronutrient deficiency with malnutrition. Weight regain or failure to lose adequate weight is less common with the BPD-DS. Overall, the incidence of BPD-DS revision is reported to be about 5%.[1,2] However, it is unclear whether this lower incidence is secondary to a lack of indication or surgeon reluctance because of the technical demands of the procedure.

Management options and operative strategy

Revision of the sleeve In patients having BPD-DS with weight regain or inadequate weight loss, an enlarged stomach, particularly the fundus, is often present because of inadequate resection or stretching. A preoperative contrast upper GI study is mandatory and helps determine the degree of excess gastric tissue present. Thus, the first approach to BPD-DS revision should be re-SG.[2] Dissection of the stomach from its adhesive attachments is performed with care not to compromise the lesser curvature blood supply. A 60-Fr bougie is passed transorally along the lesser curvature of the stomach. Using 4.8-mm staple loads, the bougie is followed proximally with transition to 3.5-mm staple loads if the more proximal gastric tissue becomes thinner. Staple line reinforcement by oversewing is recommended with care taken to avoid stricture by incorporating excessive gastric tissue.

Modifications of common channel length Occasionally performed to convert a proximal RYGB to a distal RYGB, shortening of the common channel is less commonly indicated after BPD-DS because the degree of malabsorption, by definition, is already maximized or nearly maximized. Further shortening of the common channel to less than 75 cm can lead to severe vitamin, mineral, and protein deficiencies.[36] However, approximately 5% of patients with BPD-DS require lengthening of the common channel to reverse the complications of excessive malabsorption, including severe malnutrition.[2]

Elongation of the common channel can be performed at the expense of the biliopancreatic limb length by disconnecting the alimentary limb at the ileoileostomy, followed by construction of a side-to-side functional end-to-side ileojejunostomy proximally to increase the common channel length to 250 cm.[1] Alternatively, a simple side-to-side anastomosis is constructed between the biliopancreatic limb and the alimentary limb 100 cm proximal to the ileoileostomy without division of the alimentary limb.[2]

Outcomes

There are few outcomes data addressing revision of BPD-DS. In the single study that has reported on outcomes, revision was performed a median of 17 months after BPD-DS. Indications for revision included protein malnutrition in 20 patients, diarrhea in 9 patients, metabolic abnormalities in 5 patients, and liver disease in 2 patients. At revision, the median BMI was 28 kg/m^2. Median serum albumin increased significantly from 3.6 g/dL preoperatively to 4.0 g/dL. The complication rate was 15%. There was no perioperative mortality. The median weight gain was 8.2 kg during a median follow-up of 39 months.[1]

SUMMARY

The need for revisional bariatric operations is certain to increase as the number of primary bariatric procedures increases. To formulate a successful revision strategy, it is essential to perform a thorough preoperative work-up that includes imaging, behavioral and dietary assessment, and review of the primary operative report. Outcomes vary according to the primary operation and chosen approach to revision. Initially, revisions of primary bariatric operations had a high morbidity; however, more recent studies have shown acceptably low complication rates and good weight loss with the associated health benefits. Although there is no direct evidence in the form of randomized studies indicating which patients with inadequate weight loss or weight regain will benefit most from revision or supporting one particular revision approach rather than another, based on the available studies it is possible to develop general, effective strategies.

REFERENCES

1. Hamoui N, Chock B, Anthone GJ, et al. Revision of the duodenal switch: indications, technique, and outcomes. J Am Coll Surg 2007;204(4):603–8.
2. Gagner M. Laparoscopic revisional surgery after malabsorptive procedures in bariatric surgery, more specifically after duodenal switch. Surg Laparosc Endosc Percutan Tech 2010;20(5):344–7.
3. Zingg U, McQuinn A, DiValentino D, et al. Revisional vs. primary Roux-en-Y gastric bypass–a case-matched analysis: less weight loss in revisions. Obes Surg 2010;20(12):1627–32.
4. Radtka JF 3rd, Puleo FJ, Wang L, et al. Revisional bariatric surgery: who, what, where, and when? Surg Obes Relat Dis 2010;6(6):635–42.
5. Baltasar A, Bou R, Arlandis F, et al. Vertical banded gastroplasty at more than 5 years. Obes Surg 1998;8:29–34.
6. Miller K, Pump A, Hell E. Vertical banded gastroplasty versus adjustable gastric banding: prospective long-term follow-up study. Surg Obes Relat Dis 2006;2: 570–2.
7. Van Gemert WG, van Wersch MM, Greve JW, et al. Revisional surgery after failed vertical banded gastroplasty: restoration of vertical banded gastroplasty or conversion to gastric bypass. Obes Surg 1998;8:21–8.
8. DeMaria EJ, Sugerman HJ, Meador JG, et al. High failure rate after laparoscopic adjustable silicone gastric banding for treatment of morbid obesity. Ann Surg 2001;233(6):809–18.
9. van Wageningen B, Berends FJ, Van Ramshorst B, et al. Revision of failed laparoscopic adjustable gastric banding to Roux-en-Y gastric bypass. Obes Surg 2006;16(2):137–41.
10. Moore R, Perugini R, Czerniach D, et al. Early results of conversion of laparoscopic adjustable gastric band to Roux-en-Y gastric bypass. Surg Obes Relat Dis 2009;5(4):439–43.
11. Tucker O, Sucandy I, Szomstein S, et al. Revisional surgery after failed laparoscopic adjustable gastric banding. Surg Obes Relat Dis 2008;4(6):740–7.

12. Drew RL, Linner JH. Revisional surgery for severe obesity with fascia banded stoma Roux-en-Y gastric bypass. Obes Surg 1992;2:349–54.

13. Schwartz RW, Strodel WE, Simpson WS, et al. Gastric bypass revision: lessons learned from 920 cases. Surgery 1988;104:806–12.

14. Hallowell PT, Stellato TA, Yao DA, et al. Should bariatric revisional surgery be avoided secondary to increased morbidity and mortality? Am J Surg 2009; 197(3):391–6.

15. Clapp B, Yu S, Sands T, et al. Preoperative upper endoscopy is useful before revisional bariatric surgery. JSLS 2007;11(1):94–6.

16. Burton PR, Brown WA, Laurie C, et al. Predicting outcomes of intermediate term complications and revisional surgery following laparoscopic adjustable gastric banding: utility of the CORE classification and Melbourne motility criteria. Obes Surg 2010;20(11):1516–23.

17. Shin RB. Intraoperative endoscopic test resulting in no postoperative leaks from the gastric pouch and gastrojejunal anastomosis in 366 laparoscopic Roux-en-Y gastric bypasses. Obes Surg 2004;14(8):1067–9.

18. Kligman MD. Intraoperative endoscopic pneumatic testing for gastrojejunal anastomotic integrity during laparoscopic Roux-en-Y gastric bypass. Surg Endosc 2007;21(8):1403–5.

19. Alaedeen D, Madan AK, Ro CY, et al. Intraoperative endoscopy and leaks after laparoscopic Roux-en-Y gastric bypass. Am Surg 2009;75(6):485–8 [discussion: 488].

20. Cohen R, Pinheiro JS, Corres JL, et al. Laparoscopic revisional bariatric surgery: myths and facts. Surg Endosc 2005;19:822–5.

21. Gagner M, Gentileschi P, de Csepel J, et al. Laparoscopic reoperative bariatric surgery: experience from 27 consecutive patients. Obes Surg 2002;12(2): 254–60.

22. Luján JA, Frutos MD, Hernández Q, et al. Laparoscopic versus open gastric bypass in the treatment of morbid obesity: a randomized prospective study. Ann Surg 2004;239(4):433–7.

23. Paxton JH, Matthews JB. The cost effectiveness of laparoscopic versus open gastric bypass surgery. Obes Surg 2005;15(1):24–34.

24. Ikramuddin S, Kendrick ML, Kellogg TA, et al. Open and laparoscopic Roux-en-Y gastric bypass: our techniques. J Gastrointest Surg 2007;11(2):217–28.

25. Swartz DE, Mobley E, Felix EL. Bile reflux after Roux-en-Y gastric bypass: an unrecognized cause of postoperative pain. Surg Obes Relat Dis 2009;5(1): 27–30.

26. Sugerman HJ, Starkey J, Birkenhauer R. A randomized prospective trial of gastric bypass versus vertical banded gastroplasty for morbid obesity and their effects on sweets versus non-sweets eaters. Ann Surg 1987;205:613–24.

27. Hall J, Watts JM, O'Brien PE, et al. Gastric surgery for morbid obesity. The Adelaide Study. Ann Surg 1990;211:419–27.

28. Lechner GW, Callender K. Subtotal gastric exclusion and gastric partitioning: a randomized prospective comparison of one hundred patients. Surgery 1981; 90:637–44.

29. Bessler M, Daud A, DiGiorgi MF, et al. Adjustable gastric banding as revisional bariatric procedure after failed gastric bypass–intermediate results. Surg Obes Relat Dis 2010;6(1):31–5.

30. Buchwalter JA, Herbert CA Jr, Khouri RK. Morbid obesity: second gastric operation for poor weight loss. Am Surg 1985;51:208–11.

31. MacLean LD, Rhode BM, Nohr CW. Late outcome of isolated gastric bypass. Ann Surg 2000;231(4):524–8.

32. Capella JF, Capella RF. An assessment of vertical banded gastroplasty–Roux-en-Y gastric bypass for the treatment of morbid obesity. Am J Surg 2002;183: 117–23.
33. Fobi MA, Lee H, Felahy B, et al. Choosing an operation for weight control and the transected banded gastric bypass. Obes Surg 2005;15:114–21.
34. Parikh M, Heacock L, Gagner M. Laparoscopic "gastrojejunal sleeve reduction" as a revision procedure for weight loss failure after Roux-en-Y gastric bypass. Obes Surg 2011;21(5):650–4.
35. Gobble RM, Parikh MS, Greives MR, et al. Gastric banding as a salvage procedure for patients with weight loss failure after Roux-en-Y gastric bypass. Surg Endosc 2008;22(4):1019–22.
36. Brolin RE, LaMarca LB, Kenler HA, et al. Malabsorptive gastric bypass in patients with superobesity. J Gastrointest Surg 2002;6:195–205.
37. Sugerman JH, Kellum JM, DeMaria EJ. Conversion of proximal to distal gastric bypass for failed gastric for super obesity. J Gastrointest Surg 1997;1:517–25.
38. Fobi MA, Lee H, Igwe D, et al. Revision of failed gastric bypass to distal Roux-en-Y gastric bypass: a review of 65 cases. Obes Surg 2001;11:190–5.
39. Brolin RE, Cody RP. Adding malabsorption for weight loss failure after gastric bypass. Surg Endosc 2007;21(11):1924–6.
40. Kellogg TA, Bantle JP, Leslie DL, et al. Post-gastric bypass hyperinsulinemic hypoglycemia: characterization and response to a modified diet. Surg Obes Relat Dis 2008;4(4):492–9.
41. Greenbaum DF, Wasser SH, Riley T, et al. Duodenal switch with omentopexy and feeding jejunostomy–a safe and effective revisional operation for failed previous weight loss surgery. Surg Obes Relat Dis 2011;7(2):213–8.
42. Keshishian A, Zahriya K, Hartoonian T, et al. Duodenal switch is a safe operation for patients who have failed other bariatric operations. Obes Surg 2004;14(9): 1187–92.
43. Parikh M, Pomp A, Gagner M. Laparoscopic conversion of failed gastric bypass to duodenal switch: technical considerations and preliminary outcomes. Surg Obes Relat Dis 2007;3(6):611–8.
44. Schouten R, Wiryasaputra DC, van Dielen FM, et al. Long-term results of bariatric restrictive procedures: a prospective study. Obes Surg 2010;20(12):1617–26.
45. Evans JA, Williams NN, Chan EP, et al. Endoscopic removal of eroded bands in vertical banded gastroplasty: a novel use of endoscopic scissors. Gastrointest Endosc 2006;64:801–4.
46. Balsiger BM, Murr MM, Sarr MG. Gastroesophageal reflux after intact vertical banded gastroplasty: correction by conversion to Roux-en-Y gastric bypass. J Gastrointest Surg 2000;4:276–81.
47. Bloomberg RD, Urbach DR. Laparoscopic Roux-en-Y gastric bypass for severe gastroesophageal reflux after vertical banded gastroplasty. Obes Surg 2002; 12:408–11.
48. Moreno P, Alastrue A, Rull M, et al. Band erosion in patients who have undergone vertical banded gastroplasty: incidence and technical solutions. Arch Surg 1998; 133:189–93.
49. Eckhauser FE, Knol JA, Strodel WE. Remedial surgery following failed gastroplasty for morbid obesity. Ann Surg 1998;198:585–91.
50. de Csepel J, Nahouraii R, Gagner M. Laparoscopic gastric bypass as a reoperative bariatric procedure for failed open restrictive procedures. Surg Endosc 2001; 15:393–7.

51. Sweeney JF, Goode SE, Rosemburgy AS. Redo gastric restriction: a higher risk procedure. Obes Surg 1994;4:244–7.
52. Capella RF, Capella JF. Converting vertical banded gastroplasty to a lesser curvature gastric bypass: technical considerations. Obes Surg 1998;8: 218–24.
53. Vaneerdeweg W, Hubens G, Van Gaal L, et al. Operations for failed vertical banded gastroplasty. Acta Chir Belg 1994;94:203–6.
54. Sugerman HJ, Wolper JL. Failed gastroplasty for morbid obesity: revised gastroplasty versus Roux-en-Y gastric bypass. Am J Surg 1984;148:331–6.
55. Hunter R, Watts JM, Dunstan R, et al. Revisional surgery for failed gastric restrictive procedures for morbid obesity. Obes Surg 1992;2:245–52.
56. Jones KB. Revisional bariatric surgery: safe and effective. Obes Surg 2001;11: 183–9.
57. Sugerman HJ, Kellum JM, DeMaria EJ, et al. Conversion of failed or complicated vertical banded gastroplasty to gastric bypass in morbid obesity. Am J Surg 1996;171:163–9.
58. Thoreson R, Cullen J. Indications and results of reversal of vertical banded gastroplasty. J Gastrointest Surg 2008;12:2032–6.
59. Schouten R, van Dielen FM, van Gemert WG, et al. Conversion of vertical banded gastroplasty to Roux-en-Y gastric bypass results in restoration of the positive effect on weight loss and co-morbidities: evaluation of 101 patients. Obes Surg 2007;17(5):622–30.
60. Gagné DJ, Dovec E, Urbandt JE. Laparoscopic revision of vertical banded gastroplasty to Roux-en-Y gastric bypass: outcomes of 105 patients. Surg Obes Relat Dis 2011;7(4):493–9.
61. Martikainen T, Pirinen E, Alhava E, et al. Long-term results, late complications and quality of life in a series of adjustable gastric banding. Obes Surg 2004; 4:648–54.
62. Gagner M, Gumbs AA. Gastric banding: conversion to sleeve, bypass, or DS. Surg Endosc 2007;21:1931–5.
63. Weber M, Muller MK, Michel JM, et al. Laparoscopic Roux-en-Y gastric bypass, but not rebanding, should be proposed as rescue procedure for patients with failed laparoscopic gastric banding. Ann Surg 2003;238:827–33.
64. Suter M. Laparoscopic band repositioning for pouch dilatation/slippage after gastric banding: disappointing results. Obes Surg 2001;11:507–12.
65. Westling A, Ohrvall M, Gustavsson S. Roux-en-Y gastric bypass after previous unsuccessful gastric restrictive surgery. J Gastrointest Surg 2002;6(2): 206–11.
66. Mognol P, Chosidow D, Marmuse JP. Laparoscopic conversion of laparoscopic gastric banding to Roux-en-Y gastric bypass: a review of 70 patients. Obes Surg 2004;14(10):1349–53.
67. Calmes JM, Giusti V, Suter M. Re-operative laparoscopic Roux-en-Y gastric bypass: an experience with 49 cases. Obes Surg 2005;15(3):316–22.
68. Neto MP, Ramos AC, Campos JM, et al. Endoscopic removal of eroded adjustable gastric band: lessons learned after 5 years and 78 cases. Surg Obes Relat Dis 2010;6(4):423–7.
69. Zundel N, Hernandez JD. Revisional surgery after restrictive procedures for morbid obesity. Surg Laparosc Endosc Percutan Tech 2010;20(5):338–43.
70. Foletto M, Prevedello L, Bernante P, et al. Sleeve gastrectomy as revisional procedure for failed gastric banding or gastroplasty. Surg Obes Relat Dis 2010;6(2): 146–51.

71. Iannelli A, Schneck AS, Ragot E, et al. Laparoscopic sleeve gastrectomy as revisional procedure for failed gastric banding and vertical banded gastroplasty. Obes Surg 2009;19(9):1216–20.
72. Ardestani A, Lautz DB, Tavakkolizadeh A. Band revision versus Roux-en-Y gastric bypass conversion as salvage operation after laparoscopic adjustable gastric banding. Surg Obes Relat Dis 2011;7(1):33–7.
73. Topart P, Becouarn G, Ritz P. Biliopancreatic diversion with duodenal switch or gastric bypass for failed gastric banding: retrospective study from two institutions with preliminary results. Surg Obes Relat Dis 2007;3:521–5.

Future Directions in Bariatric Surgery

Sean M. Lee, MD[a], Aurora D. Pryor, MD[b],*

KEYWORDS

- Bariatric surgery • Obesity • Metabolic surgery
- Endoscopic suturing • Endoscopy

Bariatric surgery is a field in rapid evolution, and the speed of this evolution has been accelerating over the last several decades. Predicting the future is always fraught with difficulties, but a thorough understanding of past developments is crucial to anticipating the future intelligently. The trends that have driven evolution historically often persist, and continue to be influential in the future. With this in mind, this article outlines the historical and current trends in bariatric surgery, and follows the trajectory of these trends into the future to anticipate the technologies and techniques that will be most important to the field in the coming years.

THE EVOLUTION OF BARIATRIC SURGERY

Over the last two decades, bariatric surgery has seen a steep increase in popularity in the United States. Between 1990 and 2000 the prevalence of bariatric procedures increased nearly sixfold from 2.4 to 14.1 per 100,000,[1] and these numbers continue to increase.[2,3] A conservative estimation for the total number of bariatric procedures performed in the United States each year is 200,000 to 300,000. Several factors have played a role in this increase, including a worsening epidemic of obesity and its accompanying comorbidities; improvements in the efficacy, tolerability, and safety of bariatric procedures; and an improved understanding of the financial benefits of these procedures.

The first procedure designed to affect weight loss was jejunoileal bypass (**Fig. 1**A) a procedure aimed at inducing malabsorption. Originally described in the United States by Varco in 1953[4] and subsequently modified,[5–8] this procedure relied on pure malabsorption and was plagued by problems with either too much or too little

S. Lee has nothing to disclose. A. Pryor has an ownership interest in TransEnterix and Barosense. She is a speaker or consultant for Covidien, Gore, and Olympus. Covidien provides research and fellowship support.

a Department of Surgery, Duke University Medical Center, Box 3443, Durham, NC 27710, USA
b Division of General Surgery, Department of Surgery, Stony Brook University Medical Center, HSC 18-043, Stony Brook, NY 11794-8191, USA
* Corresponding author.
E-mail address: aurora.pryor@sbumed.org

Surg Clin N Am 91 (2011) 1373–1395
doi:10.1016/j.suc.2011.08.016
0039-6109/11/$ – see front matter © 2011 Elsevier Inc. All rights reserved.

surgical.theclinics.com

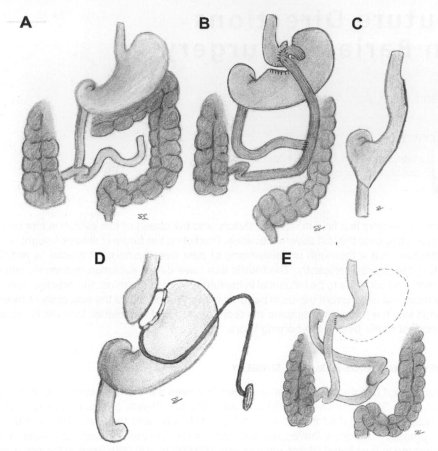

Fig. 1. Traditional bariatric procedures. (*A*) Jejunoileal bypass. (*B*) Roux-en-Y gastric bypass. (*C*) Sleeve gastrectomy. (*D*) Adjustable gastric band. (*E*) Duodenal switch.

weight loss; vitamin deficiencies; protein malnutrition; kidney stones; and bacterial overgrowth with toxin production in the bypassed segment that could cause skin problems, severe arthritis, and even liver failure. In 1966, Mason and Ito[9] introduced the gastric bypass, and their original operation evolved to include a 15- to 30-mL gastric pouch[10] and a Roux-en-Y configuration of the gastrojejunal reconstruction.[11] The resulting roux-en-Y gastric bypass (RYGB; **Fig. 1**B) is both restrictive and malabsorptive, and has become the most commonly performed bariatric procedure in the United States, with approximately 177,00 operations performed in 2006.[12] The biliopancreatic diversion (BPD) was first described in 1979 by Scopinaro and coworkers,[13] and attempted to produce malabsorption and gastric restriction while maintaining flow in all segments of the bowel and thus avoiding the more severe side effects of jejunoileal bypass. This procedure involved partial gastrectomy with closure of the duodenal stump, creation of a Roux limb 250 cm from the ileocecal valve, and anastomosis of the biliopancreatic limb to the Roux limb 50 cm from the ileocecal valve. Although early permutations were plagued by complications related to malabsorption, the procedure evolved over time to minimize these complications while remaining highly effective even after long-term follow-up.[14] In 1986, Hess and Hess[15] added a sleeve gastrectomy and modified the anastomosis to a duodenojejunal configuration, thus preserving the pylorus. The resulting procedure, the duodenal switch (DS, **Fig. 1E**), is a better restrictive procedure and minimizes dumping and stomal ulceration. It is currently the most efficacious procedure available for weight loss and for comorbidity improvement.

Multiple restrictive procedures have also evolved, starting in the early 1970s with the common tenet of reducing gastric volume. The conceptually simple gastroplasties have seen much evolution, from horizontal gastroplasty[16] through vertical banded gastroplasty.[17–20] Vertical banded gastroplasty became the standard procedure for weight loss surgery in the 1980s. Further evolution led to adjustable gastric banding and sleeve gastrectomy (see **Fig. 1C, D**), the current mainstays of restrictive weight loss procedures.[21–23]

The development and refinement of these procedures came just in time for the United States obesity epidemic. Between 1980 and 2007, the prevalence of obesity in the United States increased from 15% to 34% among adults and from 5% to 17% among children and adolescents.[24–26] In 1985 no state reported an obesity rate more than 15%, whereas in 2009 only Colorado and the District of Columbia reported rates less than 20% and in nine states more than 30% of adults are obese.[27] Similarly, in 2002 18.2 million people had diabetes in the United States, approximately 6.3% of the population. That number increased to 25.8 million, or 8.3% of the population by 2010 and the Centers for Disease Control and Prevention estimates that as many as 33% of the United States population will have diabetes by 2050.[28] The increased number of patients enticed more surgeons into the field, and competition to provide the best care for these patients drove the field into several rapid adaptations. After the first laparoscopic general surgical procedures in the late 1980s, laparoscopy was quickly adopted in bariatric procedures. The year 1993 saw the first laparoscopic vertical banded gastroplasty, laparoscopic RYGB (LRYGB), and the first laparoscopic gastric band and laparoscopic adjustable gastric band (LAGB) placement.[29–32] By 2003, 65% of all bariatric surgery was performed laparoscopically,[33] and the reduced risk of wound infection, earlier ambulation, decreased rate of respiratory complications, and decreased length of stay seen with laparoscopic bariatric procedures have helped to form the current state of bariatric surgery where average hospital stays are 1 to 3 days and mortality rates are less than 1%. New types of open or laparoscopic procedures continue to be developed aiming at better efficacy and safety,[34–38] and most recently endoscopy has been eyed as an even less invasive means of affecting weight loss and metabolic normalization through a variety of innovative techniques.[39,40]

Also important in the rise of bariatric surgery has been the financial impact of these procedures on patients, providers, and insurers. Coverage for bariatric surgery has often been challenging for patients to come by, and thus many have paid out-of-pocket. Before 2004, coverage required demonstration of significant comorbidities. In July 2004, Medicare officially recognized obesity as a disease in its own right, and coverage for bariatric procedures became somewhat easier to obtain. In 2006, Medicare officially recognized specific bariatric procedures and required patients to be treated at American Society for Metabolic and Bariatric Surgery or American College of Surgeons approved centers of excellence. Recent years have also seen more and more private insurers initiating coverage for bariatric surgery. Several international studies have demonstrated cost-savings or at least cost effectiveness of bariatric surgery,[41,42] and recent studies within the United States have shown bariatric surgery to be cost effective,[43] and in certain populations, the costs of surgery can be recouped within 25 months by healthcare savings resulting from weight loss and resolution of comorbidities.[44] Still, with up-front costs between $10,000 and $40,000, bariatric surgery has remained financially untenable for those insurers with shorter-term financial goals or more rapid customer turnover. However, as the field continues to develop, costs may decrease. Studies comparing LRYGB with open bypass reveal similar complication rates, but significantly shorter hospital stay after laparoscopic procedures.[45] As surgeons have become more facile with bariatric surgical techniques and perioperative care, hospital lengths of stay have decreased significantly in the last few years.[46] Such cost minimization is a factor in the currently increasing popularity of bariatric surgery, and as future procedures are developed and refined, cost will likely continue to be an important factor driving that development.

The evolution of bariatric surgery has clearly been driven by many different influences. Among these are an improved understanding of the biology of the gastrointestinal system, improved surgical technique, new surgical technologies, and financial factors. It is important to keep the history of the field and the factors that have influenced it in mind when considering which of the mechanisms aimed at surgically inducing weight loss and metabolic normalization will become predominant.

CURRENT SURGICAL PROCEDURES IN EVOLUTION
Ileal Interposition and Digestive Adaptation

First described by Mason in 1999,[47] ileal interposition aims to affect gut neurohormonal activity toward inducing weight loss by relocating a portion of the ileum to the proximal jejunum. A 170-200 cm long portion of ileum is excised leaving 30 cm of distal ileum behind, and relocated 50-cm distal to the ligament of Treitz by two jejunoileal anastomoses. Bowel continuity is restored with a third jejunoileal anastomosis to close the defect. In digestive adaptation, first described by Santoro and coworkers in 2006,[34] rather than relocating the ileum within an intact jejunum, the ileum moves proximally by resection of most of the jejunum. The bowel is divided 50 to 100 cm from the ligament of Treitz, and again 250 cm from the ileocecal valve. The intervening small intestine is removed, and the free ends are anastomosed together. It is believed that by moving a segment of ileum closer to the stomach it is exposed to more nutrients sooner after a meal. This results in a more rapid and pronounced hormonal feedback inhibition of the foregut, producing a rapid, yet enduring, satiety. This idea has been coined the "ileal brake." To augment this effect, both procedures are most often accompanied by a sleeve gastrectomy to provide a restrictive component to the operation.

Both procedures were conscientiously designed based on a modern understanding of the mechanical and neurohormonal functions of the gastrointestinal tract. Sleeve gastrectomy is designed to limit the amount of calories that can be taken in at any meal. This is both a mechanical effect and a hormonal one, because removal of most of the gastric fundus removes the primary cellular producers of ghrelin, a hormone known to increase hunger. After digestive adaptation, serum ghrelin levels are seen to decline.[34] The malabsorptive effect of these procedures is mild, because nearly all the ileum is retained, and the overall length of bowel allows for sufficient nutrient absorption. Described hormonal effects include postprandial increases in the serum levels of glucagon-like peptide 1 and polypeptide YY. Both of these hormones cause satiety, and are found to be abnormally low in most obese individuals. Some theorize that in the modern diet, nutrients are highly available and easily digested, and the distal bowel is exposed to relatively nutrient-poor material.[34] Thus, the distal bowel's response to luminal contents is minimized. After ileal interposition and digestive adaptation, the proximally located ileum is exposed to a nutrient-rich environment, and glucagon-like peptide 1 and polypeptide YY levels have been seen to increase significantly after digestive adaptation.[34] The ileal brake is thus more pronounced after these procedures.

Clinical evidence is also encouraging. Santoro and colleagues[35] reported an excess body weight (EBW) loss of 80% after 12 months in one study, and in another saw a mean body mass index (BMI) reduction of 20.1 kg/m^2, with resolution of hypertension in 87.5%, type II diabetes mellitus (DM) in 92.3%, and dyslipidemia in 75.8% of patients.[34] Similar results have been published for ileal interposition. Depaula and coworkers[48] reported an average EBW loss of 84.5%. Resolution of hypertension occurred in 88.4%, type II DM in 84.2%, and dyslipidemia in 82.3% with a mean follow-up of 38 months. When applied to a lower-weight population (mean BMI of 33.8 kg/m^2), another study found an even more pronounced metabolic effect with 100% resolution of hypertension and type II DM.[49] These procedures are gaining popularity as purely metabolic procedures in this low-BMI group.

Gastric Plication

Within the last few years, the increasing popularity of sleeve gastrectomy has led some surgeons to develop techniques aimed at narrowing the gastric lumen without gastrectomy. These procedures are termed "gastric plication" (**Fig. 2**). Multiple forms of plication have been published, and plication has been used alone or in combination with other bariatric procedures. It was initially described in 2007 by Talebpour and Amoli.[50] They detail a procedure that involves folding the greater curvature medially where it is then sutured near the lesser curvature in two layers. This partially closes the stomach from greater to lesser curvature creating a large intraluminal fold. Initial outcomes were promising. In a patient population with an average preoperative BMI of 47 kg/m^2, a durable EBW loss of 61% was seen after 12 months in 56 patients, 60% at 24 months in 50 patients, and 57% at 36 months in 11 patients.[50] Similar results were found in a study by Brethauer and colleagues[51] who reported an average EBW loss of 53.4% in a six-patient series with a mean starting BMI of 43.3 kg/m^2 and 12-month follow-up. In the same study, a different technique termed "anterior plication" showed a more modest weight reduction (23.3% EBW loss). Ramos and coworkers[52] published a series of greater curvature plication in 15 patients with a mean BMI of 41 kg/m^2, and after 12 months, EBW loss was 60%. In the nine patients followed for 18 months, EBW loss remained stable at 62%. In all studies, complication rates were low, and complications included gastric obstruction, vomiting, gastric leak, gastric perforation, and esophagitis. Few long-term complications have been seen, but follow-up remains limited given the relative novelty of this procedure.

Together, the data show that gastric plication is a safe and effective form of weight loss surgery, but the true durability of this procedure remains to be seen. A combined approach of gastric banding with plication with the theory that the plication helps to prevent band slippage is also being evaluated,[53] because the band may protect the gastric plication from high pressures, potentially reducing failures over time. One additional consideration with plication is eventual revision, because although theoretically reversal should be possible by releasing plication sutures, this has not been studied to date. Although gastric plication has yet to be proved in large long-term studies, it remains promising, and may well become more prevalent in the next several years.

INDICATIONS FOR BARIATRIC SURGERY

As bariatric procedures continue to evolve and improve in safety, cost, and effectiveness, the population of patients to which bariatric procedures is applied also is changing. The 1991 National Institutes of Health consensus conference on

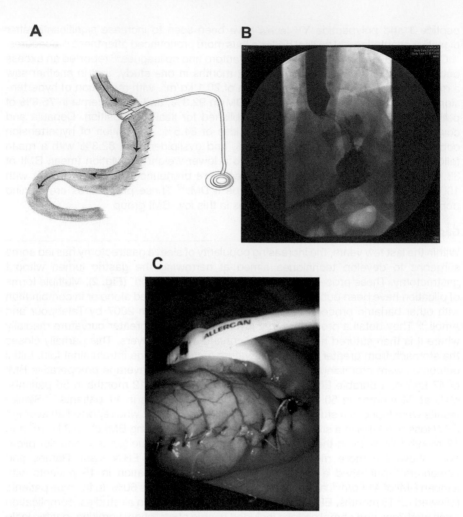

Fig. 2. Gastric plication. (*A*) Diagramatic representation of gastric plication with adjustable gastric band. (*B*) Upper gastrointestinal contrast study after combined placation and banding. (*C*) Intraoperative photo of this technique. (*Courtesy of* Dr Dana Portenier, Department of Surgery, Duke University Medical Center, Durham, NC.)

gastrointestinal surgery for severe obesity was the first clear statement of the indications for bariatric surgery.[54] In this statement, patients with a BMI greater than 40 kg/m^2 were candidates for surgical treatment, as were those with a BMI between 35 and 40 kg/m^2 with significant comorbidities interfering with their lifestyle. All patients must have also first attempted nonsurgical weight loss. This statement became the most generally accepted guide for determining the appropriateness of surgery, and has been used by several insurers to define which patients qualify for coverage.

Recently, these guidelines have been tested on several fronts given newer data suggesting a benefit of bariatric surgery to a wider range of patients. A recent study by DeMaria and colleagues[55] showed that LRYGB resulted in significant weight loss and resolution of type II DM in 76% of patients with BMI between 30 and 35 kg/m^2. Another group recently compared outcomes in patients with a BMI 30 to 40 kg/m^2 who underwent LAGB or a medical weight loss program.[56] The EBW loss for the

LAGB group was 62.5% versus 4.3% in the conventional therapy group, and the LAGB group saw significantly greater decreases in hemoglobin A_{1c} and plasma insulin and glucose levels than did the conventional group. Based on such data, an American Society for Metabolic and Bariatric Surgery consensus conference in 2004 broadened indications for bariatric surgery to include patients with BMI 30 to 34.9 kg/m^2 with a comorbid condition that can be "cured or markedly improved by substantial and sustained weight loss."[57] A recent statement of the German guidelines also included those patients with BMI 30 to 35 kg/m^2 with type II DM and eliminated previous age limitations.[58] As bariatric surgery continues to become safer, less invasive, and more effective, the indications for these procedures will continue to evolve.

NEW SURGICAL TECHNIQUES
Single-incision Laparoscopy

Single-incision laparoscopic surgery has evolved rapidly over the last 5 years. Initially envisioned as a way to minimize abdominal wall trauma during laparoscopic surgery, and to thereby reduce pain and improve cosmesis postoperatively, single-incision laparoscopy (SIL) faced numerous technical hurdles. These hurdles related to the juxtaposition of instruments at a single point in the abdominal wall. This caused significant problems with abdominal access, maintenance of pneumoperitoneum, triangulation of instruments at the operative site to permit appropriate retraction, and interference between instruments. Initial attempts at this technique used available laparoscopic tools, and were thus quite cumbersome. Still, early case series showed promise for these techniques. Single-port surgery was first reported in the urologic literature for single-access site nephrectomy in 2008.[59] Soon after, several other reports of single-access urologic procedures were published, most with encouraging outcomes.[60–63]

The first published series applying single-access techniques to bariatric surgery was that by Saber and colleagues[64] in late 2008. Their technique for single-incision sleeve gastrectomy used a 2.5-cm periumbilical incision with a 1-cm fascial incision through which a 15-mm port and two 5-mm ports were placed. They also used a subxiphoid incision for placement of a liver retractor. The procedure recapitulated that of standard laparoscopic sleeve gastrectomy, but necessitated the use of a 45-degree 5-mm laparoscope and frequent repositioning of the camera and instruments to avoid cross-interference of the instruments. In this series of seven patients with a mean preoperative BMI of 53.5 kg/m^2, all procedures were successfully completed using the single-access technique, mean operative time was 125 minutes, and there were no complications. At a mean follow-up time of 3.4 months, the mean BMI was 45.8 kg/m^2.

Since that time, several new developments have facilitated the widespread application of single-incision surgery. Various manufacturers have created single ports with multiple access lumen (eg, the SILS Port by Covidien and the TriPort by Advanced Surgical Concepts) and articulating instruments (eg, SILS hand instruments by Covidien) to facilitate triangulation during SIL procedures. Single-incision multichannel operative platforms have also been developed (**Fig. 3**).[65] Correspondingly, there has been a rapid increase in the number of published series using SIL in the last few years, and numerous publications describing innovative techniques to facilitate SIL operations.[66,67] A recent series of 140 patients undergoing either traditional five-port LRYGB or single-incision LRYGB, showed comparable complication rates and outcomes despite a longer operative time.[68] The mean EBW loss was 75.4% in the five-port group and 78.2% in the single-incision group at 12 months postoperative. The

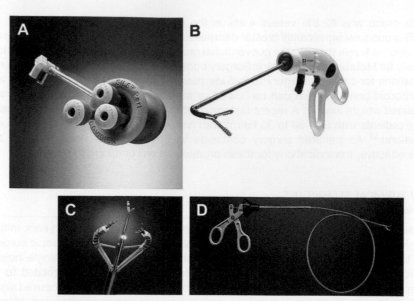

Fig. 3. Single-incision technologies. (*A*) SILS port. (*B*) SILS hand instrument. (*C*) SPIDER system head. (*D*) SPIDER system instrument. (*Courtesy of* Covidien, Inc, Mansfield, MA. Copyright © 2010 Covidien; used with permission. All rights reserved; and *Courtesy of* Trans-Enterix, Durham, NC; with permission.)

single-incision patients also reported a significantly better satisfaction with the appearance of the surgical scar. Another series used single-incision techniques to perform LRYGB and a modified version of gastric bypass termed "single loop gastric bypass."[69] In this small series BMI decreased in the two patients in the LRYGB group from 36.2 to 31.5 kg/m^2 after 2 months, and from 43.5 to 28 kg/m^2 in the single-loop gastric bypass group. Several authors have published successful results with SIL for gastric band placement, and there has been a report of SIL BPD.[70]

As SIL evolves, it is likely that improvements in technology and surgical technique will continue to simplify these procedures, making them accessible to a wider range of surgeons. Early data suggest that patients prefer the scars after SIL to conventional laparoscopy, and thus so long as the safety of these procedures continues to be equivalent to multiport laparoscopy, SIL is likely to continue to increase in popularity. Still, others have theorized[70] that SIL will eventually be replaced by "incisionless" surgery.

Natural Orifice Translumenal Endoscopic Surgery

Natural orifice surgery provides the patient with the allure of surgery without externally visible incisions. Although the theory behind such procedures originated in 1979 with the introduction of the first percutaneous endoscopic gastrostomy tube insertion,[71] the first detailed description of natural orifice surgery was presented by Kalloo and colleagues[72] in 2004 who described their experience performing transgastric peritoneoscopy in 50-kg pigs. Natural orifice translumenal endoscopic surgery (NOTES) has been applied to a variety of procedures, some of which are performed with traditional or SIL instrumentation, and some of which require the use of an endoscope. Some have applied the term to transumbilical incisions, but most minimally invasive surgeons consider NOTES to apply only to transoral, transvaginal, and trananal procedures. The term "natural orifice surgery" has been applied to transumbilical operations to limit confusion.

Currently, only a few centers in the world perform NOTES commonly, because there remain several major hurdles to its widespread application. These include development of an appropriate operative platform (eg, endoscopic instruments small and flexible enough to be safely inserted into the stomach, vagina, or colon, yet strong enough to allow surgical manipulation of tissues), and safe techniques for opening and closing the stomach, colon, and vagina. Additional concerns include the cost of these procedures and whether reimbursement will match these costs. Several advances have been made, because there are data supporting the reliability of various visceral closure devices[73,74] and techniques,[75,76] and the ability of transendoscopically delivered pressure transducers to monitor pneumoperitoneum.[77]

The application of NOTES to bariatric procedures has been limited, suffering mainly from the lack of a reliable operative platform. Hybrid procedures, however, have been published as case reports. Lacy and colleagues[78] reported performing a NOTES/minilaparoscopic sleeve gastrectomy on a 67-year-old woman with a BMI of 37 kg/m^2, hypertension, and diabetes. Transvaginal access was used for visualization with a flexible gastroscope, a 12-mm transumbilical port was used for dissecting instruments and endoscopic staplers, and two 2-mm needle ports were used for retraction. Operative time was 150 minutes, there were no complications, and the patient did well postoperatively leaving the hospital 3 days after surgery. Transvaginal sleeve gastrectomy has also been safely used by other groups. Hybrid[79] and pure[80] NOTES RYGB have been described in human cadaver models, and a porcine model for transgastric gastrojejunostomy has also been reported.[81] Endoscopic adjuncts also may provide a useful adjunct to NOTES. For example, in two separate porcine systems, endoscopically introduced magnets have been used to reliably form gastrojejunal anastomoses with or without the assistance of external magnets.[82,83] Progress in NOTES continues, and as new instruments and techniques are developed it will likely play an increasing role in the treatment of bariatric patients. This may come in the form of pure NOTES procedures, but more likely NOTES will provide a set of new tools that can be used as adjuncts to currently used procedures.

Robotics

Approved by the Food and Drug Administration in 2001, the da Vinci surgical robot (Intuitive Surgical) has become the standard robotic system for surgeons in a variety of specialties (**Fig. 4**). Although some general surgeons have adopted this robot for specific procedures, use of the robot by general surgeons has been less common than among urologic and gynecologic surgeons. The reasons for the cooler response to the da Vinci from general surgeons are multiple, but include cost, limitations of the system, and that some general surgical procedures lack the complexity and thus length to justify the added time required for positioning the robot.[84] Still, robotically assisted procedures may offer some advantages in bariatric surgery.

Robotic LAGB, sleeve gastrectomy, LGBP, and DS have all been reported.[85–96] Results on operative times have been mixed, with some series reporting increased operative times using the robot,[85] and some showing a decrease.[86] The prolongation of operative time may have reflected the learning curve of the operative team, because the authors report an average of 30 minutes for trocar and robotic arm placement. A survey of all bariatric surgeons using the da Vinci system in 2003 revealed an average set-up time of 17.7 minutes in the first 20 cases, but only 7.7 minutes in their last 20 cases.[87] Complication rates and weight loss were similar for robotic-assisted LAGB (EBW loss of 34.2% for robotic and 34.2% for standard laparoscopic after 1 year).[88] Snyder and coworkers[92] reported a series of 320 sequential robotic-assisted RYGB and compared outcomes with their series of 356 LRYGB procedures, which is one

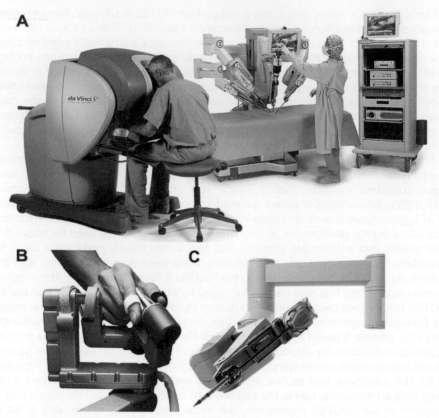

Fig. 4. da Vinci robotic systems. (*A*) da Vinci S robot complete system. (*B*) Detail of hand controls. (*C*) Detail of instrument arm with instrument loaded. (*Courtesy of* Intuitive Surgical, Inc, Sunnyvale, CA. Copyright © 2011. Intuitive Surgical, Inc.)

of the few studies showing an outcome benefit with robotic-assisted laparoscopic bariatric surgery, showing a lower leak rate for the robotic procedure (0% vs 1.7%). Complications were otherwise similar, with only nonspecific abdominal pain being more frequent in the robotic group.[92] No significant weight loss differences have been reported with robotic procedures.

Robotics offers another set of tools to the minimally invasive surgeon. Given the cost and set-up time involved in use of the da Vinci robot, it is likely to continue to be mainly used in longer, more complex procedures that can benefit most from the better visualization and type of dexterity the robot affords. Robotic advocates argue that the true cost of these systems actually remains controversial when one considers cost savings from decreased morbidities, decreased operative times for experienced users, and increased market shares and revenues for healthcare systems that make robotic procedures available to those patients who are drawn to the latest technology.[91,94–96] With the continued refinements in microprocessors and progress in robotic technology within numerous industries, it is likely that robotics will play a significant role in the future of all surgical fields. From improvements in the current master-slave type surgical systems, to robotically enhanced laparoscopic and endoscopic tools, and possibly even nanorobots that can be implanted in the abdomen or injected intravenously and carry out specific functions, the possible surgical use of robotics is expansive.

ENDOSCOPIC BARIATRIC PROCEDURES
Intragastric Balloon

The first intragastric balloon widely used in the United States was the Garren-Edwards bubble (GEB). Introduced in 1982 and FDA approved in 1985, the theory behind the balloon was that increased gastric distention would increase satiety, delay gastric emptying, and lead to reduced caloric intake and weight loss. Conceptually simple, the GEB was deployed by an endoscope into the stomach, and through a self-sealing valve, an air insufflation catheter could be inserted to fill the polyurethane cylinder to a volume of 220 mL. The bubble was then detached and allowed to float freely in the stomach. It could be recovered endoscopically by puncturing the bubble and then grasping or looping it for removal. Unfortunately, the GEB was shown in several studies to provide no weight loss benefit compared with life-style modification controls[97,98] and was inferior to bariatric surgery.[99] It also had a dismal side effect profile; in one study the GEB caused gastric erosions in 26% of patients, gastric ulcers in 14%, Mallory-Weiss tears in 11%, small bowel obstruction in 2%, and esophageal lacerations in 1%.[98] The GEB was withdrawn from the market in 1988.

Given the failure of the GEB, an expert panel was convened in 1987 in Florida, and guidelines for future intragastric space-occupying devices were devised.[100] These guidelines included a smooth soft surface to avoid gastric injury; soft and pliable deflated form to facilitate safe and simple deployment and recovery; and that devices should be fluid-filled, not air-filled. After this conference, several iterations of intragastric balloon, most notably the Taylor intragastric balloon (made of silicone and filled with 550 mL of saline) and the Ballobes intragastric balloon, failed to demonstrate efficacy.

In 1999 the BioEnterics intragastric balloon (BIB) was introduced by Allergan (**Fig. 5**). A spherical balloon made of silicone elastomer, it is filled with 400 to 700 mL of saline by a silicone catheter that is placed through the endoscope. The filling catheter is attached to a radiopaque self-sealing valve, and is detachable. The balloon volume can be adjusted endoscopically depending on the patient's clinical response. It is designed to be left in place for up to 6 months. Complications are similar, but less frequent, than earlier balloons and include gastric erosions, gastric ulcers, gastric perforation, gastric obstruction, spontaneous deflation, small bowel obstruction, vomiting, and abdominal pain. The balloon can be easily removed endoscopically by puncturing and grasping with foreign body graspers. One technique used to alert the patient of rupture is to mix methylene blue into the saline used to fill the balloon. If rupture occurs, the patient's urine is turned green.[101]

Although not available in the United States, international experience with the BIB has been well-documented. Genco and colleagues[40] reported their experience in Italy involving 2515 patients with an average BMI of 44.4 kg/m^2. After 6 months of therapy with the BIB, mean EBW loss was 33.9%, and of the 1394 patients with obesity-related comorbidities, 89% (1242 patients) saw significant improvement in their comorbidities. The most common complications were esophagitis (1.27%); gastric obstruction (0.76%); balloon rupture (0.36%); gastric ulcer (0.19%); and gastric perforation (0.19%). A Brazilian study of 483 overweight and obese patients (mean BMI 38.2 kg/m^2) treated for 6 months with BIB, revealed an average EBW loss of 48.3%.[102] Interestingly, weight loss was better in younger patients, with a trend for decreasing EBW seen in each successive age category. Longer-term follow-up revealed that at

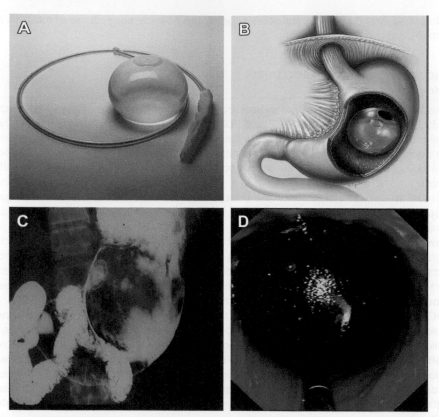

Fig. 5. Intragastric balloon. (*A*) BioEnterics intragastric balloon. (*B*) Diagram of BioEnterics intragastric balloon. (*C*) Upper gastrointestinal images with BioEnterics intragastric balloon in place. (*D*) Endoscopic appearance of BioEnterics intragastric balloon. (*Courtesy of Allergan, Irvine, CA; with permission.*)

1 year an average of more than 90% of initial weight loss was maintained, and at 2 years, 89% of weight loss persisted. The major limitation of these studies is that a significant benefit over the sham group was not proved.

Newer devices aimed at causing gastric distention include ingestible pills that swell once in the stomach. BaroNova is working on the development of what they term a "transpyloric shuttle," a pill that swells once in the stomach and then degrades over a week such that it can pass through the gastrointestinal tract. Gelesis is developing a similar technology. They are testing a pill that contains hundreds of superabsorbent hydrogel particles made from food components. When exposed to water these particles swell and form a gelatinous material. Although neither of these technologies has been tested in large-scale trials, the technology remains promising.

Endoluminal Sleeve

The EndoBarrier gastrointestinal liner is a 60-cm long impermeable fluoropolymer tube with a nitinol anchor that is endoscopically placed at the duodenal bulb (**Fig. 6**). Developed by GI Dynamics, the EndoBarrier was developed to mimic duodenojejunal bypass by preventing contact between the food bolus and the duodenal mucosa or mixing with biliary and pancreatic secretions until well into the jejunum. The nitinol

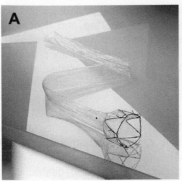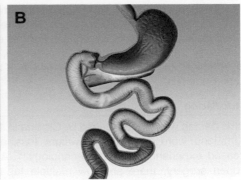

Fig. 6. Endoluminal sleeve. (*A*) Photograph of EndoBarrier gastrointestinal liner. (*B*) Diagram of EndoBarrier position within the gastrointestinal tract showing food bolus within the sleeve and bioliopancreatic secretions outside the sleeve. (*Courtesy of* GI Dynamics, Lexington, MA; with permission.)

anchor was designed to be self-expanding, placing barbs within the proximal (0.5 cm from the pylorus) duodenum to prevent migration. Recovery is facilitated by proximal drawstrings that cause the anchor to collapse and then retract into a retrieval hood that also helps protect the gastrointestinal tract from the device as it is removed through the mouth. Animal tests were promising for safety and efficacy,[103] and initial human studies demonstrated safe delivery and retrieval of the device.[104]

The first prospective human study, reported by Rodriguez-Grunert and colleagues,[105] revealed an average EBW loss of 23.6% after retrieval of the device 12 weeks after placement. Ten sleeves were placed successfully in 12 patients, and two were removed early because of abdominal pain. All patients experienced at least 10% EBW loss. A larger trial was recently reported by Schouten and coworkers.[106] A total of 41 patients participated. Thirty received the sleeve and 11 served as a diet-only control group. The average BMI in the sleeve group was 48.9 kg/m^2 and 49.2 kg/m^2 in the control group. After 12 weeks the average EBW loss was 19% in the sleeve group and 6.9 % in the control group. After 24 weeks, the EBW loss was 24.3 % in the sleeve group. Adverse events occurred in 26 of the 30 patients in the device group, and included nausea, abdominal pain, pseudopolyp formation on retrieval, and implant site inflammation, but no patient experienced a "severe" complication. Only three patients completed the 24-week arm of the study because there was a single device migration at 4 months, and the remainder of devices was removed at 4 months. This study also looked at the metabolic effects of the EndoBarrier. Type II DM was present in 8 of the 30 patients in the sleeve group, and medication use, serum glucose, and hemoglobin A_{1c} improved in seven of those eight. Average hemoglobin A_{1c} decreased from 8.8% to 7.7% at 12 weeks postoperative.

The EndoBarrier now has approval and is being used in the United Kingdom, the Netherlands, and Chile, and trials are currently underway within the United States. However, the use of the device is limited in that it is currently approved only for a limited duration.

The ValenTx endoscopically placed sleeve is a similar device, but is anchored in the esophagus and extends through the stomach and duodenum into the proximal jejunum. It provides an endoscopic bypass, potentially affecting both restriction and malabsorption. Initial trials with this device demonstrated an average EBW loss of 39.7% in the 17 patients who completed the trial, and improvement in hemoglobin A_{1c} levels in all four patients with preoperatively elevated hemoglobin A_{1c} levels during the 12-week trial period.[107] The starting population included 24 patients with a mean BMI of 42 kg/m^2, but two attempted placements were aborted and five patients required device removal for dysphagia. Further experience with endoluminal sleeves will certainly provide further insight into its use, but these devices may prove to be safe, effective, and minimally invasive means of treating obesity, diabetes, and associated conditions.

Gastric Pacing

Gastric pacing was first described by Cigaina in 1995,[36] and although initial studies of weight loss were inconsistent, weight loss after gastric pacing improved with increased experience with this technology.[37] Although early systems were placed by open surgery, there are now multiple laparoscopically placed gastric pacing systems. The Implantable Gastric Stimulation by Medtronic Transneuronix has been shown to be safe and more effective than medical weight loss programs alone.[108] The Tantalus System by MetaCure USA is a laparoscopically placed meal-sensing system that uses a technology termed "gastric contractility modulation," which refers to the device's ability to deliver stimulating electrical signals to the stomach synchronized with the intrinsic electrical activity of the stomach.[109] Another intelligent gastric pacing system is being developed by IntraPace and is currently in early clinical trials in Europe. Endoscopically placed pacing systems are a logical next step.

Another neuromodulating technology is vagal blockade. This technology derived from the observation that patients with peptic ulcer disease temporarily lose weight after gastrectomy or truncal vagotomy, and subsequently, that ghrelin levels and the appetite-stimulating function of ghrelin is reduced in these patients.[110] The vagal blocking system developed by EnteroMedics has been tested in a three-center open-label trial involving 31 patients.[111] With a mean preoperative BMI of 41.2 kg/m^2, the average EBW loss was 7.5%, 11.6%, and 14.2% at 6 weeks, 12 weeks, and 6 months, respectively. However, 25% of patients had an EBW loss greater than 25%, and one had an EBW loss of 36.8%. Three patients had significant adverse events requiring hospitalization. Although this system is implanted laparoscopically, an endoscopically placed vagal blockade device is being developed by EndoVx. Given the relative invasiveness and modest efficacy of these technologies, neuromodulation remains controversial and will likely require significant refinement before being widely applied.

Endoscopic Suturing Platforms

A multitude of endoscopic devices capable of placing sutures or tissue fasteners within the esophagus, stomach, and proximal small bowel have been developed, but few have yet to demonstrate efficacy in bariatric procedures. One of the first endoscopic suturing devices is the endoscopic sewing machine by C.R. Bard. The device is fixed to the end of a flexible endoscope and used to first attach a 3-cm ring to the lesser curvature of the stomach in line with and 8 cm distal to the gastroesophageal junction. The anterior and posterior walls of the stomach are then sutured together over the ring, and the suturing then progresses proximally to the level of the esophagus. This creates a 3- to 4-cm diameter gastroplasty. A technical feasibility study of this procedure was reported using a cadaveric porcine specimen in 2002,[112] but has not been reported since. Another early endoscopic suturing platform is the Eagle Claw endoscopic suturing device by Olympus. The first publication of this device reported its use to create a 100-mL gastric pouch in a porcine model,[113] a pouch size that was likely too large to facilitate significant weight loss. It was also used for suturing a gastrojejunal anastomosis in a porcine model.[81] It was thereafter redesigned, and the Eagle Claw VII was used in a live animal series to produce 30-mL gastric pouches.[114] This was also a limited feasibility study, and no further data have been published with this system.

Another device continues to show promising early results. C. R. Bard's EndoCinch Suturing System is a suction and suture device that attaches to a standard endoscope. The system was designed for use in fundoplication for reflux disease, but was later applied to bariatric procedures. A large-scale human trial of this device in a weight loss procedure was reported by Fogel and colleagues[115] in 2008. The study involved 64 patients with a mean BMI of 39.9 kg/m^2, and resulted in a mean EBW loss of 21.1% at 1 month, 39.6% at 3 months, 58.1% at 12 months, and 92% of patients after 12 months. Interestingly, more profound weight loss was seen in patients with lower BMIs (85% EBW loss in those patients with a BMI <35 kg/m^2) than higher BMIs (48.9% EBW loss for those with a BMI >40 kg/m^2). Fourteen endoscopies were performed during the 3- to 12-month period for change in satiety or poor weight loss. Six of these patients were found to have a loosely intact gastroplasty, and three had a disrupted gastroplasty. This device has been updated, and has been renamed the Restore Suturing System. A feasibility study using this system in 18 patients to perform restrictive gastric plication revealed an average procedure time of 125 minutes, and no significant complications.[116] Data on durability and efficacy for weight loss and comorbidity resolution are forthcoming, but some surgeons question whether these plications will be durable, because many sutures with the system are not full thickness.

Another product with promising early results is the transoral gastroplasty system by Satiety. This system created a series of stapled transmural folds by suctioning anterior and posterior gastric mucosa into a suction chamber and then firing the stapler. Several rows of staples are used to create a restrictive pouch along the lesser curvature of the stomach. The first study of this device involved 21 patients.[117] No serious complications were seen, and EBW loss at 6 months was 24.4%. During this trial, gaps were seen to develop between the superior portion of the staple lines and the angle of His, and between the first two staple lines. The device was thus redesigned to create overlapping staple lines to eliminate these gaps. A second study of 11 patients showed even better average EBW loss of 46%, but two patients had large outlets seen on 3-month follow-up endoscopy, and failed to have any significant weight loss despite repeat treatment.[118] A large-scale, multicenter trial was subsequently undertaken using a control group that received a sham endoscopy. Although the results have not been released publically, the New York Times has reported that the trial failed to show a significant benefit of transoral gastroplasty versus control, and that study and control groups lost much less weight than patients in previous trials.[119] These results led to the FDA's recent decision to not approve the device, and the subsequent withdrawal of venture capital funding from Satiety.

Another new system aimed at inducing weight loss through endoscopic manipulation of the stomach is the Trans-oral Endoscopic Restrictive Implant System, by BaroSense. This system places a "restrictor" with a 10-mm central hole for food passage in the proximal stomach. The restrictor is secured with five anchors, each of which is passed through a full-thickness plication of gastric tissue created with a specially designed endoscopic stapler. The anchors are placed sequentially, and then the restrictor is attached. A single clinical trial involving 13 morbidly obese patients with a median BMI of 42.1 kg/m^2 has been completed, and revealed a 28% EBW loss at 3 months.[120] The procedure was not completed in three patients, one because of stapler malfunctioning and two because of the development of pneumoperitoneum. Longer-term follow-up has not yet been reported, and the system continues to undergo refinement. Other endoscopic devices for suturing or plication that have yet to report clinical trial data for bariatric applications include the SafeStitch device by SafeStitch Medical; the NDO plicator by NDO Surgical (IP now owned by Johnson & Johnson); and the Endoscopic Suturing Device by Wilson-Cook Medical. The Incisionless Operating Platform and G-Prox device (USGI Medical) have also been proposed for bariatric applications. Most proposals for these devices focus on either endoluminal restriction by volume reduction or fundic ablation to improve satiety.

Still other devices have been designed and marketed for revisional bariatric surgery. Multiple studies have been published using the EndoCinch device by Bard for revision after gastric bypass.[121,122] In a study by Thompson and colleagues,[122] eight patients with failed RYGB with a mean weight regain of 27 kg resulting in a mean BMI of 40.5 kg/m^2 underwent plication of the gastrojejunostomy using the EndoCinch device, reducing the pouch diameter from a mean of 25 mm to 10 mm. The resulting average EBW loss was 23.4%, with mean BMI of 37.7 kg/m^2 4 months postprocedure. The long-term durability of these results is unknown. The StomaPhyx device from Endo-Gastric Solutions has also shown promising results in revision after failed RYGB. This device is placed over an endoscope, and uses H-fasteners to introduce endoluminal plications that reduce overall pouch and stoma size. In a recent study of 39 patients with a mean BMI of 39.8 kg/m^2, the procedure resulted in EBW loss of 10.6% at 1 month, 13.1% at 3 months, 17% at 6 months, and 19.5% at 12 months.[123] There were no major complications, and the most common minor complications included sore throat and mild epigastric pain, both lasting only a few days. The Restorative Obesity Surgery, Endoluminal procedure is performed using the Incisionless Operating Platform by USGI Medical. Similar to StomaPhyx, the device creates tissue folds and secures them with anchors using the fully endoscopic Incisionless Operating Platform. By placing folds circumferentially, the lumen is narrowed and the pouch made smaller. Borao and colleagues[124] used the device in 21 patients with more than 50% EBW loss after their primary bariatric surgery and an average of 59 lb of regained weight, to affect a 53% reduction in stomal diameter and 41% reduction in pouch size, which in turn resulted in a mean regained weight loss of 72%.

The continued evolution of these devices will likely result in increasingly safe, effective, and usable tools for minimally invasive bariatric procedures. Although continued trials and product development are costly, a simple, safe, and easy to use endoscopic suturing platform would have broad applications in bariatric surgery and reflux procedures, other gastric operations, and NOTES procedures. If past trends hold true, it is likely that if an effective and safe endoscopic bariatric procedure is developed, patient preferences would likely turn quickly to the less invasive operation. Incentive is thus strong in this field, and potential pay-offs will continue to entice the necessary scientific and capital resources even in the face of numerous previous corporate failures in the field.

SUMMARY

The field of bariatric surgery has seen rapid evolution over the last 30 years and this evolution seems to be accelerating. The four most common bariatric procedures at present (LRYGB, LAGB, sleeve gastrectomy, and BPD with DS) are all safe, effective, minimally invasive, and relatively cost-effective. These state-of-the-art procedures continue to be perfected, and improved training and regulation of the field is facilitating better access to these procedures nationally as demand is increasing sharply with a worsening obesity epidemic. As the safety and efficacy of bariatric surgery continues to improve, the indications have been broadened to more patients who can now expect a significant benefit with less risk.

The focus continues to be on reducing the invasiveness of these procedures. NOTES and fully endoscopic procedures are being developed, and as appropriate tools are developed, such procedures will likely become increasingly efficacious and simple to perform. Because these procedures have been associated with less pain, shorter hospital stays, and may well not require general anesthesia, the overall cost of these operations is likely to be significantly less than those currently available. Although financial pressures might eventually ensure the safety of these procedures given the significant costs associated with complications of gastrointestinal surgery, the surgical community must be diligent to ensure trials continue to be performed appropriately to prevent any avoidable injury. It is an exciting time for bariatric surgeons, because with each new technologic step they are able to offer patients safer, less painful, less costly, and more efficacious options for weight loss and metabolic normalization.

REFERENCES

1. Trus TL, Pope GD, Finlayson SR. National trends in utilization and outcomes of bariatric surgery. Surg Endosc 2005;19(5):616–20.
2. Hinojosa MW, Varela JE, Parikh D, et al. National trends in use and outcome of laparoscopic adjustable gastric banding. Surg Obes Relat Dis 2009;5(2):150–5.
3. Smoot TM, Xu P, Hilsenrath P, et al. Gastric bypass surgery in the United States, 1998-2002. Am J Public Health 2006;96(7):1187–9.
4. Saber AA, Elgamal MH, McLeod MK. Bariatric Surgery: The Past, Present, and Future. Obes Surg 2008;18(1):121–8.
5. Payne JH, Dewind LT, Commons RR. Metabolic observations in patients with jejunocolic shunts. Am J Surg 1963;106:273–89.
6. Scott HW Jr, Sandstead HH, Brill AB, et al. Experience with a new technique of intestinal bypass in the treatment of morbid obesity. Ann Surg 1971;174(4):560–72.
7. Sherman CD Jr, May AG, Nye W, et al. Clinical and metabolic studies following bowel by-passing for obesity. Ann N Y Acad Sci 1965;131(1):614–22.
8. Buchwald H, Varco RL. A bypass operation for obese hyperlipidemic patients. Surgery 1971;70(1):62–70.
9. Mason EE, Ito C. Gastric bypass in obesity. Surg Clin North Am 1967;47(6): 1345–51.
10. Alder RL, Terry BE. Measurement and standardization of the gastric pouch in gastric bypass. Surg Gynecol Obstet 1977;144(5):762–3.
11. Griffen WO Jr, Young VL, Stevenson CC. A prospective comparison of gastric and jejunoileal bypass procedures for morbid obesity. Ann Surg 1977;186(4): 500–9.
12. 2005. Available at: www.asbs.org/html/patients/bypass.html. Accessed May 3, 2011.
13. Scopinaro N, Gianetta E, Civalleri D, et al. Bilio-pancreatic bypass for obesity: II. Initial experience in man. Br J Surg 1979;66(9):618–20.
14. Scopinaro N, Adami GF, Marinari GM, et al. Biliopancreatic diversion. World J Surg 1998;22(9):936–46.
15. Hess DS, Hess DW. Biliopancreatic diversion with a duodenal switch. Obes Surg 1998;8(3):267–82.
16. Printen KJ, Mason EE. Gastric surgery for relief of morbid obesity. Arch Surg 1973;106(4):428–31.
17. Gomez CA. Gastroplasty in morbid obesity: a progress report. World J Surg 1981;5(6):823–8.

18. Pace WG, Martin EW Jr, Tetirick T, et al. Gastric partitioning for morbid obesity. Ann Surg 1979;190(3):392–400.
19. Long M, Collins JP. The technique and early results of high gastric reduction for obesity. Aust N Z J Surg 1980;50(2):146–9.
20. Mason EE. Vertical banded gastroplasty for obesity. Arch Surg 1982;117(5): 701–6.
21. Wilkinson LH, Peloso OA. Gastric (reservoir) reduction for morbid obesity. Arch Surg 1981;116(5):602–5.
22. Kuzmak LI, Thelmo W, Abramson DL, et al. Reversible adjustable gastric banding. Surgical technique. Eur J Surg 1994;160(10):569–71.
23. DeMaria EJ, Jamal MK. Laparoscopic adjustable gastric banding: evolving clinical experience. Surg Clin North Am 2005;85(4):773–87.
24. Flegal KM, Carroll MD, Kuczmarski RJ, et al. Overweight and obesity in the United States: prevalence and trends, 1960-1994. Int J Obes Relat Metab Disord 1998;22(1):39–47.
25. Flegal KM, Carroll MD, Ogden CL, et al. Prevalence and trends in obesity among US adults, 1999-2008. JAMA 2010;303(3):235–41.
26. Ogden CL, Carroll MD, Curtin LR, et al. Prevalence of high body mass index in US children and adolescents, 2007-2008. JAMA 2010;303(3):242–9.
27. Centers for Disease Control and Prevention. Available at: www.cdc.gov/obesitydata/trends.html. Accessed May 3, 2011.
28. Available at: www.cdc.gov/diabetes/pubs/factsheets.htm.
29. Chua TY, Mendiola RM. Laparoscopic vertical banded gastroplasty: the Milwaukee experience. Obes Surg 1995;5(1):77–80.
30. Wittgrove AC, Clark GW. Laparoscopic gastric bypass, Roux-en-Y- 500 patients: technique and results, with 3-60 month follow-up. Obes Surg 2000;10(3): 233–9.
31. Catona A, Gossenberg M, La Manna A, et al. Laparoscopic gastric banding: preliminary series. Obes Surg 1993;3(2):207–9.
32. Belachew M, Belva PH, Desaive C. Long-term results of laparoscopic adjustable gastric banding for the treatment of morbid obesity. Obes Surg 2002;12(4): 564–8.
33. Buchwald H, Williams SE. Bariatric surgery worldwide 2003. Obes Surg 2004; 14(9):1157–64.
34. Santoro S, Malzoni CE, Velhote MC, et al. Digestive adaptation with intestinal reserve: a neuroendocrine-based operation for morbid obesity. Obes Surg 2006;16(10):1371–9.
35. Santoro S, Velhote MC, Malzoni CE, et al. Preliminary results from digestive adaptation: a new surgical proposal for treating obesity, based on physiology and evolution. Sao Paulo Med J 2006;124(4):192–7.
36. Cigaina V. Gastric pacing as therapy for morbid obesity: preliminary results. Obes Surg 2002;12(Suppl 1):12S–6S.
37. Cigaina V. Long-term follow-up of gastric stimulation for obesity: the Mestre 8-year experience. Obes Surg 2004;14(Suppl 1):S14–22.
38. Miller K, Hoeller E, Aigner F. The implantable gastric stimulator for obesity: an update of the European experience in the LOSS (Laparoscopic Obesity Stimulation Survey) study. Treat Endocrinol 2006;5(1):53–8.
39. Evans JD, Scott MH. Intragastric balloon in the treatment of patients with morbid obesity. Br J Surg 2001;88(9):1245–8.
40. Genco A, Bruni T, Doldi SB, et al. BioEnterics intragastric balloon: the Italian experience with 2,515 patients. Obes Surg 2005;15(8):1161–4.

41. Ackroyd R, Mouiel J, Chevallier JM, et al. Cost-effectiveness and budget impact of obesity surgery in patients with type-2 diabetes in three European countries. Obes Surg 2006;16(11):1488–503.
42. Anselmino M, Bammer T, Fernandez Cebrian JM, et al. Cost-effectiveness and budget impact of obesity surgery in patients with type 2 diabetes in three European countries(II). Obes Surg 2009;19(11):1542–9.
43. Ikramuddin S, Klingman D, Swan T, et al. Cost-effectiveness of Roux-en-Y gastric bypass in type 2 diabetes patients. Am J Manag Care 2009;15(9): 607–15.
44. Cremieux PY, Buchwald H, Shikora SA, et al. A study on the economic impact of bariatric surgery. Am J Manag Care 2008;14(9):589–96.
45. Courcoulas A, Perry Y, Buenaventura P, et al. Comparing the outcomes after laparoscopic versus open gastric bypass: a matched paired analysis. Obes Surg 2003;13(3):341–6.
46. dos Santos Moraes I Jr, Madalosso CA, Palma LA, et al. Hospital discharge in the day following open Roux-en-Y gastric bypass: is it feasible and safe? Obes Surg 2009;19(3):281–6.
47. Mason EE. Ileal [correction of ilial] transposition and enteroglucagon/GLP-1 in obesity (and diabetic?) surgery. Obes Surg 1999;9(3):223–8.
48. Depaula AL, Stival AR, Halpern A, et al. Surgical treatment of morbid obesity: mid-term outcomes of the laparoscopic ileal interposition associated to a sleeve gastrectomy in 120 patients. Obes Surg 2011;21(5):668–75.
49. Kumar KV, Ugale S, Gupta N, et al. Ileal interposition with sleeve gastrectomy for control of type 2 diabetes. Diabetes Technol Ther 2009;11(12):785–9.
50. Talebpour M, Amoli BS. Laparoscopic total gastric vertical plication in morbid obesity. J Laparoendosc Adv Surg Tech A 2007;17(6):793–8.
51. Brethauer SA, Harris JL, Kroh M, et al. Laparoscopic gastric plication for treatment of severe obesity. Surg Obes Relat Dis 2011;7(1):15–22.
52. Ramos A, Galvao Neto M, Galvao M, et al. Laparoscopic greater curvature plication: initial results of an alternative restrictive bariatric procedure. Obes Surg 2010;20(7):913–8.
53. Hussain A, Mahmood H, El-Hasani S. Gastric plication can reduce slippage rate after laparoscopic gastric banding. JSLS 2010;14(2):221–7.
54. Gastrointestinal surgery for severe obesity. Consensus statement 1991;9(1): 1–20.
55. DeMaria EJ, Winegar DA, Pate VW, et al. Early postoperative outcomes of metabolic surgery to treat diabetes from sites participating in the ASMBS bariatric surgery center of excellence program as reported in the bariatric outcomes longitudinal database. Ann Surg 2010;252(3):559–66 [discussion: 566–7].
56. Dixon JB, O'Brien PE, Playfair J, et al. Adjustable gastric banding and conventional therapy for type 2 diabetes: a randomized controlled trial. JAMA 2008; 299(3):316–23.
57. Buchwald H. Consensus conference statement bariatric surgery for morbid obesity: health implications for patients, health professionals, and third-party payers. Surg Obes Relat Dis 2005;1(3):371–81.
58. Runkel N, Colombo-Benkmann M, Huttl TP, et al. Evidence-based German guidelines for surgery for obesity. Int J Colorectal Dis 2011;26(4):397–404.
59. Ponsky LE, Cherullo EE, Sawyer M, et al. Single access site laparoscopic radical nephrectomy: initial clinical experience. J Endourol 2008;22(4):663–6.
60. Goel RK, Kaouk JH. Single port access renal cryoablation (SPARC): a new approach. Eur Urol 2008;53(6):1204–9.

61. Kaouk JH, Haber GP, Goel RK, et al. Single-port laparoscopic surgery in urology: initial experience. Urology 2008;71(1):3–6.
62. Kaouk JH, Palmer JS. Single-port laparoscopic surgery: initial experience in children for varicocelectomy. BJU Int 2008;102(1):97–9.
63. Rane A, Rao P. Single-port-access nephrectomy and other laparoscopic urologic procedures using a novel laparoscopic port (R-port). Urology 2008; 72(2):260–3 [discussion: 263–4].
64. Saber AA, Elgamal MH, Itawi EA, et al. Single incision laparoscopic sleeve gastrectomy (SILS): a novel technique. Obes Surg 2008;18(10):1338–42.
65. Pryor AD, Tushar JR, DiBernardo LR. Single-port cholecystectomy with the TransEnterix SPIDER: simple and safe. Surg Endosc 2010;24(4):917–23.
66. Huang CK, Lo CH, Asim S, et al. A novel technique for liver retraction in laparoscopic bariatric surgery. Obes Surg 2011;21(5):676–9.
67. Thanakumar J, John PH. One-handed knot tying technique in single-incision laparoscopic surgery. J Minim Access Surg 2011;7(1):112–5.
68. Huang CK, Lo CH, Houng JY, et al. Surgical results of single-incision transumbilical laparoscopic Roux-en-Y gastric bypass. Surg Obes Relat Dis 2010. [Epub ahead of print].
69. Tacchino RM, Greco F, Matera D, et al. Single-incision laparoscopic gastric bypass for morbid obesity. Obes Surg 2010;20(8):1154–60.
70. Huang CK. Single-incision laparoscopic bariatric surgery. J Minim Access Surg 2011;7(1):99–103.
71. Gauderer MW, Ponsky JL, Izant RJ Jr. Gastrostomy without laparotomy: a percutaneous endoscopic technique. J Pediatr Surg 1980;15(6):872–5.
72. Kalloo AN, Singh VK, Jagannath SB, et al. Flexible transgastric peritoneoscopy: a novel approach to diagnostic and therapeutic interventions in the peritoneal cavity. Gastrointest Endosc 2004;60(1):114–7.
73. McGee MF, Marks JM, Onders RP, et al. Complete endoscopic closure of gastrotomy after natural orifice translumenal endoscopic surgery using the NDO Plicator. Surg Endosc 2008;22(1):214–20.
74. Mellinger JD, MacFadyen BV, Kozarek RA, et al. Initial experience with a novel endoscopic device allowing intragastric manipulation and plication. Surg Endosc 2007;21(6):1002–5.
75. Moyer MT, Pauli EM, Haluck RS, et al. A self-approximating transluminal access technique for potential use in NOTES: an ex vivo porcine model (with video). Gastrointest Endosc 2007;66(5):974–8.
76. Cios TJ, Reavis KM, Renton DR, et al. Gastrotomy closure using bioabsorbable plugs in a canine model. Surg Endosc 2008;22(4):961–6.
77. McGee MF, Rosen MJ, Marks J, et al. A reliable method for monitoring intraabdominal pressure during natural orifice translumenal endoscopic surgery. Surg Endosc 2007;21(4):672–6.
78. Lacy AM, Delgado S, Rojas OA, et al. Hybrid vaginal MA-NOS sleeve gastrectomy: technical note on the procedure in a patient. Surg Endos 2009;23(5): 1130–7.
79. Hagen ME, Wagner OJ, Swain P, et al. Hybrid natural orifice transluminal endoscopic surgery (NOTES) for Roux-en-Y gastric bypass: an experimental surgical study in human cadavers. Endoscopy 2008;40(11):918–24.
80. Madan AK, Tichansky DS, Khan KA. Natural orifice transluminal endoscopic gastric bypass performed in a cadaver. Obes Surg 2008;18(9):1192–9.
81. Kantsevoy SV, Jagannath SB, Niiyama H, et al. Endoscopic gastrojejunostomy with survival in a porcine model. Gastrointest Endosc 2005;62(2):287–92.

82. Myers C, Yellen B, Evans J, et al. Using external magnet guidance and endoscopically placed magnets to create suture-free gastro-enteral anastomoses. Surg Endosc 2010;24(5):1104–9.
83. Ryou M, Cantillon-Murphy P, Azagury D, et al. Smart Self-Assembling MagnetS for ENdoscopy (SAMSEN) for transoral endoscopic creation of immediate gastrojejunostomy (with video). Gastrointest Endosc 2011;73(2):353–9.
84. Wilson EB. The evolution of robotic general surgery. Scand J Surg 2009;98(2):125–9.
85. Muhlmann G, Klaus A, Kirchmayr W, et al. DaVinci robotic-assisted laparoscopic bariatric surgery: is it justified in a routine setting? Obes Surg 2003;13(6):848–54.
86. Edelson PK, Dumon KR, Sonnad SS, et al. Robotic vs. conventional laparoscopic gastric banding: a comparison of 407 cases. Surg Endosc 2011;25(5):1402–8.
87. Jacobsen G, Berger R, Horgan S. The role of robotic surgery in morbid obesity. J Laparoendosc Adv Surg Tech A 2003;13(4):279–83.
88. Horgan S, Vanuno D. Robots in laparoscopic surgery. J Laparoendosc Adv Surg Tech A 2001;11(6):415–9.
89. Mohr CJ, Nadzam GS, Curet MJ. Totally robotic Roux-en-Y gastric bypass. Arch Surg 2005;140(8):779–86.
90. Ali MR, Bhaskerrao B, Wolfe BM. Robot-assisted laparoscopic Roux-en-Y gastric bypass. Surg Endosc 2005;19(4):468–72.
91. Hubens G, Balliu L, Ruppert M, et al. Roux-en-Y gastric bypass procedure performed with the da Vinci robot system: is it worth it? Surg Endosc 2008;22(7):1690–6.
92. Snyder BE, Wilson T, Leong BY, et al. Robotic-assisted Roux-en-Y gastric bypass: minimizing morbidity and mortality. Obes Surg 2010;20(3):265–70.
93. Diamantis T, Alexandrou A, Nikiteas N, et al. Initial experience with robotic sleeve gastrectomy for morbid obesity. Obes Surg 2011;21(8):1172–9.
94. Murphy D, Challacombe B, Khan MS, et al. Robotic technology in urology. Postgrad Med J 2006;82(973):743–7.
95. Sanchez BR, Mohr CJ, Morton JM, et al. Comparison of totally robotic laparoscopic Roux-en-Y gastric bypass and traditional laparoscopic Roux-en-Y gastric bypass. Surg Obes Relat Dis 2005;1(6):549–54.
96. Moser F, Horgan S. Robotically assisted bariatric surgery. Am J Surg 2004;188(Suppl 4A):38S–44S.
97. Hogan RB, Johnston JH, Long BW, et al. A double-blind, randomized, sham-controlled trial of the gastric bubble for obesity. Gastrointest Endosc 1989;35(5):381–5.
98. Benjamin SB, Maher KA, Cattau EL Jr, et al. Double-blind controlled trial of the Garren-Edwards gastric bubble: an adjunctive treatment for exogenous obesity. Gastroenterology 1988;95(3):581–8.
99. Kirby DF, Wade JB, Mills PR, et al. A prospective assessment of the Garren-Edwards Gastric Bubble and bariatric surgery in the treatment of morbid obesity. Am Surg 1990;56(10):575–80.
100. Schapiro M, Benjamin S, Blackburn G, et al. Obesity and the gastric balloon: a comprehensive workshop. Tarpon Springs, Florida, March 19-21, 1987. Gastrointest Endosc 1987;33(4):323–7.
101. Bernante P, Francini F, Zangrandi F, et al. Green urine after intragastric balloon placement for the treatment of morbid obesity. Obes Surg 2003;13(6):951–3.
102. Sallet JA, Marchesini JB, Paiva DS, et al. Brazilian multicenter study of the intragastric balloon. Obes Surg 2004;14(7):991–8.

103. Tarnoff M, Shikora S, Lembo A, et al. Chronic in-vivo experience with an endoscopically delivered and retrieved duodenal-jejunal bypass sleeve in a porcine model. Surg Endosc 2008;22(4):1023–8.

104. Gersin KS, Keller JE, Stefanidis D, et al. Duodenal- jejunal bypass sleeve: a totally endoscopic device for the treatment of morbid obesity. Surg Innov 2007;14(4):275–8.

105. Rodriguez-Grunert L, Galvao Neto MP, Alamo M, et al. First human experience with endoscopically delivered and retrieved duodenal-jejunal bypass sleeve. Surg Obes Relat Dis 2008;4(1):55–9.

106. Schouten R, Rijs CS, Bouvy ND, et al. A multicenter, randomized efficacy study of the EndoBarrier Gastrointestinal Liner for presurgical weight loss prior to bariatric surgery. Ann Surg 2010;251(2):236–43.

107. Sandler BJ, Rumbaut R, Paul Swain C, et al. Human experience with an endoluminal, endoscopic, gastrojejunal bypass sleeve. Surg Endosc 2011;25(9): 3028–33.

108. Shikora SA, Storch K. Implantable gastric stimulation for the treatment of severe obesity: the American experience. Surg Obes Relat Dis 2005;1(3):334–42.

109. Sanmiguel CP, Haddad W, Aviv R, et al. The TANTALUS system for obesity: effect on gastric emptying of solids and ghrelin plasma levels. Obes Surg 2007;17(11):1503–9.

110. le Roux CW, Neary NM, Halsey TJ, et al. Ghrelin does not stimulate food intake in patients with surgical procedures involving vagotomy. J Clin Endocrinol Metab 2005;90(8):4521–4.

111. Camilleri M, Toouli J, Herrera MF, et al. Intra-abdominal vagal blocking (VBLOC therapy): clinical results with a new implantable medical device. Surgery 2008; 143(6):723–31.

112. Awan AN, Swain CP. Endoscopic vertical band gastroplasty with an endoscopic sewing machine. Gastrointest Endosc 2002;55(2):254–6.

113. Hu B, Chung SC, Sun LC, et al. Transoral obesity surgery: endoluminal gastroplasty with an endoscopic suture device. Endoscopy 2005;37(5):411–4.

114. Kantsevoy SV, Hu B, Jagannath SB, et al. Technical feasibility of endoscopic gastric reduction: a pilot study in a porcine model. Gastrointest Endosc 2007; 65(3):510–3.

115. Fogel R, De Fogel J, Bonilla Y, et al. Clinical experience of transoral suturing for an endoluminal vertical gastroplasty: 1-year follow-up in 64 patients. Gastrointest Endosc 2008;68(1):51–8.

116. Brethauer SA, Chand B, Schauer PR, et al. Transoral gastric volume reduction for weight management: technique and feasibility in 18 patients. Surg Obes Relat Dis 2010;6(6):689–94.

117. Deviere J, Ojeda Valdes G, Cuevas Herrera L, et al. Safety, feasibility and weight loss after transoral gastroplasty: first human multicenter study. Surg Endosc 2008;22(3):589–98.

118. Moreno C, Closset J, Dugardeyn S, et al. Transoral gastroplasty is safe, feasible, and induces significant weight loss in morbidly obese patients: results of the second human pilot study. Endoscopy 2008;40(5):406–13.

119. Pollack A. Hoping to avoid the knife. The New York Times; March 17, 2011. p. B1.

120. de Jong K, Mathus-Vliegen EM, Veldhuyzen EA, et al. Short-term safety and efficacy of the trans-oral endoscopic restrictive implant system for the treatment of obesity. Gastrointest Endosc 2010;72(3):497–504.

121. Schweitzer M. Endoscopic intraluminal suture plication of the gastric pouch and stoma in postoperative Roux-en-Y gastric bypass patients. J Laparoendosc Adv Surg Tech A 2004;14(4):223–6.
122. Thompson CC, Slattery J, Bundga ME, et al. Peroral endoscopic reduction of dilated gastrojejunal anastomosis after Roux-en-Y gastric bypass: a possible new option for patients with weight regain. Surg Endosc 2006; 20(11):1744–8.
123. Mikami D, Needleman B, Narula V, et al. Natural orifice surgery: initial US experience utilizing the StomaphyX device to reduce gastric pouches after Roux-en-Y gastric bypass. Surg Endosc 2010;24(1):223–8.
124. Borao F, Gorcey S, Capuano A. Prospective single-site case series utilizing an endolumenal tissue anchoring system for revision of post-RYGB stomal and pouch dilatation. Surg Endosc 2010;24(9):2308–13.

Index

Note: Page numbers of article titles are in **boldface** type.

Surg Clin N Am 91 (2011) 1397–1408
doi:10.1016/S0039-6109(11)00137-X
0039-6109/11/$ – see front matter © 2011 Elsevier Inc. All rights reserved.

surgical.theclinics.com

Moving?

Make sure your subscription moves with you!

To notify us of your new address, find your **Clinics Account Number** (located on your mailing label above your name), and contact customer service at:

Email: journalscustomerservice-usa@elsevier.com

800-654-2452 (subscribers in the U.S. & Canada)
314-447-8871 (subscribers outside of the U.S. & Canada)

Fax number: 314-447-8029

Elsevier Health Sciences Division
Subscription Customer Service
3251 Riverport Lane
Maryland Heights, MO 63043

*To ensure uninterrupted delivery of your subscription, please notify us at least 4 weeks in advance of move.

Printed and bound by CPI Group (UK) Ltd, Croydon, CR0 4YY

03/10/2024

01040459-0010